Psychopathology in
Later Adulthood

WILEY SERIES ON ADULTHOOD AND AGING

Michael Smyer, Editor

Psychopathology in Later Adulthood

Edited by
SUSAN KRAUSS WHITBOURNE

John Wiley & Sons, Inc.

New York • Chichester • Weinheim • Brisbane • Singapore • Toronto

Library of Congress Cataloging-in-Publication Data:

Psychopathology in later adulthood / [edited by] Susan Krauss Whitbourne.
    p.   cm.
  Includes bibliographical references and index.
  ISBN 0-471-19359-3 (cloth : alk. paper)
  1. Geriatric psychiatry. 2. Aged—Mental health. 3. Aged—Psychology. 4. Psychology, Pathological. I. Whitbourne, Susan Krauss.
  [DNLM: 1. Aged. 2. Mental Disorders. 3. WT 150 P97427 2000]
  RC451.4.A5 P7777 2000
  618.97'689—dc21

00-039894

10 9 8 7 6 5 4 3 2 1

Contributors

Editor
Susan Krauss Whitbourne, PhD
Department of Psychology
University of Massachusetts—
    Amherst
Amherst, Massachusetts

Claudia Avina, BA
Department of Psychology
University of Nevada—Reno
Reno, Nevada

Yeates Conwell, MD
Department of Psychiatry
University of Rochester
School of Medicine and Dentistry
Rochester, New York

Frederick L. Coolidge, PhD
Department of Psychology
University of Colorado at Colorado
    Springs
Colorado Springs, Colorado

Jody Corey-Bloom, MD, PhD
Department of Neurosciences
University of California—San Diego
La Jolla, California

Leah P. Dick-Sisken, PhD
Hillside Hospital
Glen Oaks, New York

Paul R. Duberstein, PhD
Department of Psychiatry
University of Rochester
School of Medicine and Dentistry
Rochester, New York

Barry A. Edelstein, PhD
Department of Psychology
West Virginia University
Morgantown, West Virginia

Jane E. Fisher, PhD
Department of Psychology
University of Nevada—Reno
Reno, Nevada

Mark Floyd, PhD
Department of Psychology
University of Nevada—Las Vegas
Las Vegas, Nevada

Jennifer Forde, MA
Department of Psychology
University of Alabama
Tuscaloosa, Alabama

Edith S. Lisansky-Gomberg, PhD
Professor Emerita
Department of Psychiatry
School of Medicine
Alcohol Research Center
University of Michigan
Ann Arbor, Michigan

Dee A. Haynie, PhD
Department of Human and Family
    Studies
Pennsylvania State University
University Park, Pennsylvania

Gregory A. Hinrichsen, PhD
Hillside Hospital
Glen Oaks, New York

Deborah A. King, PhD
Department of Psychiatry
University of Rochester
School of Medicine and Dentistry
Rochester, New York

Kenneth L. Lichstein, PhD
Department of Psychology
University of Memphis
Memphis, Tennessee

Howard E. Markus, PhD
Department of Psychiatry
University of Rochester
School of Medicine and Dentistry
Rochester, New York

Ronald R. Martin, MA
Department of Psychology
West Virginia University
Morgantown, West Virginia

Deborah R. McKee, MA
Department of Psychology
West Virginia University
Morgantown, West Virginia

Suzanne Meeks, PhD
Department of Psychological and
    Brain Sciences
University of Louisville
Louisville, Kentucky

William T. O'Donohue, PhD
Department of Psychology
University of Nevada—Reno
Reno, Nevada

Brant W. Riedel, PhD
Department of Psychology
University of Memphis Prevention
    Center
Memphis, Tennessee

Erlene Rosowsky, PsyD
Department of Psychiatry
Harvard Medical School
Cambridge, Massachusetts

Forrest Scogin, PhD
Department of Psychology
University of Alabama
Tuscaloosa, Alabama

Daniel L. Segal, PhD
Department of Psychology
University of Colorado at Colorado
    Springs
Colorado Springs, Colorado

Steven H. Zarit, PhD
Department of Human and Family
    Studies
Pennsylvania State University
University Park, Pennsylvania

Contents

Preface

With the growth of the aging population, the field of clinical geropsychology is becoming a major area of research, theory, and practice. This volume is intended to contribute scholarly and applied perspectives to this expanding field. It is organized according to standard classifications used in the *Diagnostic and Statistical Manual of Mental Disorders*, 4th edition *(DSM-IV)*, with specific chapters focusing on particular disorders as they appear in the later adult years. The intention is to present a state-of-the-art text and reference work that can guide clinical training and practice. Each chapter provides a clinical case at the outset, which is then integrated into the substantive content relevant to the disorder. Through these cases, the reader can gain a sense of the complex ways in which psychological disorders unfold in the latter years of the life span. Epidemiology and relevant research and theory are also discussed for each of the specific disorders as they appear in older adults.

The opening chapters present general perspectives on theory and clinical practice. Chapter 1, "Introduction to Clinical Issues," by Steven H. Zarit and Dee A. Haynie, contains an overview of the field of clinical geropsychology. In addition to presenting a life span approach to understanding psychological disorders in later life, the authors provide an overview of *DSM-IV* and, in particular, illustrate its relevance to older adults. Principles of assessment and treatment are discussed in broad terms, setting the stage for fuller discussions in later chapters. Issues in research on the psychology of aging are also presented as these relate to an understanding of the causes and treatments of disorders in the older adult years. Chapter 2, "The Normal Aging Process," written by the editor, provides a summary of the expectable changes that occur in middle and later adulthood, ranging from physical changes to patterns of cognitive and personality development. In Chapter 3, "Assessment of Older Adult Psychopathology," by Barry A. Edelstein, Ronald R. Martin, and Deborah R. McKee, a thorough review is provided of the major assessment tools and their applicability to this population. A consistent theme throughout these opening chapters is the need to distinguish between normal aging and diseases that are prevalent in later life, particularly dementia.

Chapter 4, "Personality Disorders," by Daniel L. Segal, Frederick L. Coolidge, and Erlene Rosowsky, discusses the personality disorders as they are observed in older adults. Adaptations of assessment and treatment methods for older adults with these disorders are presented. In Chapter 5, "Anxiety in Older Adults," Forrest Scogin, Mark Floyd, and Jennifer Forde review the available literature on anxiety disorders. In addition to discussing the major disorders, the authors relate these phenomena as observed in older adults to dementia and other medical conditions found in this population. Chapter 6, "Mood Disorders in Older Adults," by Deborah A. King and Howard E. Markus, reviews the major mood disorders as they appear in later life. Chapter 7, "Sexual Dysfunctions in Later Life," by Claudia Avina, William T. O'Donohue, and Jane E. Fisher includes a discussion of the major disorders within this spectrum.

In Chapter 8, "Schizophrenia and Related Disorders," Suzanne Meeks provides a comprehensive review of the available literature on the course and treatment of this disorder. Relationships to cognitive deficits are also discussed. Chapter 9, "Dementia," by Jody Corey-Bloom, describes in depth the symptoms, epidemiology, treatment, and current understanding of Alzheimer's disease. Suicide is discussed in Chapter 10 by Paul R. Duberstein and Yeates Conwell. Relationships to other disorders observed in later adulthood are also examined. Edith S. Lisansky-Gomberg presents an overview of substance abuse disorders in later life in Chapter 11, focusing on the range of disorders most likely to be observed in this population. A wide range of theories and treatment is presented and applied to the variety of substance abuse disorders found in older adults. The topic of sleep disorders in later adulthood is covered in Chapter 12, "Insomnia in Older Adults," by Brant W. Riedel and Kenneth L. Lichstein. Because insomnia is the major sleep disorder observed in this age group, focus is given entirely to this problem.

Chapter 13, "General Principles of Therapy," written by Gregory A. Hinrichsen and Leah P. Dick-Siskin, integrates many of the treatment issues presented in earlier chapters. Models relevant to the psychological treatment of older adults, in addition to other forms of therapeutic intervention, are contrasted and applied to a specific case. As in earlier chapters, the case is used to highlight critical issues and concerns in dealing with people of advanced years.

It is very rewarding to be able to contribute a volume of this scope and depth to this developing field. The authors have done a commendable job in integrating theory, research, and treatment within an overall developmental perspective. Pedagogical tools are available to assist both the professional and student reader. Study questions and recommended readings provide the basis for further exploration and discussion of the many fascinating topics explored throughout the chapters. Ultimately, it is my hope that this book will not only inform the psychologists who read the material contained between its covers, but will provide the basis for more humane and educated clinical approaches to the treatment of individuals in later life.

SUSAN KRAUSS WHITBOURNE

CHAPTER 1

Introduction to Clinical Issues

STEVEN H. ZARIT AND DEE A. HAYNIE

CASE STUDY

Mrs. Frieda Baker was a 69-year-old woman who was referred because of depression to the psychological service of a vision rehabilitation program. She had multiple health problems, which resulted in her becoming socially isolated and which contributed to her depression. She had poor vision due to cataracts and glaucoma and was virtually blind in bright sunlight. In addition, she had chronic back problems that limited how far she could walk. Because she could no longer walk outside safely, she had become a virtual prisoner in her apartment, going outdoors only when a van from the senior service center took her shopping.

Fortunately, Mrs. Baker had been referred to a rehabilitation program for people with serious vision loss. As a first step, she was fitted with special wrap-around sunglasses that improved her ability to see in sunlight, and she received mobility training so that she could use her remaining vision to cross streets safely. She was still obviously depressed, and so she was referred to the psychological service for assessment and possible therapy.

Mrs. Baker described a pattern of extreme social isolation that resulted from her vision and back problems. Unable to work or even get around, she had remained in her apartment nearly all of the past two years. Her only son was an alcoholic, from whom she was estranged. A behavior treatment for depression, developed by Lewinsohn and colleagues (e.g., Lewinsohn, Muñoz, Youngren, & Zeiss, 1992), which has had good success with older adults (Zeiss & Steffen, 1996), was undertaken. Behind this approach is the idea that people who are depressed typically find themselves in a vicious cycle: feeling depressed, decreasing pleasant activities, feeling more depressed, and so on. The therapist helps to break this cycle by having clients identify and then schedule activities that they enjoy. Engaging in pleasant events improves mood, which can lead to a focus on other problems or difficulties that might have been contributing to the person's depression.

In this case, Mrs. Baker's search for pleasant events took on an almost existential quality. Her life had previously revolved around her work and the few friendships she had through her job. She could no longer work due to her disability, and, as a result, she had lost touch with most of her friends. She faced the problem of creating a life that would accommodate her pronounced disabilities. She gradually became more active, including

1

coming to the rehabilitation center as a volunteer. Her mood improved as she engaged in more pleasant activities, but she felt there was still something missing, an activity that would give meaning to her life. Some possible avenues were closed to her because of her disabilities. She considered taking classes at the local community college, but getting there involved walking uphill one block from the bus stop. She could not do that because of her back problems.

Finally, Mrs. Baker decided on an activity that she had wanted to do all her life but had never gotten around to: painting. She located a painting class for senior citizens and found that she enjoyed it greatly and had a flair for it, despite her vision problems. She set up an easel in her kitchen and began spending mornings painting when the light was right. Painting invigorated her and gave her life meaning. Her depression decreased and she even won a prize for her paintings in a citywide arts contest for disabled artists.

PRINCIPLES OF GEROPSYCHOLOGY

This case example is remarkable in some ways but also typical, illustrating major features of geropsychology. The most important aspect of this case is that it demonstrates the possibility for growth and change in later life. Decline and disability are, of course, very real possibilities in old age. Most older people experience relatively benign psychological changes compared to when they were younger and can function well in their daily lives. When people develop disabilities such as Mrs. Baker's, many retain a resiliency that makes it possible for them to adapt to their losses. At one time, psychologists might have viewed a woman like Mrs. Baker as a hopeless case due to her age and depression. She might even have been confined to a mental institution or nursing home where she would aimlessly wait out the rest of her days. Instead, she was able to find meaning and fulfillment in her life when given appropriate rehabilitation services for her disabilities.

AGING FROM A LIFE SPAN PERSPECTIVE

The ability to work with older clients and to identify treatable aspects of their problems requires an understanding of the aging process, including the potential for decline and disability, as well as the possibilities for continued growth and change. We have organized the growing literature on aging into several key points that capture the dynamic interplay of growth and decline in later life. In doing so, we have drawn heavily on the life span developmental theory developed by Paul Baltes (1987, 1997).

Aging as a Multidimensional Process

Aging can best be viewed as the interaction of biological, psychological, and social processes. We typically think of aging as a biological process marked by outward signs such as gray hair and wrinkles, but aging also can occur in psychological and social realms. Psychologically, the ways people learn and process information change, though, as we will see, not always for the worse. Likewise, people move through social roles and transitions such as having children and seeing them mature, leave home, and have children of their own. These types of psychological and social changes have a profound effect on what we think of as aging.

Consistent with this multidimensional perspective, clinical work with older people is carried out best by multidisciplinary teams that pay attention to the whole person, and not just to one symptom or system. In Mrs. Baker's case, for example, several professionals were involved in the rehabilitation effort, including mobility trainers, optometrists, low-vision technicians who trained her to use optical aids, and a psychologist.

Age or Disease?

It is important to distinguish aging from disease. The normal aging process, whether viewed at a biological, psychological, or social level, is relatively benign and does not lead to catastrophic changes. Rather, dramatic decline occurs as a result of disease. As an example, at one time, it was believed that aging eventually led to senility and that everyone would become senile if they lived long enough. We now know that the syndrome of severe, progressive memory and intellectual decline that we call senility or senile dementia results from several different diseases, such as Alzheimer's, but is not a universal part of growing older. The risk of Alzheimer's disease, like that of many other illnesses, increases with advancing age, but a majority of people at 80, 90, and even 100 do not suffer from this type of mental decline (Johansson & Zarit, 1997). Aging is associated with an increased risk of developing Alzheimer's disease and various other diseases, but the aging process is not inherently pathological.

This distinction between normal aging and disease has much practical significance. There has been a tendency to view all older people as experiencing negative changes (e.g., senility, rigidity), but that is not the case. Older people who suffer from diseases that impair their functioning should get appropriate care. The majority of older people, however, are relatively healthy and should not be construed as having diminished capacity in their ability to carry out everyday activities. In other words, we should not view all older people as having changes typical of dementia or other diseases. And as the case example illustrated, even in the face of some chronic diseases, older people may retain the resiliency to make creative adaptations.

Development as an Ongoing Process

As the term "life span development" implies, development and aging are a continuing process. Development does not stop at a particular age, but continues throughout life. Although there can be decline, there is also the possibility of continued growth. People do not lose the capacity to grow or change at a particular age, whether at 50, 60, 70, or even 80. There are certainly considerable individual differences in the degree of openness to new ideas and change. Some people at 20 or 30 are rigid and fixed in their ways, whereas others, like Mrs. Baker, can draw on their creative potential despite their advanced age.

Continuities in Development

As we observe people over time, we find evidence for both continuity and change in psychological functioning. How people function in the present is usually consistent with how they performed in the past. People do not take on a different persona or different qualities when they get old. There is no single or universal pattern of mental decline, nor do people enter a stage of life in which their behavior can be explained by a simple precept or formula. Rather, as people grow older, there is continuity with their previous life. An older person who is demanding and angry is likely to have been so when younger. Likewise, someone who is vitally involved in everyday life in all likelihood was like that earlier in life. In fact, personality characteristics are "age blind"; that is, they remain relatively stable throughout adulthood (Costa & McCrae, 1988). People continue to be recognizable as themselves, despite outward physical changes.

These findings of continuity have practical importance for people who work with older adults. Understanding an older person means finding out about that person's past, including experiences, preferences, values, beliefs, hopes, and fears. Even when working with someone with severe disabilities such as Alzheimer's disease, finding out about the person's past is key to developing a good relationship and providing good care.

Patterns of Change with Aging

There can also be change throughout the life span. The changes that occur with aging can be viewed in two ways: as *interindividual* differences and as *intra-individual* differences. Interindividual differences refer to the ways that people differ from one another. There are many sources of interindividual differences, including aging. People may also differ from one another on some ability due to their education, cultural background or ethnicity, prior experience or other factors. The rate at which abilities change can also vary from one person to the next. Intra-individual changes refer to the changes an individual experiences over time. People experience age-related changes at different rates for different abilities. As an example, someone may experience a decline in cardiovascular fitness, which leads to limited mobility, but can still perform well at intellectual tasks. In other words, changes in abilities are often specific rather than global.

Compensation for Decline

One of the most important facets of aging is the ability to compensate for decline by utilizing functions that have not declined. Baltes (1987) calls this process "selective optimization with compensation." The best example of this type of compensation comes from Salthouse's (1984) classic study of older typists. One of the earliest and most predictable changes with aging is a decline in reaction time, which typically begins around age 20. Although there are considerable interindividual differences in the rate of change in reaction time, older people consistently perform worse on speeded tasks than younger people. Salthouse observed that older expert typists were still able to maintain a high rate of typing speed compared to younger typists. He found that they were able to maintain their productivity despite declines in reaction time by anticipating the upcoming text better than younger typists. In other words, older typists were able to draw on their experience to offset an age-related decline in reaction time.

We see evidence of compensation in many different realms. An older tennis player who has slowed down a step and lost some power may compensate by using better strategies, such as placing a bewildering array of spins on the ball that keep a younger player off balance. Older people maintain expert performance in a variety of areas, ranging from chess to law, suggesting that selective optimization with compensation is a common process (Salthouse, 1990).

Improving with Age: Plasticity and Training

Another important consideration is that change does not always involve decline. People can improve their performance on particular abilities through experience and training. It was once thought that intellectual abilities peaked in the 20s and then gradually declined. Longitudinal studies that have followed people through their adult years have demonstrated that many intellectual abilities, especially verbal abilities that benefit from experience, increase into the 40s and 50s and do not decline until the 60s or even later (Schaie, 1996).

A portion of the decline that we ascribe to aging may be due to a lack of practice or fitness. Regarding physical parameters such as endurance and strength, a sedentary lifestyle may result in some of the changes we call aging, and these changes can be reversed with appropriate training (Evans, 1996; Evans & Cyr-Campbell, 1997). It is widely believed that improved physical fitness has made it possible for people to live longer and healthier lives. Similarly, it has been hypothesized that at least some portion of intellectual decline may be the result of a lack of practice or of exercising these intellectual abilities. A variety of cognitive training studies have demonstrated that older people can make improvements in their intellectual functioning (e.g., Baltes & Kliegl, 1992; Floyd & Scogin, 1996; Hill, Sheikh, & Yesavage, 1988).

Training can be used to overcome decline due to inactivity or lack of practice. It can also be used to demonstrate plasticity, that is, the capacity for new growth (Staudinger, Marsiske, & Baltes, 1995). Plasticity was long regarded as a quality of the young. A young person who suffers a brain injury, for example, will have more recovery of function than an older person, as the brain is able to form more new connections to overcome the effects of the injury. But there remains some potential for plasticity with aging. As an example, animals placed in enriched laboratory environments where there is ample stimulation show development of more neural connections than animals living in standard, unstimulating environments (Diamond, Johnson, Protti, Ott, & Kajisa, 1985; Rosenzweig & Bennett, 1996).

A similar capacity for growth has been demonstrated in humans. In an interesting series of training studies with older people, Willis and colleagues (Willis, Blieszner, & Baltes, 1981; Willis & Nesselroade, 1990) found clear evidence of plasticity in cognitive abilities. People were trained in skills that would help their performance on either a fluid intelligence task, which is generally affected more by aging, or a crystallized intelligence task, which tends to be stable with age. The average age of people in the sample was 70 years. Following training, people showed improvement on the test related to the skills they learned, though not on the other test. These results demonstrated that training in underlying skills could improve intellectual performance, even on a fluid intelligence task that typically declines with aging. More impressively, a follow-up seven years later indicated that the benefits of training were largely maintained (Raykov, 1997; Willis & Nesselroade, 1990).

The possibility for plasticity and its limits can be demonstrated by testing the limits, that is, pushing people to high levels of performance until they cannot respond further (Baltes, 1987). In testing the limits, we can see both the possibilities for development and the boundaries created by aging. As an example, if we observe a younger and an older person walk a certain distance, we are not likely to find much difference (Baltes, 1987). If we look at marathon runners, however, we find clear differences. Some older people can run marathons, which demonstrates the possibility of maintaining a high level of functioning in later life. At the same time, the best older runner will run a marathon in a slower time than good younger runners. Of course, an older person who can run a marathon is in better shape than many younger people who lead largely sedentary lives, but there is a limit imposed by aging.

Baltes and colleagues (Baltes & Kliegl, 1992; Kliegl, Smith, & Baltes, 1989) have examined the effects of testing the limits for cognitive performance. Older and younger people participated in an experiment in which they learned a strategy for remembering long lists of items, called the method of loci. This method involves associating something you want to remember with a particular place or location, such as a room in your house or a familiar place in the city where you live. Older people were able to learn and use this memory technique. When tested on word lists, older people learned more slowly and could only manage shorter lists than younger people (15 words compared to 30), but they were still able to increase the number of words recalled on average from 6 prior to training to 15 after training. In testing the limits, then, we can see how much potential there is for growth, as well as the limits to plasticity imposed by the aging process.

IMPLICATIONS OF A LIFE SPAN PERSPECTIVE FOR PSYCHOPATHOLOGY IN LATER LIFE

These perspectives on the normal aging process contribute to a better understanding of psychopathology in later life in several ways. First, aging is not by itself a pathological process. Although aging or age-related issues such as the death of a spouse may play a role in the development of a psychological problem, age is not the sole cause, nor does it preclude the possibility for recovery.

Second, there is considerable variability among older people. The many different pathways and experiences people have had during their lives contribute to these individual differences. Further, age-related changes occur at different times and in varying degrees from one person to the next, increasing individual differences further. Finally, the social and ethnic backgrounds of older people are another source of variability.

Assessment Issues with Older Adults

There are similarities but also some important differences in clinical practice with older adults (Zarit & Zarit, 1998). Assessment takes a more central place in clinical work with older people than it does with younger people. In particular, three assessment issues are of paramount importance when working with an older client.

First, many referrals for assessment have either an explicit or implicit request to determine if a person is suffering from dementia. Although most older people do not have dementia, the association of dementia and old age in the minds of family members, physicians, and even older clients themselves makes it important to establish if the person may be suffering from this type of progressive decline.

Second, assessment of an older person more often has to deal with the issue of the comorbidity of health problems; that is, the person is suffering both from mental health and medical problems. The example of Mrs. Baker illustrated a typical pattern of comorbidity of depression and medical problems, in her case, vision loss and back problems.

Psychiatric symptoms can be both a primary and a secondary consequence of medical problems. Some illnesses have a direct or primary effect on neurobiological systems that make psychiatric symptoms more likely. An example is Parkinson's disease, which is associated with a loss of the neurotransmitter dopamine. Dopamine is also implicated in depression, and, as a result, depression is a common correlate of Parkinson's disease. Of course, the pain, threat, and/or disability associated with an illness can lead to anxiety, depression, or other problems.

An important part of assessment is to identify when an illness might be implicated in the etiology of psychopathology. In those cases, treatment of the medical problem can lead to a reduction of psychiatric symptoms. Conversely, it is often necessary to treat a psychiatric problem so that a person can more fully comply with medical or rehabilitation efforts. Rather than assuming that disability inevitably causes people to feel depressed, it is important to identify ways that the person might be able to compensate better through physical or psychological means. People who have disabilities due to illness or disease can often learn new techniques to help them recover the ability to perform some tasks. In Mrs. Baker's case, she was taught how to get around safely outdoors and also how to use visual aids such as high-powered magnifiers that helped her read and carry out other visual tasks. Depression, however, can often get in the way of learning these types of strategies. A coordinated program that emphasizes multifaceted and multidisciplinary efforts to restore function, such as the one Mrs. Baker participated in, is more likely to be successful in sorting out the comorbidity of chronic illness and emotional distress.

Not only are the illnesses of older people a possible source of psychiatric symptoms, so are the medications they take for those illnesses. Medication-related problems are very common among older people. One reason is that rates of prescription drug use are very high. Most older people are taking one or more prescription medications, and it is not uncommon to find people on 10 or more medications. At the same time, older individuals are more susceptible to adverse effects from medications. As we grow older, the ways our bodies process medications change. In particular, older people absorb, metabolize, and excrete medications more slowly (Beizer, 1994). This means that it takes longer for a medication to reach to a therapeutic dosage, but then the medication may remain in the body longer, causing it to build up to toxic levels. A related problem is when a person takes multiple medications, because there can be harmful interactions between two or more of them. It is also very common for prescription drugs to have harmful interactions with alcohol as well as with nonprescription drugs or with foods (Adams, 1997). Of course, the more medications one takes, the more possibilities for harmful interactions among them. Thus, the potential that medications might cause adverse reactions and lead to an increase in psychiatric symptoms is much stronger among older people than among younger people. Assessment of medications needs to be an important focus when evaluating symptoms in an older adult.

A common comorbidity problem is that many illnesses, as well as the medications used to treat them, can lead to a loss of memory and other cognitive problems that resemble dementia (see Zarit & Zarit, 1998, for a review). For that reason, it is strongly urged that people suspected of suffering from Alzheimer's disease or other dementing illnesses receive a thorough physical examination to rule out potentially treatable causes due to other illnesses and/or medications.

The third assessment issue concerns the family of the older person. Family members are more likely to be involved in bringing the older person in for an assessment. When an older person is experiencing serious memory problems that make it impossible to get a complete picture of the history, it can be very helpful to enlist the assistance of a spouse, child, or other relative who knows the person well and who can fill in the missing information. When a family member accompanies the designated patient, the clinician conducting the assessment must ask the question, "Who *is* the patient?" In some cases, the older person neither wants nor will benefit from help. The family member, however, is struggling with the stresses involved in caring for a frail or difficult older person and may respond to treatment to help him or her cope more effectively with the situation (Zarit & Zarit, 1998). When involving other people, the clinician should respect the confidentiality of the client and not seek out other information or divulge material told in confidence by that client without explicit consent (Zarit & Zarit, 1998).

Implications for Treatment of Older People
There are several challenges in planning and implementing treatment for older people. A major consideration is to identify treatable aspects of the problem. As we have stressed, older people retain the capacity to change even in the face of significant illnesses. Yet, because of prevailing stereotypes about aging, older people are often regarded as undesirable clients who cannot respond to treatment. Sometimes, the gains will be limited but important. It may not be possible to restore someone to a prior level of functioning, but treatment can nonetheless make the situation significantly better. For people suffering from dementia, it is currently not possible to do much to reverse the underlying illness, but we can

make changes in psychological and social aspects of the problem. Family caregivers can learn more effective strategies for managing behavior problems associated with dementia or identify more support and assistance so that the care demands falling on them become more manageable (Zarit & Zarit, 1998). The person with dementia may benefit indirectly from these types of interventions or more directly from treatments such as support groups, which have been reported to be very helpful to people in the early stages of their illness (Yale, 1999).

Another issue in the treatment of older adults is the more complex use of medications for psychiatric problems. Changes in how older people process medications in their body result in a more unpredictable response to psychotropic medications (Beizer, 1994). It can be difficult to find a dosage that is neither too low nor too high. In addition, there may be medical reasons why an older person may not be able to take a particular medication.

Finally, just as family members can play a role in assessment, they may also be a valuable part of treatment. Many older people have concerns about their family that can be addressed more directly by bringing in the people involved. This can be done in a couple of sessions and does not require longer-term family therapy (Zarit & Zarit, 1998).

CLASSIFYING LATE LIFE DISORDERS: THE *DSM-IV*

The fourth edition of the American Psychiatric Association's *Diagnostic and Statistical Manual of Mental Disorders (DSM-IV,* 1994) evolved primarily to provide a guide for reliable diagnosis in clinical practice (*DSM-IV*, American Psychiatric Association, 1994). Other objectives included facilitating research through the use of operational criteria for diagnosis that could be replicated from one study to the next and improving communication between clinicians and researchers by adopting a common terminology (*DSM-IV*, 1994). Age-related characteristics, however, have only partly been incorporated into diagnostic criteria, and so an ongoing concern is whether at least some diagnostic approaches need to be modified for older adults.

The *DSM-IV* (1994) classification system has five axes, each of which refers to a different domain of information that may help the clinician plan treatment and predict outcome. The axes provide information about various mental disorders and general medical conditions, psychosocial and environmental problems, and level of functioning.

The first axis consists of clinical disorders and usually can be thought of as the reason the person is seeking help (reason for the visit). A person can have more than one Axis I disorder, and all should be reported. The first diagnosis listed is then considered to be the principal diagnosis or reason for the visit.

The second axis, or Axis II, is where personality disorders and mental retardation are reported. A personality disorder (there are 10 specific disorders) is an enduring pattern of inner experience and behavior that deviates markedly from the expectations of the person's culture, is pervasive and inflexible, has an onset in adolescence or early adulthood, is stable over time, and leads to distress or impairment (DSM-IV, 1994). Mental retardation involves subaverage intellectual functioning accompanied by significant limitations in adaptive functioning, and onset must occur before the age of 18 years.

Axis III is for reporting current general medical conditions that might reveal how the person's mental disorder is being affected by his or her physical health. General medical disorders can be related to mental disorders in a number of ways. For instance, the general medical condition may be the direct cause of the development or worsening of mental symptoms and so the mechanism for this effect is physiological (DSM-IV, 1994). In this case, when the mental disorder is a consequence of a general medical condition, a "mental disorder due to a general medical condition" should be diagnosed on Axis I, and the general medical condition should be recorded on both Axis I and Axis III. An Axis I mental disorder may also be present as a reaction to a medical condition (e.g., depression as a reaction to a diagnosis of cancer). Some general medical conditions may not be directly related to the mental disorder but nevertheless be important when decisions about treatment and prognosis are being made.

Psychosocial and environmental problems are reported on Axis IV. Usually, the psychosocial and environmental problems occurring within a year of the current assessment are listed. Examples include life events, a lack of social support or personal resources, interpersonal difficulties, or other problems associated with a person's current difficulties. In some instances, a psychosocial and environmental problem may be the primary focus of clinical attention. In this situation, the psychosocial or environmental problem should also be recorded on Axis I, coded "other conditions that may be a focus of clinical attention."

Overall level of functioning is reported on Axis V and is useful in treatment planning and predicting the efficacy of treatment. Overall functioning is assessed using the Global Assessment of Functioning (GAF) scale. This scale is used to rate only psychological, social, and occupational functioning, not physical or environmental limitations. The ratings of overall psychological functioning are on a scale of 100 to 0, with 100 indicating superior functioning with no symptoms and 10 or lower indicating persistent danger of severely hurting self or others.

In the DSM-IV, V Codes are sometimes used to indicate other conditions that may be a focus of clinical attention. An example of a V Code is a situation in which there is not enough information to know whether a presenting problem is attributable to a mental disorder (e.g., V62.82, Bereavement). A V Code may also be used to indicate that there is no diagnosis or condition on Axis I or no diagnosis on Axis II (V71.09).

The DSM-IV was produced by 13 work groups comprised of experts in their respective fields. In turn, the work groups reported to the Task Force on DSM-IV, which consisted of 27 members, many of whom were chairs of their work groups (DSM-IV, 1994). An attempt was made to ensure that diverse clinical and research disciplines and settings were represented. Many of the participants were international experts and people with different ethnic backgrounds in the United States, which allowed cultural diversity issues to be addressed. The Task Force on DSM-IV communicated openly with many components of the American

Psychiatric Association and with more than 60 organizations, including the American Psychological Association *(DSM-IV,* 1994*).*

A major strength of the *DSM-IV* lies in the consideration of extensive empirical evidence in defining disorders and their characteristics. In the past, psychiatric diagnosis was characterized by vague definitions of disorders that led to unreliable diagnosis. The *DSM-IV* is built on empirical studies that identify which symptoms and characteristics typically are present in a disorder. The authors of the *DSM-IV* also stressed constructing clear and precise definitions of disorders and symptoms so that clinicians will interpret the definitions in similar ways and make more accurate diagnoses.

For diagnosis of psychopathology in older adults, the *DSM-IV* has strengths and weaknesses. The main strength is improvement of those categories that mainly include older people, namely, dementia and delirium. The *DSM-IV* also added two new categories specifically for older adults, age-related cognitive decline and mild neurocognitive disorder. The main weakness is that the *DSM-IV* largely does not address the issue of criteria for diagnosis of older people with other disorders. Should the criteria for depression, for example, be the same or different for an older person compared to a younger person? In fairness, there is little research available to guide questions like this. The larger issue, however, is that we do not know to what extent many common disorders look different in later life than earlier in life. This question is important, because accurate diagnostic criteria for older people will lead to better diagnosis and improved access to treatment.

In the sections that follow, we first look at the diagnoses specific to later life and then turn to other categories of disorders that are commonly found among older people.

DISORDERS OF LATER LIFE

DELIRIUM

Delirium is a particularly troubling category, because it is frequently overlooked or misdiagnosed, with sometimes severe consequences. Previous editions, the *DSM-III* (1980) and *DSM-III-R* (1987), replaced an older category of acute brain syndrome with delirium and developed diagnostic criteria for it. These criteria were based on the clinical experience of expert psychiatrists and represented an improvement over the previous classification scheme. However, they were not based on systemic empirical data and were not adequately field-tested (Liptzin & Levkoff, 1994). These problems are largely corrected in the *DSM-IV.*

In the *DSM-IV* (1994), delirium is characterized by a disturbance of consciousness and a change in cognition that develop over a short period of time, usually hours to days. There should be evidence that the delirium is a direct physiological consequence of a general medical condition, substance intoxication or withdrawal, use of a medication, toxin exposure, or a combination of these factors. The disorders that make up the delirium section are distinguished by etiology, for instance, delirium due to a general medical condition or substance-induced delirium (including medication side effects). According to *DSM-IV*, associated features (common symptoms but not part of the actual criteria) may include a disturbance in the sleep-wake cycle, disturbed psychomotor behavior, and emotional disturbances, or no diagnosis on Axis II (V71.09).

Reviewing alternative classification schemes such as the tenth edition of the *International Classification of Diseases (ICD-10)* as well as empirical studies of delirium, Liptzin and Levkoff (1994) recommended criteria that focus on the core symptoms of impairment of consciousness/attention along with a change in cognition. The symptoms of sleep and psychomotor disturbances were felt to be associated features, and it was recommended that these be included in the text rather than the criteria. Subtypes of delirium such as hyperactive, hypoactive, or mixed states were considered to be interesting but premature and requiring further research. Liptzin and Levkoff determined that the category of dementia with delirium was not viable because there was not anything unique about delirium with or without dementia. These two conditions should be diagnosed independently.

DEMENTIA

The dementia section of the *DSM-IV* (1994) is made up of disorders that are characterized by the development of multiple cognitive deficits (including memory impairment) that are due to the direct physiological effects of a general medical condition, to the persisting effects of a substance, or to multiple etiologies (e.g., the combined effects of cerebrovascular disease and Alzheimer's disease). Criteria for the diagnosis of dementia include demonstrable impairment of short-term and long-term memory and at least one of the following: impaired abstract thinking, impaired judgment, disturbance of higher cortical functions (e.g., aphasia, agnosia, apraxia), or personality change. These impairments must not occur exclusively during the course of delirium and must significantly interfere with work or usual social activities or relationships. To meet the criteria for dementia, a person needs to be evaluated through a neurological examination, neuropsychological testing, and an assessment of functioning in activities of daily living (Salmon, Butters, Thal, & Jeste, 1994).

The *DSM-IV* criteria represent some modifications from previous editions that bring the classification of dementia in line with current empirical evidence. There is more attention to subtypes of dementia: dementia of the Alzheimer's type (DAT), vascular dementia, dementia due to other general medical conditions, dementia due to multiple etiologies, and dementia not otherwise specified.

The findings of the study by Salmon et al. (1994) are an example of how the criteria in the *DSM-IV* are derived from research. For instance, progressive decline in multiple cognitive areas (particularly memory) and in functional abilities are warranted for a diagnosis of dementia. Personality change was not seen as an effective criterion, and neurological signs play an important supporting role in the diagnosis of DAT but are not effective on their own.

AGE-RELATED COGNITIVE DECLINE AND MILD NEUROCOGNITIVE DISORDER

Rediess and Caine (1997) discuss the addition of two new designations in the *DSM-IV* (1994) of age-related cognitive decline (ARCD) and mild neurocognitive disorder. ARCD is a V Code indicating that although it may not be indicative of a disease diagnosis, it is a condition that may be a focus of clinical attention. Mild neurocognitive disorder is proposed as a research diagnosis in need of further study and appears in Appendix B of the *DSM-IV*. Rediess and Caine state that these two terms together reflect a trend toward representing age-associated cognitive changes across a continuum from normal functioning to dementia.

These new categories were developed based on clinical observations that patients often exhibit neurocognitive symptoms (mild cognitive impairment) that do not meet the criteria for dementia but that nonetheless affect daily functioning. The main feature of the new diagnostic guidelines is decline in cognitive performance that can include memory impairment and learning or concentration difficulties. The main difference between the two categories is that ARCD is not associated with any specific medical disorder, whereas mild neurocognitive disorder can be the beginning of a progressive decline toward dementia.

The category mild neurocognitive disorder is particularly interesting because it reflects that cognitive changes can be caused by many different factors. The criteria were developed from three sources: the literature on alcohol and substance abuse and dependence, the literature on neurological disorders, and the literature on medical disorders with central nervous system complications (Gutierrez, Atkinson, & Grant, 1994). Persons with alcoholism could experience neuropsychological problems such as disturbances in learning recall, abstracting ability, and complex conceptual motor skills that exist in the context of relatively preserved IQ (Gutierrez et al., 1994). Mild neurocognitive problems can also occur in people involved in polysubstance abuse (Gutierrez et al., 1994). There is abundant evidence that certain medical conditions such as chronic obstructive pulmonary disease and autoimmune diseases produce mild neurobehavioral disturbances (Gutierrez et al., 1994). The treatment of these diseases with medication can reverse the neurocognitive disorder in some cases or prevent further deterioration. Both these new V Code categories may also include people in the early stages of progressive dementing disorders such as Alzheimer's disease and Parkinson's disease, where there can be a prolonged period of mild neurocognitive impairment that is clinically significant but fails to meet the *DSM-IV* (1994) criteria for dementia.

DIAGNOSES NOT SPECIFIC TO LATER LIFE

We now consider categories of disorders that are not specific to later life. We have been selective, because virtually any problem that occurs earlier in life can persist or reoccur in late life, and have highlighted some key categories that are particularly important for later life. In each case, the main issue is to what extent current definitions reflect an understanding of how a particular disorder is manifested in later life, and if diagnostic criteria should be similar or different for older people.

Substance-Related Disorders

The *DSM-IV* (1994) category of substance-related disorders includes abuse of specific substances such as alcohol and 10 other classes of drugs, the side effects of medications, and the exposure to toxins. The substance-related category is further broken down into substance use disorders (substance use and dependence) and substance-induced disorders (including disorders resulting from misuse of medications). According to Allen and Landis (1997), the available literature suggests that substance use disorders decrease with increasing age and that the prevalence is higher in men than in women. Certain groups of older adults have higher rates of substance use disorders, such as hospitalized patients (alcohol abuse) and older people living in the community who abuse prescription drugs, especially sedative-hypnotics, antianxiety agents, and analgesics (Allen & Landis, 1997).

As in many of the *DSM-IV* categories, the diagnostic criteria for substance abuse were not developed with older adults in mind and are not adequately validated with older people, which could lead to an underestimation of these disorders. There are two main concerns about the present criteria. First, they do not reflect a greater susceptibility to medications among older adults. An older individual who is dependent on alcohol may drink less yet continue to become intoxicated because of physiological changes in the way alcohol is absorbed, metabolized, and excreted. Older people are also more likely to be taking prescription medications, which can increase the effects of alcohol and other substances or lead to toxic interactions with these substances. Second, one part of the diagnostic criteria of substance abuse is poor work performance (i.e., an adverse consequence of drinking), which may not be applicable for the older person (Allen & Landis, 1997). The effects of substance abuse may be less obvious, such as when an older person with a drinking problem rarely ventures outside the house. This invisibility of the problem may lead to underdiagnosis. Further research and clinical data in regard to substance-related disorders and aging are needed to substantiate and improve *DSM* diagnostic criteria.

Mood Disorders

The *DSM-IV* (1994) can be viewed as a categorical approach to the diagnosis of depression and other affective disorders in late life. As Blazer and Koenig (1996) point out, older people often suffer from depressive symptoms that do not meet diagnostic criteria for major depression, yet these symptoms adversely affect their quality of life. In contrast to the *DSM-IV*, the *ICD-10* allows for diagnosis of mild, moderate, or severe depression. This type of approach would encompass many older people who are omitted by the main *DSM-IV* criteria but who could benefit from treatment.

In addition, depression may present in some unusual ways in later life (Blazer & Koenig, 1996). For many of today's older adults, it is more acceptable to have a medical than a mental health problem. As a result, depression may be manifested by somatic complaints or apathy but with no overt complaints about feeling sad or blue. A variation on this pattern is pseudodementia, in which the person complains of excessive memory loss but has little or no objective memory impairment and improves with treatment for depression.

Bereavement is a V Code in the *DSM-IV* that becomes the focus of clinical attention when there are symptoms of depression during the first two months after the loss of a loved one. Symptoms that are not considered part of a "normal" grief reaction include extreme feelings of worthlessness and active suicidal ideation. Any person fulfilling the criteria for major depression at or beyond two months from the death should be recognized as having a major depressive episode (Blazer & Koenig, 1996).

Anxiety Disorders

Anxiety disorders are another category where diagnostic criteria may not reflect important differences in older people. Older people may express anxiety in terms of physiologic arousal (panic attacks, motor tension or restlessness, autonomic hyperactivity, or sleep disturbance) or overt behavioral responses (compulsive behaviors or exaggerated startle response) (Palmer, Jeste, & Sheikh, 1997). In fact, it has been suggested that older adults are more likely than younger adults to exhibit a mixture of anxiety and depression. The diagnosis of mixed anxiety-depressive disorder is included in the *DSM-IV* appendix to guide further study.

Palmer et al. (1997) raise the question of whether physical and psychosocial changes associated with aging change the way anxiety symptoms cluster for older people when compared to younger patients. An example of such a change is a decrease in physical abilities such as vision, which might result in an older person's being hesitant to go out at night. Palmer et al. point out the importance of making the distinction of whether or not this behavior is a phobic response or an adaptive one.

Anxiety states and many medical conditions have often been found to be associated in younger and older adults (Palmer et al., 1997). A number of factors may be attributed to the high comorbidity of anxiety and medical problems. Anxiety as well as depression can be a psychological response to the onset of a medical problem and/or a side effect of prescribed or over-the-counter medications used to treat the medical problem. In turn, some medications, such as beta blockers, used in the treatment of hypertension may have anxiolytic effects, which may mask the existence of an anxiety disorder. Physical illnesses such as hyperthyroidism and cardiac arrhythmia may present clinically as anxiety. The opposite may also be true: symptoms of anxiety such as palpitations, sweating, and dizziness may be expressed by the older adult as physical symptoms. In considering the *DSM-IV* diagnostic criteria for an anxiety disorder, it is necessary to rule out any direct physiological effects of a general medical condition. Due to the high comorbidity of anxiety and medical problems in older adults, this differentiation can be especially complex. Palmer et al. conclude that research is needed to determine the diagnostic accuracy for specific anxiety disorders as outlined in the *DSM-IV* and whether revision or reclustering of symptoms is necessary to describe better the anxiety syndrome in older adults.

Personality Disorders

Personality disorders, which by their definition have an onset in late adolescence or early adulthood, often persist into old age. There is little information, however, on how these syndromes change as people age or if the same or different criteria should be used for their diagnosis in later life (Camus, Augusto de Mendonça Lima, Gaillard, Simeone, & Wertheimer, 1997).

The comorbidity of personality disorders and problems such as depression and anxiety may be fairly common in later life (Camus et al., 1997). Treatment of a person with depression and a long-standing personality disorder will be more difficult, and may result in only partial alleviation of symptoms. Failure to recognize this comorbidity may cause the clinician to become extremely frustrated over the lack of response to usual treatment. As we have stressed, this lack of response is often due more to the type of disorder than to the age of the person.

CASE DIAGNOSIS

In concluding this section on classifying late life disorders, we illustrate how the case of Mrs. Baker can be conceptualized using the *DSM-IV* as a framework. Using the multiaxial format, a *DSM-IV* evaluation of Mrs. Baker when she first sought help is presented in Table 1.1.

Axis I designates the clinical disorder that was the reason Mrs. Baker was referred for psychological services (reason for the visit). It was determined that Mrs. Baker was experiencing a major depressive disorder (first 3 digits are 296). The clinician would gather additional background information to ascertain whether Mrs. Baker had any previous history of depressive illnesses. This is indicated in the fourth digit of the diagnostic code, either 2 (if there is only a single major depressive episode) or 3 (if there are recurrent major depressive episodes). The fifth digit in the diagnostic code for major depressive disorder indicates the current state of the disturbance. In Mrs. Baker's case, her depression was quite severe.

There was nothing in Mrs. Baker's background information that warranted a diagnosis on Axis II indicating a personality disorder (mental retardation is also reported here). A V Code was used to indicate that there is no diagnosis

Table 1.1 Example of *DSM-IV* evaluation.

Axis I	296.23	Major depressive disorder, single episode, severe without psychotic features.
Axis II	V71.09	No diagnosis.
Axis III	366.9	Cataract.
	365.9	Glaucoma.
	369.9	Visual loss.
		Back pain.
Axis IV		Extreme social isolation, estranged from only son.
Axis V	GAF = 50	(prior to treatment.)

(V71.09). On Axis III, several medical conditions were noted. Mrs. Baker's poor vision was due to cataracts and glaucoma, and she had chronic back problems. The listing of these medical conditions allows the clinician to understand better how Mrs. Baker's mental condition was being affected by her physical health. From the scenario presented in this chapter, it is very likely that Mrs. Baker's psychological distress was a reaction to her physical disabilities.

Psychosocial and environmental problems for Mrs. Baker, which are reported on Axis IV, consisted of her being socially isolated and estranged from her only son. Her overall level of functioning (GAF = 50) was assessed on Axis V. Mrs. Baker was exhibiting serious symptoms as evidenced by her extreme social isolation.

Although one might be inclined to argue that Mrs. Baker's distress was a result of her physical limitations, a principle of geropsychology was confirmed: her case demonstrated the possibility for growth and change in later life. With a behavioral therapeutic intervention, Mrs. Baker's mood improved significantly. She became more socially engaged and found an activity that made her life meaningful despite her physical limitations. It should be noted that when using the *DSM-IV* multiaxial evaluation, the strengths of the individual, such as useful coping skills, are not at the forefront. This is a clinical issue regardless of the person's age.

RESEARCH ISSUES IN THE PSYCHOPATHOLOGY OF LATER LIFE

Research on issues of aging is complex because it involves devising strategies to estimate changes that have occurred over relatively long periods of time and to differentiate effects due specifically to aging from change resulting from other influences on people's lives. As an example, people may grow older in different ways in societies that venerate and respect elders compared to those that place a higher value on youth. The influence of the social position of older people in a particular society is important, but should not be mistaken for a universal pattern of aging.

The research issues involved in studying psychopathology in later life are similar to research on normal processes of aging. (Schaie & Willis, 1996 provide a comprehensive introduction to research methods for studying aging.) We examine some of the key issues as well as the implications for understanding psychopathology in old age.

RESEARCH DESIGN: CROSS-SECTIONAL, LONGITUDINAL, AND SEQUENTIAL STUDIES

Most research on aging is conducted by comparing old and young people. This type of research is called *cross-sectional*. According to Schaie and Willis (1996), cross-sectional research reveals age differences, that is, how old and young people differ on a particular characteristic at a particular point in time. These findings, however, do not indicate whether these differences are due to aging or to other influences. In particular, cohort or generational differences can contribute to differences between old and young. Young and old people may differ on a particular characteristic not because the older group has changed, but because each generation started out with different levels of that characteristic. For example, older people may hold certain beliefs that differ from the young because they have always held those beliefs, not because they have become more rigid or conservative with age. There is evidence of generation differences on a number of characteristics, such as intelligence (Schaie, 1996), personality (Whitbourne, Zuschlag, Elliot, & Waterman, 1992), and even rates of depressive symptoms (Roberts, Lee, & Roberts, 1991).

Specific historical events can also contribute to age differences. The passage of Medicare in 1965, which provides comprehensive health insurance for everyone 65 and older, has probably been one of the major factors associated with improved health among subsequent cohorts of people turning 65. It is no accident that today's older people are healthier and have better functioning than previous generations.

An alternative to cross-sectional studies is *longitudinal* research. In a longitudinal study, the researcher follows the same people over time. This type of design makes it possible to observe how people change. Often, these changes reflect at least in part the effects of aging, but they can also be related to other factors. A particular cohort, such as baby boomers, may age in a unique way. Likewise, a specific historical event can lead to changes in the cohort being followed but not other cohorts in the population.

To overcome these problems, Schaie (1996; Schaie & Willis, 1996) has proposed conducting different types of *sequential* studies. In a cohort sequential study, for example, several cohorts of people are followed over time. This design makes it possible to examine whether the changes occurring in one cohort are specific to that generation or are replicated in the next cohort. Likewise, it is possible to consider whether changes in one time period are related to events that occurred during that era or if a similar pattern of change is observed in successive cohorts at the same time in their lives.

Using this design, Schaie (1996) has found that age differences in intelligence are due more to cohort differences than to aging. Younger cohorts have had successively higher initial levels of intelligence on many abilities compared to older cohorts. Furthermore, most dimensions of intelligence continue to rise during the adult years, with decline occurring only by the decade of the 60s or 70s. Even then, some people remain stable over time in most or all dimensions of intelligence, or even increase. These findings contrast sharply with cross-sectional research on intelligence, which has emphasized age differences between young and old. Those age differences, however, were due mainly to cohort effects.

There is a place for each type of research design in studying aging. Cross-sectional research is quicker and less expensive to conduct than longitudinal research and can provide useful information on how old and young people may differ. This can be important for planning programs and policies, as long as cross-sectional differences are not interpreted as indicating age changes.

Longitudinal research provides a better estimate of the changes that may be occurring with aging, but it can take a long time to conduct. Researchers must also address problems of sample attrition due to dropping out or death. Sequential studies also suffer from the same drawbacks as longitudinal research, although Schaie (1996) uses the strategy of adding new subjects over time to estimate for the specific effects of attrition.

PROBLEMS IN EVALUATING OLDER PEOPLE

Another important research issue is that it is more difficult to assess functioning and performance among older compared to younger people (Zarit & Zarit, 1998). Older people may tire more quickly and need frequent breaks to perform at their maximum ability. As a result, it may be necessary to space out testing or assessment sessions across multiple days to avoid confounding the test results with the effects of fatigue. The pace of testing also needs to be slower; the tester needs to read instructions to present material at a slower pace. It is simply not possible to test an older person at the same quick pace as with a younger person. Failure to take this slowing of response into account may produce test results that indicate a decrement in performance for the older person that is attributable to the pace of the tester rather than the person's ability.

Older people also may have hearing and vision problems that make assessment more difficult. It is important when assessing older people to make sure they have brought along eyeglasses, hearing aids, or other sensory aids. Assessments need to be conducted in settings in which there is good lighting and acoustics. Background noise and other distractions will interfere with test performance.

IMPLICATIONS OF RESEARCH ISSUES FOR STUDYING PSYCHOPATHOLOGY IN LATER LIFE

These research issues have three important implications for the study of psychopathology in later life. First, it cannot be assumed that the psychological problems an older person experiences are associated with aging. These problems may have originated in later life, or they may be part of a long-standing pattern. In other words, we need to distinguish between the age of the person and the age of his or her problem. Just as we need longitudinal or sequential research to uncover the effects of aging, we need to take a longitudinal perspective when viewing psychopathology.

It is generally useful to take this type of developmental perspective on psychopathology, that is, determining at what age a disorder typically has its onset and how it changes over time. With schizophrenia, for example, most forms have their onset in adolescence and young adulthood. Following people over time, we find that some have a complete remission of symptoms, some have partial remission or suffer from intermittent episodes, and some have an apparently unwavering course (Ciompi, 1987). There is much that can be learned by studying these different developmental trajectories. By contrast, if we study schizophrenia and aging by obtaining a sample of older people who currently meet the criteria for a schizophrenic disorder, we need to be careful not to draw incorrect inferences about either schizophrenia or aging. A group of older schizophrenics may contain people who had more severe or treatment-resistant forms of the disorder to start with, so that their symptoms have persisted to late life. Aging may play some role in worsening or alleviating some types of symptoms, as well as introducing new stresses. An older person with schizophrenia may have fewer social supports and suffer more from the deaths of parents and other family members than someone with a better social network. On the other hand, a lessening of social demands in later life may lead to better functioning for some people with chronic mental disorders. Overall, the key to understanding the etiology of schizophrenia and other chronic mental illnesses lies in the period of life when the disorder has its onset and in the factors that influence the subsequent course of symptoms. Aging does not lead to these chronic and immutable conditions, though aging issues may play some role in an individual's current problems and concerns.

This developmental perspective on psychopathology suggests the importance of taking a careful history of an individual suffering from psychological symptoms. When symptoms have occurred previously in the person's life, we can identify which treatments had been effective before. If a particular treatment was helpful once, it is likely to be helpful again. We can also determine if there are some specific effects of aging that may be contributing to the current episode. Often, social losses, such as the death of a close relative or friend, or financial problems can trigger a new episode of a disorder such as depression. Rather than ascribing these problems solely to aging, and then feeling hopeless because the effects of aging cannot be reversed, we can uncover evidence of which treatments had previously been effective.

Some disorders have their first onset in later life, and so aging can be presumed to have a more central role. These processes may be biological, such as the onset of a major illness, but they can also be psychological and social. Depression and anxiety disorders typically have an onset earlier in life, but symptoms can occur for the first time in later life. There is also a disorder considered to be a late-onset schizophrenia, which is usually characterized by paranoid symptoms (Zarit & Zarit, 1998). The most common problem that has a late-life onset is dementia, which occurs only rarely before age 60 and is quite common after age 75. Treatment of late-onset disorders involves identifying sources of resiliency from earlier in the person's life and helping the person reestablish these more effective patterns of coping. Taking a careful history of the person, then, is also important both in recurrent disorders and in those that have a first onset in old age. Even in cases of people suffering from dementia, there may be resources used earlier in life that can be drawn on, including the person's social network, that may partly alleviate the effects of the disorder.

A second implication of research methods for studying psychopathology in later life is the importance of cohort or generational differences. People's behavior and beliefs have been shaped to a large extent by their background and past experiences. Today's older people who grew up during the Great Depression of the 1930s, for example, have a different attitude about money than do more recent cohorts who have lived through a period of unprecedented prosperity. As a result, a young therapist may have a difficult time understanding why a relatively wealthy older person is unwilling to spend money on something that would make his or her life easier. This reluctance is not a sign of pathology; it is a strongly ingrained habit. We can better understand how problems develop and can be treated in later life by becoming familiar with the generational influences that shaped this cohort of older people.

The third issue is the considerable diversity in aging. This diversity is due to many sources. Older people do not all change at the same rate or at the same chronological age. Some people experience decline in an ability relatively early in life, whereas others continue to show improvements in that same ability until relatively late in life. There is no single universal pattern of aging, nor is there a single organizing psychological principle. Older people are very different from each other because of the variety of their life experiences as well as the varying rates of aging.

An important source of diversity in aging is ethnicity and social class. People in disadvantaged racial and ethnic groups have been described as experiencing double jeopardy; that is, they are faced with negative stereotypes about their ethnic group and about aging. Perhaps the most dramatic evidence of these negative effects is on life expectancy. African American men have a life expectancy seven years lower than that of White men, and the difference for women is over four years (Hayward & Heron, 1999). Likewise, the difference for Hispanics is almost six years for men and three years for women.

These negative effects may be partly offset by social resources within minority communities. For many African Americans, for example, their families are a source of support and strength in later life, and older people are treated with respect and care. Many continue to play important roles in their families, for example, taking an active part in raising grandchildren. How we grow older is influenced by social conditions, so factors such as race, ethnicity, and social class need to be taken into account.

Another major source of diversity in aging is gender. Women and men have different life experiences, which influence how they grow older. Today's generation of older people was raised during a period when there was great differentiation of roles and responsibilities between men and women. The changing roles of men and women in society may be a source of bewilderment and resentment to some older people or lead to regrets about lost opportunities among others.

Gender is also important for its strong relation to life expectancy. Women live longer than men in virtually every country (Kinsella & Taeuber, 1993). In the United States, the average difference in life expectancy is seven years: women can expect to live 79 years; men's life expectancy is 72 years (Treas, 1995).

These differences in life expectancy have important social implications for the lives of older people. First, it means that communities of older people are predominantly women. Among people aged 65, women outnumber men by a ratio of 3 to 2. By very late life, the proportion of women is even greater: at age 80, there are only 43 men for every 100 women (U.S. Bureau of the Census, 1992).

Second, these differences in life expectancy affect marriage rates in later life. Older men are more likely to be married and older women more likely to be widows. Among people 65 and older, 77% of men but only 42% of women are married (U.S. Bureau of the Census, 1992). Several factors account for these marriage rates. Men tend to marry women younger than themselves, and so their wives outlive them. If a man outlives his wife, there will be many single women he might remarry who are his age or younger. For a woman whose husband dies, the odds are different: there will be relatively fewer men her age or older, because men have a shorter life expectancy, and fewer still will be single. Because of social traditions, it is relatively rare for a woman to marry a man who is younger than she.

CONCLUSION

This chapter provided a comprehensive overview of how clinical work with an older person might be conceptualized and implemented. The objective was to walk through a clinical case coupled with clinical and empirical considerations as a heuristic method of working with older adults. Presentation of various principles of geropsychology allows the clinician to begin assimilating a theoretical basis for understanding emotion and behavior in later life. Classifying late life disorders using the *DSM-IV* introduced how this version of the manual was refined using empirically derived findings and some of the limitations imposed when considering the gerontological literature. The disorders presented in this chapter, although not exhaustive, were attempts to acquaint the reader with the more common disorders that a clinician might encounter in a therapeutic setting.

Because one of the primary goals of the *DSM-IV* is to facilitate research, the section concerning research issues in the psychopathology of later life questioned the assumption that psychological problems an older person may be experiencing are associated with aging. The importance of considering cohort or generational differences and the considerable diversity in aging were pointed out. By linking clinical practice and research findings, better diagnostic criteria can be developed as well as better guidelines for therapeutic interventions.

STUDY QUESTIONS

1. In what ways does the clinical vignette about Mrs. Baker illustrate major features of geropsychology?
2. Give a brief description and example of the process Baltes (1987) calls "selective optimization with compensation."

3. Willis and her colleagues (Willis, Blieszner, & Baltes, 1981; Willis & Nesselroade, 1990) found evidence of plasticity or the capacity for growth in cognitive abilities. Describe what these authors found.
4. Give an example of a limitation to plasticity imposed by the aging process.
5. In what ways can the normal aging process contribute to a better understanding of psychopathology in later life?
6. When working with an older client there are several assessment issues that need to be taken into account. Describe two of these assessment issues.
7. Describe briefly the two new designations specific to late life that were included in the *DSM-IV*.
8. Discuss a major limitation of the *DSM-IV* diagnostic criteria when considering its use with elderly people.
9. Cross-sectional research provides what kind of information? What is a potential problem with using this kind of research?
10. What is an alternative to cross-sectional research? What are the advantages? Disadvantages?
11. Illustrate an important source of diversity in aging.

SUGGESTED READING

Busse, E.W., & Blazer, D.G. (Eds.). (1996). *Textbook of geriatric psychiatry* (2nd ed.). Washington, DC: American Psychiatric Press, Inc.

REFERENCES

Adams, W.L. (1997). Interactions between alcohol and other drugs. In A.M. Gurnack (Ed.), *Older adults' misuse of alcohol, medicines, and other drugs* (pp. 185–205). New York: Springer.

Allen, D.N., & Landis, R.K.B. (1997). Substance abuse in elderly individuals. In P.D. Nussbaum (Ed.), *Handbook of neuropsychology and aging: Critical issues in neuropsychology* (pp. 111–137). New York: Plenum Press.

American Psychiatric Association. (1994). *Diagnostic and statistical manual of mental disorders* (4th ed.). Washington, DC: Author.

Baltes, P.B. (1987). Theoretical propositions of life-span developmental psychology: On the dynamics between growth and decline. *Developmental Psychology, 23,* 611–626.

Baltes, P.B. (1997). On the incomplete architecture of human ontogeny: Selection, optimization, and compensation as foundations of developmental theory. *American Psychologist, 52,* 366–380.

Baltes, P.B., & Kliegl, R. (1992). Further testing of limits of cognitive plasticity: Negative age differences in a mnemonic skill are robust. *Developmental Psychology, 28(1),* 121–125.

Beizer, J.L. (1994). Medications and the aging body: Alteration as a function of age. *Generations, 18,* 13–17.

Blazer, D.G., & Koenig, H.G. (1996). Mood disorders. In E.W. Busse & D.G. Blazer (Eds.), *The American Psychiatric Press textbook of geriatric psychiatry* (2nd ed., pp. 235–263). Washington, DC: American Psychiatric Press.

Camus, V., Augusto de Mendonça Lima, C., Gaillard, M., Simeone, I., & Wertheimer, J. (1997). Are personality disorders more frequent in early onset geriatric depression? *Journal of Affective Disorders, 46,* 297–302.

Ciompi, L. (1987). Review of follow-up studies on long-term evolution and aging in schizophrenia. In N.E. Miller & G.D. Cohen (Eds.), *Schizophrenia and aging* (pp. 37–51). New York: Guilford Press.

Costa, P.T., Jr., & McCrae, R.R. (1988). Personality in adulthood: A six-year longitudinal study of self-reports and spouse ratings on the NEO personality inventory. *Journal of Personality and Social Psychology, 54,* 853–863.

Diamond, M.C., Johnson, R.E., Protti, A.M., Ott, C., & Kajisa, L. (1985). Plasticity in the 904-day-old male rat cerebral cortex. *Experimental Neurology, 87,* 309–317.

Evans, W.J. (1996). Reversing sarcopenia: How weight training can build strength and vitality. *Geriatrics, 51*(5), 46–53.

Evans, W.J., & Cyr-Campbell, D. (1997). Nutrition, exercise, and healthy aging. *Journal of the American Dietetic Association, 97,* 632–638.

Floyd, M., & Scogin, F. (1996). Effects of memory training on the subjective memory functioning and mental health of older adults: A meta-analysis. *Psychology and Aging, 12,* 150–161.

Gatz, M. (Ed.). (1995). *Emerging issues in mental health and aging.* Washington, DC: American Psychological Association.

Gutierrez, R., Atkinson, J.H., & Grant, I. (1994). Mild neurocognitive disorder: A needed addition to the nosology of cognitive impairment (organic mental) disorders? In T.A. Widiger, A.J. Frances, H.A. Pincus, M.B. First, R. Ross, & W. Davis (Eds.), *DSM-IV sourcebook* (pp. 287–317). Washington, DC: American Psychiatric Association.

Hayward, M.D., & Heron, M. (1999). Racial inequality in active life among adult Americans. *Demography, 36,* 77–91.

Hill, R.D., Sheikh, J.I., & Yesavage, J.A. (1988). Pretraining enhances mnemonic training in elderly adults. *Experimental Aging Research, 14*(4), 207–211.

Johansson, B., & Zarit, S.H. (1997). Early cognitive markers of the incidence of dementia and mortality: A longitudinal population-based study of the oldest old. *International Journal of Geriatric Psychiatry, 12,* 53–59.

Kinsella, K., & Taeuber, C.M. (1993). An aging world II. *International Population Reports.* (IPR Publication NO. P95/92-3). Washington, DC: U.S. Department of Commerce.

Kliegl, R., Smith, J., & Baltes, P.B. (1989). Testing the limits and the study of adult age differences in cognitive plasticity of a mnemonic skill. *Developmental Psychology, 25,* 247–256.

Lewinsohm, P.M., Muñoz, R.F., Youngren, M.A., & Zeiss, A.M. (1992). *Control your depression* (Rev. ed.). New York: Simon & Schuster.

Liptzin, B., & Levkoff, S. (1994). Analysis of data on a large geriatric hospitalized population relevant to the *DSM-IV* criteria for delirium. In T.A. Widiger, A.J. Frances, H.A. Pincus, M.B. First, R. Ross, & W. Davis (Eds.), *DSM-IV sourcebook* (pp. 87–90). Washington, DC: American Psychiatric Association.

Nussbaum, P.D. (Ed.). (1997). *Handbook of neuropsychology and aging.* New York and London: Plenum Press.

Palmer, B.W., Jeste, D.V., & Sheikh, J.I. (1997). Anxiety disorders in the elderly: *DSM-IV* and other barriers to diagnosis and treatment. *Journal of Affective Disorders, 46,* 183–190.

Raykov, T. (1997). Growth curve analysis of ability means and variances in measures of fluid intelligence of older adults. *Structural Equation Modeling, 4,* 283–319.

Rediess, S., & Caine, E.D. (1997). Aging, cognition, and *DSM-IV*. *Aging Neuropsychology & Cognition, 3*, 105–117.

Roberts, R.E., Lee, E.S., & Roberts, C.R. (1991). Changes in prevalence of depressive symptoms in Alameda County. *Journal of Aging and Health, 3*, 66–86.

Rosenzweig, M.R., & Bennett, E.L. (1996). Psychobiology of plasticity: Effects of training and experience on brain and behavior. *Behavioural Brain Research, 78*, 57–65.

Salmon, D.P., Butters, N., Thal, L., & Jeste, D.V. (1994). Alzheimer's disease: Data analysis for the *DSM-IV* Task Force. In T.A. Widiger, A.J. Frances, H.A. Pincus, M.B. First, R. Ross, & W. Davis (Eds.), *DSM-IV sourcebook* (pp. 91–107). Washington, DC: American Psychiatric Association.

Salthouse, T.A. (1984). Effects of age and skill in typing. *Journal of Experimental Psychology: General, 113*, 345–371.

Salthouse, T.A. (1990). Cognitive competence and expertise in aging. In J.E. Birren & K.W. Schaie (Eds.), *Handbook of the psychology of aging* (3rd ed., pp. 310–391). New York: Academic Press.

Schaie, K.W. (1996). *Intellectual development in adulthood: The Seattle Longitudinal Study.* Cambridge, England: Cambridge University Press.

Schaie, K.W., & Willis, S.L. (1996). *Adult development and aging* (4th ed.). New York: HarperCollins.

Staudinger, U.M., Marsiske, M., & Baltes, P.B. (1995). Resilience and reserve capacity in later adulthood: Potentials and limits of development across the life span. In D. Cicchetti & D.J. Cohen (Eds.), *Developmental psychopathology: Vol. 2. Risk, disorder, and adaptation* (pp. 801–847). New York: Wiley.

Treas, J. (1995). Older Americans in the 1990s and beyond. *Population Bulletin, 50*(2). Washington, DC: Population Reference Bureau.

U.S. Bureau of the Census (1992). Sixty-five plus in America. *Current Population Reports, Special Studies* (Series No. P23-178). Washington, DC: U.S. Government Printing Office.

Whitbourne, S.K., Zuschlag, M.K., Elliot, L.B., & Waterman, A.S. (1992). Psychosocial development in adulthood: A 22-year sequential study. *Journal of Personality and Social Psychology, 63*, 260–271.

Willis, S.L., Blieszner, R., & Baltes, P.B. (1981). Intellectual training research in aging: Modification of performance on the fluid ability of figural relations. *Journal of Educational Psychology, 73*, 41–50.

Willis, S.L., & Nesselroade, C.S. (1990). Long-term effects of fluid ability training in old-old age. *Developmental Psychology, 26*(6), 905–910.

Yale, R. (1999). Support groups and other services for individuals with early stage Alzheimer's disease. *Generations, 23*, 57–61.

Zarit, S.H., & Zarit, J.M. (1998). *Mental disorders in older adults: Fundamentals of assessment and treatment.* New York: Guilford Press.

Zeiss, A.M., & Steffen, A. (1996). Behavioral and cognitive-behavioral treatments: An overview of social learning. In S.H. Zarit & B.G. Knight (Eds.), *A guide to psychotherapy and aging* (pp. 35–60). Washington, DC: American Psychological Association.

CHAPTER 2

The Normal Aging Process

SUSAN KRAUSS WHITBOURNE

CASE STUDY

Mr. D. is a 78-year-old retired engineer who lives in a condominium in Florida with his wife of 50 years. He considers himself to be in good health and maintains an active lifestyle in which he combines golf, workouts at the gym, and frequent walking as ways of staying physically fit. Although his knees occasionally ache somewhat, Mr. D. takes care to stretch properly before a workout and he is considering taking a yoga class. A large part of his day is spent online as he exchanges e-mail with his children, grandchildren, and former coworkers. In addition, he enjoys playing computer games and likes to plan via the Internet the occasional trips he takes with his wife. Although he has always had an excellent memory, lately he has noticed that some things are harder to remember than they used to be, such as the e-mail address of a new acquaintance. However, Mr. D. has always felt that he could tackle any problem that came along, including this one. Now he keeps lists of important pieces of information and schedules reminders on his computer. Mr. D. has an optimistic outlook on the future and feels that the "good luck" he has had all his life will sustain him for years to come.

The physical aging process technically begins when an individual is conceived, as the passage of time is associated with changes in each cell of the body. However, for practical purposes, aging is not considered a relevant phenomenon in an individual's life until some point in adulthood. The onset of aging in adulthood does not occur at one specific point, however. Age-related changes in the body accumulate gradually and at different rates in the various bodily systems.

Although aging is essentially a biological process, the rate and timing of age-related changes interact in significant ways with psychological and sociocultural factors. There are many ways that older individuals can either accelerate or decelerate the effects of aging on their body. The extent to which adults engage in these processes is theorized to be a function, in part, of the individual's identity. Most individuals in adulthood attempt to maintain a consistent sense of the self over time (Whitbourne & Collins, 1998). Optimal aging occurs when individuals achieve a balance by maintaining their positive view of the self over time while adapting their behaviors to compensate for or prevent age-related losses. As described elsewhere in this volume, certain psychological disorders such as depression, anxiety, and exacerbation of personality disorder symptoms can interact in important ways with the identity changes associated with the aging process.

In the sections that follow, the emphasis is on explaining the most important physical and cognitive changes associated with the aging process. Interactions with personality and social context are also discussed. Preventative and compensatory measures are presented where the data permit such implications to be drawn, with a focus on the areas that clinicians can emphasize in helping their older clients to maximize their functioning.

APPEARANCE AND MOBILITY

Age changes in appearance and mobility are among the first effects of aging that individuals notice. Because the outside appearance of the individual is used by others as a social cue to age, many people in this society are sensitive to even small age-related changes. Changes in bodily systems that contribute to appearance may also have more significance in terms of general health and susceptibility to illness.

APPEARANCE

Skin

The wrinkling and sagging of the skin are processes that take on significance early in adulthood and continue throughout middle age as the skin starts to lose its firmness and elasticity. Visual changes in the appearance of skin are accounted for in part by the fact that with increasing age, the cells of the epidermis become less regular in their arrangement (Kligman, Grove, & Balin, 1985), collagen molecules undergo the deleterious changes involved in cross-linking that make them more rigid, and elastin fibers become more brittle. The result of the changes in collagen and elastin is a loss of the skin's flexibility and ability to conform to the changing shape of the skin as the limbs move. Contributing to changes in the skin's appearance and function is lowered activity of sweat and sebaceous glands. The layer of subcutaneous fat begins to thin in middle adulthood, and fat shifts to collect as fatty deposits around the torso.

Other changes in the coloring of the skin occur due to the development of *arcus senilus* ("age spots"), pigmented outgrowths, greater visibility of capillaries and arteries in the skin, and varicose veins. The nails also start to show signs of aging as their growth rate slows and they take on a yellowish appearance. Facial appearance is affected by tooth discoloration, tooth loss, the wearing of eye-glasses, and the accumulation of fat, fluid, and dark pigmentation under the eyes.

Many of the changes in the skin are due to photoaging, age changes caused by exposure to the sun's harmful radiation. Parts of the body that are more exposed to the sun, such as the face and arms, are more likely to show the changes described here than are parts of the body that are not exposed (Takema, Yorimoto, Ohsu, Osanai, & Kawai, 1997). Sunscreen that effectively blocks the rays of the sun is the most effective prevention (Farmer & Naylor, 1996). Cigarettes should also be avoided, as smoking is harmful to the skin. Some compensation for changes that have already occurred can be attained through facial massages (Iida & Noro, 1995), skin emollients, and the application of vitamin E (Nachbar & Korting, 1995).

Hair

Changes in the color of the hair are a universal age-related process that occur due to loss of pigmentation in the hairs that remain on the head as melanin production ceases. The actual shade of gray that develops is the result of the mixture of the white (unpigmented) hairs with the remaining pigmented hairs. Eventually, for most people, all the hairs are unpigmented and the overall hair color is white. Less universal, but also frequent in occurrence, is a thinning of the hair on the head. The thinning of the hair, although more obvious in men, actually occurs in both sexes. Hair loss in general results from the destruction of the germination centers that produce the hair. In the form of hair loss that is specific to males and is genetically determined, called male pattern baldness, the hair follicles continue to produce very fine hair, almost invisible vellus hair. Although hair stops growing or becomes less visible where it is desired, it may appear in larger amounts in places where it is not welcome, such as the chin on women, the ears, and in thicker clumps around the eyebrows.

Body Build

Beginning in middle adulthood, individuals show significant changes in height and weight. A decline in height, which continues well into the 70s and 80s, is consistently demonstrated both in cross-sectional and longitudinal studies, and is more pronounced in women (de Groot, Perdigao, & Deurenberg, 1996; Suominen, 1997). Changes in height occur due to loss of bone material in the vertebrae, which collapse and thereby shorten the length of the spine. Total body weight increases from early adulthood until the mid-50s and then declines after that. Most of the weight gain that occurs through the years of middle adulthood is due to an accumulation of body fat in the torso. When weight loss occurs after the 50s, this is due to loss of lean body mass, that is, muscle and bone (Baumgartner, Heymsfield, & Roche, 1995).

There are significant preventative and compensatory measures that individuals can take to offset the aging of body build. Involvement in aerobic exercise leads to improved muscle tone and reductions in fat. Resistance training can help to offset age losses in bone content that contribute to the loss of height. The average middle-aged and older adult can see positive results within two to three months by engaging in vigorous walking, jogging, or cycling for 30 to 60 minutes a day, for three to four days a week (Vitiello et al., 1997).

MOBILITY

The structures that support mobility are the bones, joints, tendons and ligaments that connect the muscles to the bones, and the muscles that control flexion and extension. Beginning in the 40s, or earlier in the case of injury, each component of mobility undergoes significant age-related losses. Consequently, there is a gradual reduction of walking speed (Bohannon, 1997) and a development of joint pain leading to restriction of movement in daily activities (Grimby & Wiklund, 1994).

Muscles

The adult years are characterized by a progressive loss of muscle mass, a process known as sarcopenia. Accompanying sarcopenia is a loss of strength beginning in the 40s to 50s, with a decline thereafter of 12% to 15% per decade (Hurley, 1995). By contrast, isometric strength is generally maintained (Bemben, Massey, Bemben, Misner, & Boileau, 1996).

Strength training is the chief preventative and compensatory measure for sarcopenia (McCartney, Hicks, Martin, & Webber, 1995, 1996). Using either progressive or high-intensity resistance training, adults can more than double their maximum muscle strength. Effective training typically involves 8 to 12 weeks, three to four times per week, at 70% to 90% of the one repetition maximum. Even if an individual takes a break from an exercise program, the lost strength can quickly be regained once exercise is resumed (Taaffe & Marcus, 1997).

Bones

The general pattern of bone development in adulthood involves an increase in the rate of bone destruction compared to renewal and greater porosity of the calcium matrix leading to loss of bone mineral content. Estimates of the decrease in bone mineral content over adulthood are 5% to 12% per decade from the 20s through the 90s (McCalden, McGeough, Barker, & Court-Brown, 1993), with an accompanying decrease in strength of 8.5% per decade (McCalden, McGeough, & Court-Brown, 1997). Part of the increased susceptibility to fracture of older bone can be accounted for by a loss of elasticity, meaning that bone breaks rather than bends when pressure is applied (Zioupos & Currey, 1998). The rate of bone loss is greater in women, particularly those who are past reproductive age and are no longer producing the hormone estrogen in monthly cycles (Garnero, Sornay Rendu, Chapuy, & Delmas, 1996). Heavier people in general have higher bone mineral content, and so they lose less in adulthood, particularly in the weight-bearing limbs that are involved in mobility (Edelstein & Barrett-Connor, 1993).

Among women, African American women have higher bone mineral content than do Whites (Perry et al., 1996), and among Whites, bone loss is greater in those with fair skin (May, Murphy, & Khaw, 1995). Still, bone loss is generally higher in women of all races studied (Krall et al., 1997), including Whites, African Americans (Perry et al., 1996), and Chinese (Xu, Huang, & Ren, 1997). Hispanic women show patterns of bone loss similar to non-Hispanic Whites, even though the risk of hip fracture among Hispanic women is lower (Villa, Marcus, Ramirez Delay, & Kelsey, 1995).

Smoking, alcohol use, and poor diet exacerbate bone loss in later adulthood, but bone loss can be slowed by aerobic activity, resistance training with weights, increased calcium intake prior to menopause, and use of vitamin D (Dawson-Hughes et al., 1995; S. Murphy, Khaw, May, & Compston, 1994; Sinaki, 1996; Welten, Kemper, Post, & van Staveren, 1995).

Joints

Structural changes occur with age in virtually every component of the joint. By the 20s and 30s, the arterial cartilage that protects the joints begins to degenerate, and as it does so, the bone underneath begins to wear away. At the same time, outgrowths of cartilage begin to develop that further interfere with the smooth movement of the bones against each other. The fibers in the joint capsule become less pliable, reducing flexibility (Ralphs & Benjamin, 1994).

Unlike muscles, joints do not benefit from constant use. On the contrary, these deterioration processes are directly related to the amount of stress placed on the joints. Exercise cannot compensate for or prevent age-related changes. However, precautions taken in early adulthood can reduce the chance of losses in middle age. Most important is proper footwear, particularly during exercise. People who engage in occupational activities that involve repetitive motions of the wrist can minimize damage by the use of ergonomically designed accessories. Exercise that strengthens the muscles supporting the joint also helps to improve its functioning (Blanpied & Smidt, 1993). Both kinds of exercise have the additional benefit of stimulating circulation to the joints, thereby enhancing the blood supply that promotes repair processes in the tendons, ligaments, and surfaces of the exercising areas.

VITAL BODILY FUNCTIONS

Age-related changes in the bodily systems that support life ultimately determine the individual's survival. Along with the nervous system, the functioning of these vital organs determines the length and the quality of life. Changes in the vital bodily systems can also have important psychological consequences.

CARDIOVASCULAR SYSTEM

The component of the heart that has the most relevance to aging is the left ventricle, which loses muscle mass and strength and increases in fat and connective tissue. The wall of the left ventricle becomes thicker and less compliant during each contraction, leading the left ventricle to lose its effectiveness as a pumping mechanism. Therefore, less blood is ejected into the aorta with each contraction of the heart. The arteries become less able to accommodate the flow of blood that spews from the left ventricle. This loss of flexibility in the arteries is referred to as vasculopathology of aging (Bilato & Crow, 1996). Adding to these changes is the continuing deposit of plaque along the arterial walls of fatty substances, consisting of cholesterol, cellular waste products, calcium, and fibrin (a clotting material in the blood). Although theoretically distinct from atherosclerosis, there is a resemblance between some of the normal structural changes that begin in middle age and those associated with this arterial disease.

The primary indicators of cardiovascular efficiency are aerobic capacity, the maximum amount of oxygen that can be delivered through the blood, and cardiac output, the amount of blood that the heart pumps per minute. Both indices decline consistently at a rate of about 10% per decade from age 25, so that the average 65-year-old has 40% lower cardiovascular efficiency.

Exercise is a primary form of prevention against age-related cardiovascular changes. To be effective, exercise must stimulate the heart rate to rise to 60% to 75% of maximum capacity, and this training must take place three to four times a week. The specific effects of exercise on heart muscle vary by gender. For men, exercise strengthens the myocardial muscle, causing it to be more effective in exerting pressure on the left ventricle to contract and leading ultimately to more blood reaching the body's cells. For women, however, exercise does not have the same effects on ventricular dynamics (Spina, Miller, Bogenhagen, Schechtman, & Ehsani, 1996). Clearly, more data are needed to understand these apparent gender differences in the relationship between exercise and cardiovascular functioning. Exercise must also be combined with a diet that is low in saturated fats. Most of the adult population must carefully monitor cholesterol levels, particularly from middle age and upward. Although total cholesterol level decreases during this period, this decline includes a lowering of the HDL cholesterol (Ferrara, Barrett-Connor, & Shan, 1997; Wilson, Anderson, Harris, Kannel, & Castelli, 1994), which can result in an increase in the individual's risk of heart disease (Stampfer et al., 1996).

The consequences of age-related changes in the arteries include an increasing probability from middle adulthood on in developing hypertension. Although normal aging is not associated with increased blood pressure, hypertension rates rise in older populations. For males, the risk increases from 22% to 32% of the population between the ages of 45 to 64 and 64 and over; the rates for females are 23% and 40% (Statistics, 1997). A lowering of both saturated fat and salt are known to prevent or reduce hypertension. Exercise further contributes to the effects of diet on hypertension. In addition to its physiological effects, exercise can also provide an avenue of stress reduction that can contribute to lowered blood pressure.

RESPIRATORY SYSTEM

Aging affects the process of respiration in part through a reduction in the strength of the respiratory muscles and in part through an increase in rigidity of the connective tissue in the chest wall to be expanded during inspiration and contracted during expiration. These changes have the effect of reducing the amount of air that can be pumped in and out of the lungs (Teramoto, Fukuchi, Nagase, Matsuse, & Orimo, 1995). Aging is also associated with a "failing lung" (Rossi, Ganassini, Tantucci, & Grassi, 1996) that causes the lung tissue itself to lose expandability. Consequently, all measures of lung functioning in adulthood show age-related losses from about 40 years and on (Rossi et al., 1996).

Exercise can strengthen the chest wall and thereby compensate for some loss of pumping capacity of the respiratory muscles. However, there is no measure available to offset changes that occur in the lung tissue itself. The best that can be hoped for is to minimize the effects of aging on the lungs, and this is done by not smoking cigarettes (Rossi et al., 1996). The cessation of smoking is clearly associated with improvements in lung functioning in adults over 50. In a large-scale study of almost 1,400 adults from age 51 to 95 years, lung functioning was significantly lower in smokers than nonsmokers across the entire age range (Frette, Barrett-Connor, & Clausen, 1996).

URINARY SYSTEM

Studies dating back to the late 1940s showed that loss of the nephron (the basic unit of the kidney) occurs consistently throughout adulthood at a rate of 6% per decade and that virtually all measures of renal efficiency show a steady and consistent drop-off over time (Davies & Shock, 1950). This view has been challenged by more refined studies which indicate that normal aging is not associated with impaired kidney functioning (Epstein, 1996; Fliser et al., 1997). However, when the kidney is placed under stress, such as during illness, extreme exertion, or a heat wave, declines in functioning become evident. Because of the risk of lower excretion rates, medication levels must be carefully monitored in middle-aged and older adults who are at risk of such conditions (Montgomery, 1990).

Changes with aging may also occur in the elastic tissue of the bladder such that it cannot as efficiently retain or expel urine. Despite these changes, the majority of older adults do not experience significant problems in the area of bladder functioning, as only 2% of men and 5% of women report bladder problems as a chronic condition (National Center for Health Statistics, 1997). Estimates of the prevalence of urinary incontinence among the over-65 population range from a low of 6% to 8% of those living in the community to a high of 20% to 30% or more of those living in institutions (Iqbal & Castleden, 1997). Stress incontinence, which is loss of urine during a sudden physical action, is more likely to occur in women due the effects of childbirth or age-related decreases in estrogen. Urge incontinence, which involves loss of control over urinary sphincters, is associated with prostate disease in men. Behavioral controls are often successful in treating incontinence (Burgio & Engel, 1990; Burns et al., 1993), and Kegel exercises can help prevent stress incontinence in women.

DIGESTIVE SYSTEM

Although the normal aging process may in and of itself contribute little to changes in the gastrointestinal system, reduced functioning may still occur for other reasons, such as abnormal feelings of fullness (Clarkston et al., 1997) and health conditions that can interfere with absorption of nutrients (Lovat, 1996). Many lifestyle factors that change in middle and later adulthood also contribute to digestive functioning. These factors include family composition, financial resources, and age-related mobility and cognitive problems. Other factors reflect the exposure that individuals have through the media to the need to use dietary supplements, digestive aids, and laxatives after the age of 40 or 50. Despite the image portrayed by the media, problems such as fecal incontinence affect only a small fraction of even the over-65 population (3% of men and 7% of women) (National Center for Health Statistics, 1997).

BODILY CONTROL SYSTEMS

Changes in the processes that regulate metabolism, reproduction, and control against infection interact with those that control appearance, mobility, and the vital life functions just discussed.

ENDOCRINE SYSTEM

For centuries, scientists have been fascinated with the prospect that the cause of aging will someday be linked to the functions of the endocrine system. In recent years, additional interest in this system was fostered by recognition of the importance of hormones in determining the amount and proportions of muscle, bone, and fat in the body. The potential relevance of sex hormones to this important area of functioning, and possibly to other physical and psychological functions as well, also creates heightened interest in the endocrine system in general.

Growth Hormone

There is a consistently documented decline estimated at 14% per decade over adulthood in the secretion of growth hormone (GH) (Kern, Dodt, Born, & Fehm, 1996; Toogood, O' Neill, & Shalet, 1996). A related hormone produced by the liver, IGF-1 (insulinlike growth factor 1), also shows an age-related decrease across adulthood. IGF-1 stimulates muscle cells to increase in size and number, perhaps by stimulating their genes to increase the production of muscle-specific proteins. The decline in what is called the somatotrophic axis (GH and IGF-1) is called "somatopause." Because GH production affects the metabolism of proteins, lipids, and carbohydrates, the somatopause is thought to account for a number of age-related changes in body composition across adulthood, including loss of bone mineral content (Boonen et al., 1996), increases in fat, and a decrease in muscle mass (Bjorntorp, 1996). Normally, GH production shows regularly timed peaks during nighttime sleep; in older adults, this peak is smaller (Prinz et al., 1995). GH also rises during heavy resistance exercise, and in adults over 70, this response is attenuated (Hakkinen & Pakarinen, 1995).

The recent media attention given to hormones and aging includes claims that GH replacement therapy is the magic potion that can stop the aging process (Taaffe et al., 1994). In addition to being extremely expensive, however, there is evidence that the side effects of this treatment outweigh any of its possible advantages (Riedel, Brabant, Rieger, & von zur Muhlen, 1994). GH is linked to joint pain, enlargement of the heart, enlargement of the bones, diabetes, and pooling of fluid in the skin and other tissues, which can lead to high blood pressure and heart failure. A safer and cheaper alternative is exercise, which can accomplish some of the positive effects of GH replacement therapy, including favorable effects on GH secretion and bodily composition (Brown, Birge, & Kohrt, 1997; Silverman & Mazzeo, 1996).

Cortisol

Cortisol production is regulated by a negative feedback loop between the adrenal gland and the pituitary gland, intended to protect the body from damage from the effects of unchecked rises. Such damage can affect the thymus gland, depress immune responses in general, and cause destruction of tissue, breakdown of proteins, and formation of fat deposits (Seaton, 1995). Increases in circulating cortisol (the "stress hormone") in the blood may also be linked to damage to cells in the hippocampus and therefore contribute to memory problems (Van Cauter, Leproult, & Kupfer, 1996).

There are many advocates of the so-called glucocorticoid cascade hypothesis of aging, which considers changes in cortisol levels to be a central mechanism in the aging process (O'Brien, Schweitzer, Ames, Tuckwell, & Mastwyk, 1994; Wilkinson, Peskind, & Raskind, 1997). Supporting this hypothesis, researchers have estimated that cortisol levels rise from 20% to 50% between the years of 20 to 80 at a rate of 5% to 7% per decade (Van Cauter et al., 1996). Adding weight to this hypothesis is evidence of heightened cortisol response of older people, particularly women, to stress or physiological stimulation (Gotthardt et al., 1995; Kelly, Hayslip, & Servaty, 1996; Peskind et al., 1995; Seeman, Singer, & Charpentier, 1995).

However, not all the data support the glucocorticoid cascade hypothesis (Gotthardt et al., 1995; Nicolson, Storms, Ponds, & Sulon, 1997). Longitudinal data based on yearly testing of healthy older adults over a three- to six-year period show that some older individuals increase, some decrease, and some remain stable in cortisol levels. Furthermore, variations in cortisol level may relate to individual differences in personality, particularly anxiety (Lupien et al., 1996). Another factor that may play a role in cross-sectional studies is obesity, which is positively related to cortisol levels in middle-aged men (Field, Colditz, Willett, Longcope, & McKinlay, 1994). Although it is not known whether obesity causes higher cortisol levels or vice versa, the existence of such data calls into question a general hypothesis about cortisol and aging.

Melatonin

The production of melatonin declines with increasing age, and circulating melatonin levels are affected by certain environmental conditions, such as food restriction, which increases melatonin levels and prevents its age-related decline. It is thought that melatonin may have beneficial effects on certain aspects of aging and age-associated diseases, especially in the brain and immune system. However, the weight of the evidence does not favor melatonin supplements (Huether, 1996). Not only are these ineffective, but they can interfere with sleep cycles if taken at the wrong time. Other side effects include confusion, drowsiness, headaches, and constriction of blood vessels, which would be dangerous in people who have high blood pressure. Finally, the dosages usually sold in over-the-counter medications may be as high as 40 times the amount normally found in the body, and the effect of such large doses taken over a long term has not been determined.

Dehydroepiandrosterone (DHEA)

This hormone is a weak male steroid (androgen) produced by the adrenal glands. It is a precursor to the sex hormones testosterone and estrogen and is believed to have a variety of functions in the body. Some of these functions include increasing production of other sex steroids and availability of IGF-1 and positively influencing some functions in the central nervous system.

DHEA, which is higher in males than in females, shows a pronounced decrease over the adult years, reducing by 80% to 90% between the years of 20 and 80. This phenomenon, termed "adrenopause" (Lamberts, van den Beld, & van der Lely, 1997), is greater in men, although men continue to have higher levels than women because they start at a higher baseline. There is some evidence that loss of DHEA is related to functional declines in various measures of physical and mental health, particularly for women (Berr, Lafont, Debuire, Dartigues, & Baulieu, 1996). Researchers have attempted to determine whether changes in DHEA are related to the reductions with age in insulin sensitivity (Denti et al., 1997) and immune system functioning (James et al., 1997). The relationship of DHEA decrease and testosterone levels in men is also being explored (Morley et al., 1997).

Although there are no definitive answers other than the fact that the decline in DHEA is probably a reliable one, DHEA replacement therapy is rivaling GH and melatonin in the anti-aging industry. There are some proponents in the scientific community for the use of DHEA supplements (Yen, Morales, & Khorram, 1995), but other researchers cast doubt on its utility (Barrou, Charru, & Lidy, 1997; R.A. Miller, 1996). Like GH therapy, there may also be some attendant risks, notably liver problems and an increase in risk of prostate and breast cancer.

Estrogen and the Menopause

The menopause is the last stage of a gradual biological process in which the ovaries slow in the production of female sex hormones. This process takes place over a three- to five-year span called the perimenopause, ending in the menopause, when the women has not had her menstrual period for one year. The average age of menopause is 50 years, but the timing varies among individuals. Menopause occurs earlier in women who are thin or malnourished or who smoke.

Although women vary considerably in their progression through the menopause (as is true during puberty), there are certain characteristic symptoms. One of the most prominent is the occurrence of "hot flashes," which are sudden sensations of intense heat and sweating that can last from a few moments to half an hour. Over half of women experience hot flashes over the course of a two-year period. These changes in perceived body temperature are the result of decreases in estrogen levels, which cause the endocrine system to release higher amounts of other hormones that affect the temperature control centers in the brain. Fatigue, headaches, night sweats, and insomnia are other physiological symptoms thought to be the result of fluctuating estrogen levels. Psychological symptoms are also commonly reported, such as irritability, mood swings, depression, memory loss, and difficulty concentrating, but the evidence regarding the connection between these symptoms and the physiological changes involved in menopause is far from conclusive.

Along with these hormonal changes are alterations in the reproductive tract. The tissues throughout the system become thinner, less elastic, and altered in position and shape. Due to lower estrogen levels, there is a reduction in the supply of blood to the vagina and surrounding nerves and glands. The tissues become thinner, drier, and less able to produce secretions to lubricate before and during intercourse. The result is the possibility of discomfort during intercourse and greater susceptibility to infection, which is more prevalent among women over 50 (Laumann, Paik, & Rosen, 1999). In addition, the woman may become more susceptible to urinary problems such as infections and stress incontinence (as discussed above).

More widespread throughout the body are other effects of menopause associated with the impact of decreasing estrogen levels on other bodily systems. Loss of bone strength in women becomes much more pronounced after menopause. Atherosclerosis and high blood pressure, as well as other cardiovascular diseases, also become more prevalent among postmenopausal women. It appears that estrogen provides a protection against these diseases during the reproductive years that is lost at menopause. There are also changes in cholesterol levels in the blood associated with menopause, causing postmenopausal women to be at higher risk of atherosclerosis and associated conditions. Estrogen is also thought to be a protective factor against Alzheimer's disease, and its diminution therefore may take away this protection.

Estrogen-replacement therapy (ERT) was introduced in the 1940s to counteract the negative effects of estrogen loss on postmenopausal women. However, this therapy increased the risk of cancer and blood clots. Currently, women receiving estrogen are given lower doses along with progestin (called hormone-replacement therapy, or HRT) to reduce cancer risk. Even this treatment, when taken over a long course, however, can increase a woman's risk of developing breast cancer. HRT can also trigger asthma and gallstones and cause blood sugar levels to change, posing a danger to women with diabetes. Some women also suffer side effects such as tenderness of the breasts and headaches from estrogen, or bloating and depression from progestin. Another alternative is a selective estrogen replacement modulaters (SERM) such as raloxifene. This form of HRT has a more targeted effect on bone loss. Other recommended approaches in addition to HRT to counteract the effect of hormonal changes include engaging in exercise, giving up smoking, lowering cholesterol intake, and having one alcoholic drink a day.

HRT is also emerging as a preventive measure for Alzheimer's disease. A number of explanations of the possible role of estrogen in preventing Alzheimer's disease have emerged, including the possibility that estrogen facilitates verbal functioning throughout life (Sherwin, 1996), perhaps by maintaining serotonergic and cholinergic pathways (McEwen, Alves, Bulloch, & Weiland, 1997). Another possibility is that estrogen improves blood flow in regions of the brain affected by Alzheimer's disease (Birge, 1997).

Testosterone

The term "andropause" was coined to refer to age-related declines in the male sex hormone testosterone, corresponding, theoretically, to declines in estrogen for women. Supposedly related to the andropause is a loss of sexual potency, although it is now recognized that changes in erectile functioning are related more to the circulatory than the endocrine system as well as to social factors and stress (Laumann et al., 1999). However, debate continues regarding the extent to which a drop in testosterone applies to normal aging. According to conventional wisdom and a number of cross-sectional studies, there is a decrease in free testosterone across progressively older age groups of men starting at the age of 40 and continuing at a rate of 1% per year after that (de Lignieres, 1993). However, not all studies show this pattern, and researchers recognize that a number of potentially confounding methodological factors exist that might account for the disparities across investigations (Maas, Jochen, & Lalande, 1997). In one rare longitudinal study, changes in testosterone levels were found to be correlated with cholesterol levels, percent of body fat, cigarette smoking, and behavioral tendencies that predispose an individual to developing cardiovascular disease. Nevertheless, taking all these factors into account, a slight testosterone decrease was noted over the 13-year period of the study in men between the age of 41 and 61 years (Zmuda et al., 1997).

Changes in testosterone in healthy aging men are only slight although detectable. Testosterone therapy is considered appropriate for men who have a clear hormonal deficiency, but it is not advisable for otherwise healthy middle-aged and older men to take externally administered testosterone. There is an increased risk associated with its use for developing cancer as well as a variety of deleterious changes, such as an enlarged prostate gland, higher cholesterol, infertility, and acne. These problems outweigh any advantages that may exist for muscle strength, sexual potency, and the prevention of frailty.

IMMUNE SYSTEM

Declines in immune system functioning have been suspected for many years based on observations of age-related increases in autoimmune diseases and the clinical observation that older adults are more vulnerable to influenza and many forms of cancer. However, there is still much that remains to be resolved, such as whether observed immune deficiencies in older adults are the result of normal aging or disease processes. In addition to the fact that the immune system is incredibly complicated, there is much disagreement in the published literature over the causes of the decline. Nevertheless, researchers feel confident enough that the observed age effects are reliable to have coined the term "immune senescence" to describe the features of the aging immune system (R.A. Miller, 1996).

The primary feature of immune senescence is the decline of T cell functioning, including a lowered proliferation of T cells during cell-mediated immunity and a lowering of helper T cells in humoral immunity. There are more memory T cells and fewer naïve T cells, and as a result, the system is less able to respond to newly encountered antigens (R.A. Miller, 1996). The ability to produce antibodies by B cells is also compromised by the aging process, but it is not clear whether this is due to a decline in the B cells themselves or to less effective action of helper T cells. There is also some evidence for changes in certain interleukins, the substances produced by T cells. One of these, interleukin-6, increases with age, which suggests the possibility that they somehow interfere with the immune response. In contrast, interleukin-2 diminishes with age, a fact that may account for decreases in T cell proliferation. The functioning of NK cells in the bloodstream is maintained in later life, but these cells may be less effective in the spleen and lymph node tissues, which is where they are most needed. There also may be important links between the immune and endocrine systems. For example, interleukin-2 is depressed when estrogen levels decrease.

The cause of immune senescence is commonly thought to be due to the involution of the thymus, which loses most of its functioning by early adulthood. Thus, the T cells that circulate in the secondary lymphoid organs are mature T cells that were produced early in the individual's life during exposure to new antigens. Countering this fact is the suggestion that the system may have more dynamic properties than would be true if anatomy were the sole determinant of immune functioning. Thus, the fact that new T cells are stimulated by existing T cells could mean that, everything else being equal, the numbers of T cells may actually remain more stable than the demise of the thymus would indicate (R.A. Miller, 1996). Furthermore, if the remaining T cells are able to retain or improve their responsiveness, this would compensate for their sheer loss of numbers (Born et al., 1995). Established wisdom nevertheless regards the immune system as a target of the aging process and, further, as a prime suspect in regulating length of life.

This being said, there are many interactions between immune system functioning and other physical and psychological processes. Diet and exercise, in particular, can either enhance or detract from various immune system indicators.

For example, additives such as zinc and vitamin E can improve immune responsiveness (Lesourd, 1997; Sone, 1995). Conversely, older people who eat low-protein diets show deficient immune functioning in addition to other serious losses in body composition (Castaneda, Charnley, Evans, & Crim, 1995). As is true for diet, exercise can influence immune responsiveness (Shinkai, Konishi, & Shephard, 1997; Venjatraman & Fernandes, 1997). Given this knowledge, it is necessary to reevaluate the existing data on aging and the immune system, in which exercise and diet were not controlled. Previous findings may have presented an overly negative picture of the effects of aging.

NERVOUS SYSTEM

Early research on the effects of the aging process on the nervous system was based on the hypothesis that, because neurons do not reproduce, there is a progressive loss of brain tissue across the adult years that is noticeable by the age of 30. The model of aging based on this hypothesis was called by some the "neuronal fallout model." However, in the years intervening since that early research, it is becoming clear that in the absence of disease, the aging brain maintains much of its structure and function. Research conducted in the late 1970s and 1980s provided the first evidence that, when given proper amounts of stimulation in the form of mental activity, aging organisms can compensate for loss of neurons by increasing the number of synapses formed by the remaining neurons (Coleman & Flood, 1987). Improvements in methods due to the availability of brain scans as well as experimental studies involving synaptic proliferation and neuron regeneration are further responsible for the current climate of greater optimism regarding age and the nervous system. Furthermore, with refinements in the definition and diagnosis of Alzheimer's disease, researchers are increasingly able to separate the effects of normal aging from the severe losses that occur in this disease and related conditions.

Recent studies using brain imaging techniques show considerable interindividual variability in patterns of brain changes across adulthood. In one large magnetic resonance imaging (MRI) study of adults, percentages of atrophy ranging from 6% to 8% per year were reported, but there was wide individual variation both in patterns of cortical atrophy and in ventricular enlargement (Coffey et al., 1992). Some of this variability may be accounted for by health status. Those in good health are spared some of the effects of aging, such as reductions in temporal lobe volume (DeCarli et al., 1994). There also may be significant gender variations, as there are larger increases for men than women in the ventricular spaces in the brain (Matsumae et al., 1996). Men show greater reductions than women in the frontal and temporal lobes (Cowell et al., 1994) as well as in the parieto-occipital area (Coffey et al., 1998). Conversely, men may be relatively spared compared to women in the case of the hippocampus and parietal lobes (D.G. Murphy et al., 1996).

In studies of the frontal lobes using both MRI and positron-emission tomography (PET) scans, age reductions appear to be more conclusively demonstrated than in studies of other cortical areas (Raz et al., 1997), with estimates ranging from a low of 1% per decade (De Santi et al., 1995) to a high of around 10% (Eisen, Entezari-Taher, & Stewart, 1996). There is also evidence for reductions in the volume of the hippocampus with increasing age in adulthood (de Leon et al., 1997; Raz, Gunning-Dixon, Head, Dupuis, & Acker, 1998). These patterns of findings are interpreted as providing a neurological basis for the behavioral observations of memory changes in later adulthood (Golomb et al., 1996; Nielsen Bohlman, & Knight, 1995).

However, there are compensating factors indicating that if older adults suffer brain deficits in one area, they make up for these by increasing the activation of other brain regions (Cabeza et al., 1997). Studies using PET scans have also shown older adults to be less able to increase the blood flow to specific parts of the brain in response to tasks that demand the use of those brain regions (Ross et al., 1997). However, they may also compensate by using other brain circuits to make up for decreases in the frontal lobes (Chao & Knight, 1997).

TEMPERATURE CONTROL

It is standard news fare in the summer and winter each year to hear that with each heat wave or cold snap, older adults are at risk of dying from hyper- or hypothermia, conditions known together as dysthermia. Heat exposure was the cause of 6,615 deaths in the United States between the years 1979 and 1995. Of the over 2,700 people whose deaths were known to be linked to weather conditions (either extreme heat or cold) 62% occurred in people over the age of 55 years and the percentages rose sharply with each age decade (Centers for Disease Control, 1998). However, researchers shed doubt on the common wisdom that age alone increases the risk of hyperthermia and hypothermia. Some of the factors known to contribute to dysthermia are amount of body fat (Inoue, Nakao, Araki, & Ueda, 1992), gender (Young, 1991), and physical fitness (Young & Lee, 1997). With regard to physical fitness, for example, it is known that older adults have an impaired ability to secrete sweat in conditions of extreme heat (Inoue, 1996). The lack of body cooling mechanisms can lead to heat exhaustion and heat stroke in extreme heat conditions. However, men in their late 50s to early 70s who have greater aerobic power have superior sweat gland functioning and blood flow to the skin, processes that improve body heat adaptation (Tankersley, Smolander, Kenney, & Fortney, 1991). More and more researchers concur that in the absence of disease, older, fit adults may have some impairment in thermal regulation, but not to the extent that was once believed.

SENSATION AND PERCEPTION

There are a variety of changes that occur in adulthood throughout individual sensory systems. These changes reduce the quality of input that reaches the brain to be integrated in subsequent stages of information processing.

Vision

It is well established that visual acuity shows a consistent drop across the years of adulthood as measured by the Snellen chart. The level of acuity in an 85-year-old is about 80% less than that of a person in the 40s, a loss that is about 2% per year. The loss of acuity is greater in African Americans than in Whites and appears to be similar for men and women (West et al., 1997). By raising the level of illumination, it is possible to compensate somewhat for this loss, but in dimly lit surroundings, older people have a great deal more trouble when they must observe details at a distance. On the other hand, adults over the age of 40 years are sensitive to glare, so sudden increases in light or exposure to bright scattered light can impair rather than improve visual acuity. Presbyopia, the second major normative age-related change in the eye, makes it more difficult to focus on near objects, a condition that must be corrected by wearing reading glasses or bifocals.

Hearing

There are two forms of hearing loss that can occur in later life, and because they are so common, they are considered a normal component of the aging process. In sensorineural hearing loss, also known as presbycusis, degenerative changes occur in the cochlea or auditory nerve leading from the cochlea to the brain. Presbycusis is most often associated with loss of high-pitched sounds. In conductive hearing loss, damage occurs in one of the structures that transmits sounds, most often the tympanic membrane. Although hereditary factors, various health problems (diabetes, heart disease, high blood pressure), and the use of some medications (aspirin, antibiotics) can contribute to hearing loss in later adulthood, exposure to loud noise is the most frequent cause. Another hearing disturbance that is relatively common in older people is tinnitus, in which the individual perceives sounds in the head or ear (such as a ringing noise) when there is no external source for it. The condition can be temporarily associated with use of aspirin, antibiotics, and anti-inflammatory agents. Changes in the bones of the skull due to trauma and the buildup of wax in the ears may also contribute to tinnitus.

With the many improvements in hearing aids, much of the age-associated hearing loss can be corrected without being forced to rely on an outwardly detectable device. There are also communication strategies that can be used by others to ensure that they are heard, such as avoiding interference, speaking in low tones, facing the person while speaking, and remaining patient.

INFORMATION PROCESSING AND MEMORY

The cognitive operations involved in attention, short-term memory, and long-term memory are the topic of considerable research in the psychology of aging. Deficits in these areas due to normal aging can have potential influences on the manifestation of psychological disorders in later life.

Information Processing

It is a well-established finding that reaction time increases with age in adulthood, at least within very short spans of time on the order of several hundreds of milliseconds. This finding is the basis for the general slowing hypothesis (Salthouse, 1996), which states that the increase in reaction time reflects a general decline of information-processing speed within the aging nervous system. A related concept is the age-complexity hypothesis, which proposes that due to slowing of central processes in the nervous system, age differences increase with increasing complexity of the task (Cerella, Poon, & Williams, 1980). Attentional deficits are thought to contribute in part to the slowing of reaction time with age. The theory of attentional resources and aging proposes that older adults have a limited amount of energy available for cognitive operations due to reductions in central nervous system capacity (Salthouse, 1985). An alternative theory is the inhibitory deficit hypothesis, which proposes that aging involves a reduction in the cognitive resources available for controlling or inhibiting attention (Hasher & Zacks, 1988).

Memory

Age-related reductions occur in working memory, the ability to hold information in storage while simultaneously processing new information. According to the speed deficit hypothesis, age-related declines in working memory span are a result of reduced processing speed (Salthouse, 1993). As was true for attention, the inhibition deficit theory of memory proposes that older adults are more likely to activate irrelevant information and are less efficient in suppressing such information once it enters working memory (Radvansky, Zacks, & Hasher, 1996). This irrelevant information, called "mental clutter," is thought to interfere with processing in working memory and in the processes of encoding material into and retrieval from long-term memory. A more process-oriented proposal is the environmental support hypothesis, which proposes that age differences in memory occur in tasks that provide little context or support and demand high levels of self-initiated processing (Craik, 1994). When these heavy demands are placed on working memory, older adults do not have the ability to process the material as efficiently or effectively.

The theorized reduction across adulthood in processing resources and ability to engage in self-initiated mental strategies is reflected in age differences in the component of long-term memory known as episodic memory, or memory for events. Age comparisons on free recall tasks and many other laboratory tasks consistently favor young adults (Craik & Jennings, 1992; Verhaeghen, Vandenbroucke, & Dierckx, 1998). Although the vast majority of memory studies on aging are cross-sectional and hence subject to cohort effects, longitudinal data are available to confirm the general pattern of negative age effects in free recall after the age of 55 years (Zelinski & Burnight, 1997). Semantic memory, or memory for words and knowledge, by contrast, is theorized to be spared from the negative effects of the aging process (Wingfield, Lindfield, & Kahana, 1998). In the area of procedural memory, it appears that adults retain well-learned and practiced motor skills such as playing an instrument, touch typing, or riding a bicycle for as long as they are able to perform these actions. Furthermore, as was discussed in Chapter 1, the greater experience of older adults can serve to compensate for changes in working memory in areas involving procedural expertise such as playing bridge or chess, reading, cooking, gardening, and typing (Charness, 1989; Cohen, 1996). Procedural memory may also be regarded as a form of implicit memory. The results of research on age differences in implicit memory parallel the findings on procedural memory in adulthood. Tasks that involve no conscious effort at recall show no age differences (Zacks, Hasher, & Li, 1998). Similar findings are observed when individuals with amnesia are tested on implicit memory tasks (Schugens, Daum, Spindler, & Birbaumer, 1997).

Problems in retrieval from long-term memory appear in research on the tip-of-the-tongue phenomenon, an effect observed more in older adults both in laboratory and everyday life situations (Burke & Mackay, 1997). Although the information eventually can be recalled, the experience can lead to inconvenience and embarrassment, as when one cannot greet an acquaintance by name. Information that is stored and not accessed from remote memory appears to become increasingly difficult to retrieve. It is often assumed that older people can remember information from many years in the past better than they can remember recently acquired information. However, this apparent truism is not supported by data on remote memory (Squire, 1989). Over time, memory for past events becomes less vivid and loses detail (Cohen, 1996). The exception to this finding on remote memory is in the area of autobiographical memory, or recall of one's own past. Events that have a great deal of personal relevance and are rehearsed many times, such as the birth of a child or the achievement of an important career goal, do retain their clarity (Cohen, 1998).

Prospective memory is another area of interest in memory research and aging, given the common complaint of older adults that they become absent-minded. It appears there are minimal age differences across adulthood in the ability to perform tasks involving event-based prospective memory (being cued by one event with another). However, older adults are disadvantaged when they must perform time-based prospective memory tasks (such as remembering when to take medication) (Park, Hertzog, Kidder, Morrell, & Mayhorn, 1997). Age differences in prospective memory are also more likely to occur when the individual is performing a cognitive task that must be interrupted (Einstein, McDaniel, Smith, & Shaw, 1998; Kidder, Park, Hertzog, & Morrell, 1997).

Attempts to establish connections between laboratory memory tasks and brain scans are providing important data on brain-behavior connections. For example, young adults were shown to have more positive event-related potentials (indicating greater activation) than older adults during an explicit memory task (Swick & Knight, 1997). One possible area of age-related effects are the frontal lobes, which may play a role in working memory and source memory (Trott, Friedman, Ritter, & Fabiani, 1997). A second area is the hippocampus-medial temporal lobe areas that may be involved in memory encoding and retrieval from explicit memory (Henkel, Johnson, & De Leonardis, 1998; Raz et al., 1998; Smith, 1996).

Other physiological factors are also cited as possible sources of age-related memory changes. Inspired perhaps by research on possible hormonal contributions to Alzheimer's disease, investigators have examined the effects of ERT on memory functioning in older adults who do not have dementia. In one such study, scores on several standard memory measures were higher in women receiving estrogen treatment than in women who were not (Resnick, Metter, & Zonderman, 1997). A relationship also has been observed between higher levels of cortisol and lower levels of memory performance (Lupien et al., 1994; Seeman, McEwen, Singer, Albert, & Rowe, 1997). Chronically heightened blood glucose also appears to be related to memory losses in older adults, due, it is thought, to the negative effects of high levels of insulin (Vanhanen et al., 1998). On the positive side, there is evidence that older people who have high levels of aerobic fitness show a small (5%) but significant improvement on complex speed-based cognitive measures (van Boxtel et al., 1997).

Intelligence

Schaie's (1996) study of intelligence on the Seattle Longitudinal Study (SLS) has produced a compelling literature on the complex nature of intelligence in later adulthood. The overall picture in patterns of intelligence test scores as obtained longitudinally is of stability until the 50s or 60s, followed by decline through the oldest age tested. However, although some individuals may show declines in some tests of intelligence by the mid-50s, there are not significant losses until the decade of the 70s. Furthermore, none of the SLS participants showed general deterioration of functioning, even at the oldest age test of 88 years. Schaie concluded that most people are able to retain competent performance of familiar skills, particularly those that are of personal importance.

Behind the age trends are individual differences in patterns of gains and losses in adulthood, and the SLS has provided considerable data to help understand these patterns. One obvious factor that would seem to affect intelligence test scores is health status. Arthritis, cancer, and osteoporosis are health conditions shown to be associated with intelligence test scores (Schaie, 1996). Sensory functioning was shown in the SLS to be associated with intelligence test scores, findings consistent with a more recent large-scale investigation of older adults in Berlin (P.B. Baltes & Lindenberger, 1997; Lindenberger & Baltes, 1997). The SLS also documented the existence of a relationship between cardiovascular disease and declines in cognitive performance. Independently of such diseases, hypertension in middle adulthood is in itself a risk factor for poorer cognitive performance in the 70s and beyond (Launer, Masaki, Petrovitch, Foley, & Havlik, 1995). Lower limb strength, along with visual sensitivity and reaction time, emerged in one study of women over 60 as related to cognitive performance (Anstey, Lord, & Williams, 1997). Indeed, although small in magnitude, one report has emerged indicating a positive relationship in an older sample between a measure of fluid intelligence and participation in sports (Cerhan et al., 1998). Given the theoretical basis of fluid intelligence as reflective of neurological

functioning, a relationship between test scores and measures of brain functioning would be expected. Researchers are reporting that fluid intelligence seems
to be at least somewhat related to indices of frontal lobe functioning (Bigler,
Johnson, Jackson, & Blatter, 1995; Isingrini & Vazou, 1997; Robbins et al., 1998).

Individual differences in intelligence test scores were also predicted by social and cultural factors as assessed in the SLS. People with higher levels of
education are protected somewhat from the negative effects of aging on intelligence, and the same is true of being involved in a complex and stimulating
work environment. Being married to a spouse with high levels of education
and intelligence is another protective factor, as is exposure to intellectually
stimulating environments in general. Retirement has a positive effect on
maintenance of intellectual functioning as long as the individual is leaving a
boring and routine job. Those who are engaged in a complex and stimulating
occupation show a more pronounced decrement after they retire (Schaie,
1996). Taken together, these qualities add up to higher amounts of what
Schaie (1983) has called "life complexity." Other researchers have reported
similar relationships between intellectual performance and education (Elias,
Elias, D'Agostino, Silbershatz, & Wolf, 1997; Plassman et al., 1995; Smits,
Smit, van den Heuvel, & Jonker, 1997) and lifestyle (M.M. Baltes & Lang,
1997; Gold et al., 1995; Steen, Berg, & Steen, 1998).

Adding perhaps to the complexity of understanding the relationship between lifestyle factors and intellectual changes in adulthood are findings on
personality and its relationship to intellectual functioning. The personality
variable found by Schaie and colleagues to be most strongly related to aging
and intelligence is rigidity-flexibility (Schaie, Dutta, & Willis, 1991). In contrast to stereotyped views of older adults as more rigid than younger persons,
the results from the SLS on this variable indicate that people are extremely stable in the extent to which they are flexible or rigid. Instead of older people becoming more rigid, it seems that younger and younger cohorts are becoming
more flexible. Nevertheless, those older adults who are more open in attitudes
and personality style preserve their intellectual functioning over a longer period of time than their more rigid age peers (Schaie et al., 1991).

INTERACTIONS WITH PERSONALITY AND PSYCHOPATHOLOGY IN LATER LIFE

In this chapter, a number of changes in basic functioning, health, and cognitive
processes thought to be associated with aging have been described. Clinicians
need to be aware of these normal aging processes as well as the most frequently
observed chronic diseases in assessing, diagnosing, and treating older adults.
However, even though certain age changes are to be expected as more frequent
among this population, it does not follow that these should be disregarded as
targets of treatment. Age-related hearing loss may be expectable, but when it
occurs, it must nevertheless be factored in as a possible contributor to depression or exacerbation of a personality disorder. Moreover, there is no reason to

assume that once a change has occurred it is permanent. Many of the changes discussed in this chapter are, if not preventable, at least remediable. Even if a change cannot be reversed, individuals can be taught ways to overcome the physical limitations or emotional frustrations associated with that change. For example, individuals with arthritis may experience considerable pain and restriction of movement; the disease may be irreversible, but the symptoms can be managed through behavioral methods and appropriate medications.

The area of prevention is an important one, however, particularly in the provision of therapy to individuals in their 50s and 60s, when many age-related changes and health problems become increasingly apparent. In this regard, the possible existence of a relationship between personality and health in adulthood is a topic of great interest in the fields of health psychology and behavioral medicine. Since the first intriguing data supporting such a relationship were reported on the Type A personality (M. Friedman & Rosenman, 1974), investigators have sought to determine whether people with certain personality types are more susceptible to chronic or even fatal illnesses such as cardiovascular disease and cancer. There appears to be a relationship between various components of the Type A behavior pattern and cardiovascular disease risks factors, such as high serum cholesterol (the low-density lipoproteins) and the experience of angina pain (Edwards & Baglioni, 1991). In addition, high levels of hostility, part of the Type A pattern, are thought to be independent predictors of mortality (T.Q. Miller, Smith, Turner, Guijarro, & Hallet, 1996). Type A personality traits may also be part of a larger constellation of cardiovascular risk factors including smoking, body weight, leisure activities, and hormonal levels (Zmuda et al., 1997).

Additional evidence supporting the personality-health connection comes from studies showing that the overall quality of an individual's psychological adjustment can influence the subsequent development of death from both cardiovascular disease and injury. In a study of the Terman sample of gifted children, whose mental health was assessed at midlife, the chance of dying over the following 40 years was higher for those who had shown the poorest adjustment (Martin et al., 1995). The relationships may go even farther back than middle adulthood. Children high in conscientiousness had lower death rates than those with low childhood conscientiousness. It was not simply that the conscientious individuals avoided high-risk activities and therefore accidental death, or that they had better health habits. Instead, these highly conscientious individuals seemed better equipped to cope with life stress, to build stable relationships with others, and to have high "ego strength" or a "self-healing personality" (H.S. Friedman et al., 1995). Similarly, among women in a longitudinal study of personality development from college to midlife, a personality trait labeled "intellectual efficiency" was positively related to changes in health throughout midlife. Conversely, personality trait measures of hostility and anxiety were negatively related to health (Adams, Cartwright, Ostrove, Stewart, & Wink, 1998).

Although clinicians cannot turn back time or change an individual's personality trait structure (McCrae & Costa, 1990), it is possible to help middle-aged and older clients learn to recognize the potential problems associated with their particular constellation of personality traits. Modification of behaviors related to these traits may provide an important intervention strategy to prevent subsequent preventable deterioration of physical and cognitive functioning. Furthermore, older individuals may also be encouraged to take advantage of regulatory strategies that maintain positive emotions even in the face of limited physical and cognitive resources. According to socioemotional selectivity theory (Carstensen, Isaacowitz, & Charles, 1999), people who age successfully regulate their exposure to circumstances in which positive affect can be maximized. Other coping strategies involving emotional regulation, employed naturally by individuals with high levels of subjective well-being, can be taught to older individuals who are overwhelmed by physical and cognitive age-related changes (Diehl, Coyle, & Labouvie-Vief, 1996; Mroczek & Kolarz, 1998).

Clinicians must also be aware of the social context and its role in health and normal aging processes. Researchers are increasingly turning to explanations of relationships between health and personality variables such as hostility, anxiety, lowered self-esteem, and low levels of mastery, optimism, and sense of control. At every point along the social class gradient, those who are in higher positions have greater abilities to influence the outcomes of their lives. Both the possession of this power and awareness of it may play important mediating roles in affecting health (Adler et al., 1994). Unfortunately, changes in social context are outside the realm of ordinary clinicians (although see Wandersman & Nation, 1998), but continued sensitivity to the impact of cultural and socioeconomic factors can serve as important clinical tools in the intervention process.

CONCLUSION

Mr. D., who lives a relatively advantaged life in retirement, illustrates some of the common features observed in healthy and well-adjusted older individuals. A "successful ager" by any definition, Mr. D. represents the majority of the over-65 population, who are able to maintain their physical and cognitive functioning, enjoy positive relationships with family, and feel both satisfaction and challenge in their everyday lives. This model of aging is an important one to bear in mind when considering the many difficulties that can beset older individuals whose past lives and current circumstances are not so fortunate.

STUDY QUESTIONS

1. What are the major age-related changes that occur in each of the body's major organ systems?
2. Summarize the six chronic diseases discussed in this chapter and discuss their implications for mental health.
3. How might a clinician's attitudes toward aging affect how he or she relates to an older adult client?

4. What are the major effects of aging on information processing and memory? How are these related?
5. Discuss the impact of social context on health, physical functioning, and intelligence in later life.
6. Why is Mr. D. considered to be a "successful ager"? To what extent do you think his attitudes reflect his educational background and current social status?

SUGGESTED READINGS

Carstensen, L.L., Isaacowitz, D.M., & Charles, S.T. (1999). Taking time seriously: A theory of socioemotional selectivity. *American Psychologist, 54,* 165–181.

Craik, F.I.M. (1994). Memory changes in normal aging. *Current Directions in Psychological Science, 3,* 155–158.

Labouvie-Vief, G., & Diehl, M. (1999). Self and personality development. In J.C. Cavanaugh & S.K. Whitbourne (Eds.), *Gerontology: An interdisciplinary perspective* (pp. 238–268). New York: Oxford University Press.

Martin, L.R., Friedman, H.S., Tucker, J.S., Schwartz, J.E., Criqui, M.H., Wingard, D.L., & Tomlinson-Keasey, C. (1995). An archival prospective study of mental health and longevity. *Health Psychology, 5,* 381–387.

Mroczek, D.K., & Kolarz, C.M. (1998). The effect of age on positive and negative affect: A developmental perspective on happiness. *Journal of Personality and Social Psychology, 75,* 1333–1349.

Salthouse, T.A. (1996). The processing-speed theory of adult age differences in cognition. *Psychological Review, 103,* 403–428.

Schaie, K.W. (1994). The course of adult intellectual development. *American Psychologist, 49,* 304–313.

Whitbourne, S.K. (1996). *The aging individual: Physical and psychological perspectives.* New York: Springer.

REFERENCES

Adams, S.H., Cartwright, L.K., Ostrove, J.M., Stewart, A.J., & Wink, P. (1998). Psychological predictors of good health in three longitudinal samples of educated midlife women. *Health Psychology, 17,* 412–420.

Adler, N.E., Boyce, T., Chesney, M.A., Cohen, S., Folkman, S., Kahn, R.L., & Syme, S.L. (1994). Socioeconomic status and health: The challenge of the gradient. *American Psychologist, 49,* 15–24.

Anstey, K.J., Lord, S.R., & Williams, P. (1997). Strength in the lower limbs, visual contrast sensitivity, and simple reaction time predict cognition in older women. *Psychology and Aging, 12,* 137–144.

Baltes, M.M., & Lang, F.R. (1997). Everyday functioning and successful aging: The impact of resources. *Psychology and Aging, 12,* 433–443.

Baltes, P.B., & Lindenberger, U. (1997). Emergence of a powerful connection between sensory and cognitive functions across the adult life span: A new window to the study of cognitive aging? *Psychology and Aging, 12,* 12–21.

Barrou, Z., Charru, P., & Lidy, C. (1997). Dehydroepiandrosterone (DHEA) and aging. *Archives of Gerontology and Geriatrics, 24,* 233–241.

Baumgartner, R.N., Heymsfield, S.B., & Roche, A.F. (1995). Human body composition and the epidemiology of chronic disease. *Obesity Research, 3,* 73–95.

Bemben, M.G., Massey, B.H., Bemben, D.A., Misner, J.E., & Boileau, R.A. (1996). Isometric intermittent endurance of four muscle groups in men aged 20–74 years. *Medicine and Science in Sports and Exercise, 28,* 145–154.

Berr, C., Lafont, S., Debuire, B., Dartigues, J.F., & Baulieu, E.E. (1996). Relationships of dehydroepiandrosterone sulfate in the elderly with functional, psychological, and mental status, and short-term mortality: A French community-based study. *Proceedings of the National Academy of Sciences, USA, 93,* 13410–13415.

Bigler, E.D., Johnson, S.C., Jackson, C., & Blatter, D.D. (1995). Aging, brain size, and IQ. *Intelligence, 21,* 109–119.

Bilato, C., & Crow, M.T. (1996). Atherosclerosis and the vascular biology of aging. *Aging, 8,* 221–234.

Birge, S.J. (1997). The role of estrogen in the treatment of Alzheimer's disease. *Neurology, 48*(Suppl. 7), S36–S41.

Bjorntorp, P. (1996). The regulation of adipose tissue distribution in humans. *International Journal of Obesity and Related Metabolic Disorders, 20,* 291–302.

Blanpied, P., & Smidt, G.L. (1993). The difference in stiffness of the active plantarflexors between young and elderly human females. *Journal of Gerontology: Medical Sciences, 48,* M58–M63.

Bohannon, R.W. (1997). Comfortable and maximum walking speed of adults aged 20–79 years: Reference values and determinants. *Age and Ageing, 26,* 15–19.

Boonen, S., Lesaffre, E., Dequeker, J., Aerssens, J., Nijs, J., Pelemans, W., & Bouillon, R. (1996). Relationship between baseline insulin-like growth factor-1 (IGF-1) and femoral bone density in women aged over 70 years: Potential implications for the prevention of age-related bone loss. *Journal of the American Geriatrics Society, 44,* 1301–1306.

Born, J., Uthgenannt, D., Dodt, C., Nunninghoff, D., Ringvolt, E., Wagner, T., & Fehm, H.L. (1995). Cytokine production and lymphocyte subpopulations in aged humans. An assessment during nocturnal sleep. *Mechanisms of Ageing and Development, 84,* 113–126.

Brown, M., Birge, S.J., & Kohrt, W.M. (1997). Hormone replacement therapy does not augment gains in muscle strength or fat-free mass in response to weight-bearing exercise. *Journals of Gerontology. Series A, Biological Sciences and Medical Sciences, 52,* B166–B170.

Burgio, K.L., & Engel, B.T. (1990). Biofeedback-assisted behavioral training for elderly men and women. *Journal of the American Geriatrics Society, 38,* 338–340.

Burke, D.M., & Mackay, D.G. (1997). Memory, language, and ageing. *Philosophical Transactions of the Royal Society of London–Series B: Biological Sciences, 352,* 1845–1856.

Burns, P.A., Pranikoff, K., Nochajski, T.H., Hadley, E.C., Levy, K.J., & Ory, M.G. (1993). A comparison of effectiveness of biofeedback and pelvic muscle exercise treatment of stress incontinence in older community-dwelling women. *Journal of Gerontology: Medical Sciences, 38,* M167–M174.

Cabeza, R., Grady, C.L., Nyberg, L., McIntosh, A.R., Tulving, E., Kapur, S., Jennings, J.M., Houle, S., & Craik, F.I. (1997). Age-related differences in neural activity during memory encoding and retrieval: A positron emission tomography study. *Journal of Neuroscience, 17,* 391–400.

Carstensen, L.L., Isaacowitz, D.M., & Charles, S.T. (1999). Taking time seriously: A theory of socioemotional selectivity. *American Psychologist, 54,* 165–181.

Castaneda, C., Charnley, J.M., Evans, W.J., & Crim, M.C. (1995). Elderly women accommodate to a low-protein diet with losses of body cell mass, muscle function, and immune response. *American Journal of Clinical Nutrition, 62,* 30–39.

Centers for Disease Control. (1998). Heat related mortality—United States 1997. *Morbidity and Mortality Weekly Report, 47* (No. 23), 473–475.

Cerella, J., Poon, L.W., & Williams, D.M. (1980). Age and the complexity hypothesis. In L.W. Poon (Ed.), *Aging in the 1980s* (pp. 332–340). Washington, DC: American Psychological Association.

Cerhan, J.R., Folsom, A.R., Mortimer, J.A., Shahar, E., Knopman, D.S., McGovern, P.G., Hays, M.A., Crum, L.D., & Heiss, G. (1998). Correlates of cognitive function in middle-aged adults. *Gerontology, 44,* 95–105.

Chao, L.L., & Knight, R.T. (1997). Age-related prefrontal alterations during auditory memory. *Neurobiology of Aging, 18,* 87–95.

Charness, N. (1989). Age and expertise: Responding to Talland's challenge. In L.W. Poon, D.C. Rubin, & B.A. Wilson (Eds.), *Everyday cognition in adulthood and late life* (pp. 437–456). Cambridge, England: Cambridge University Press.

Clarkston, W.K., Pantano, M.M., Morley, J.E., Horowitz, M., Littlefield, J.M., & Burton, F.R. (1997). Evidence for the anorexia of aging: Gastrointestinal transit and hunger in healthy elderly vs. young adults. *American Journal of Physiology, 272,* R243–R248.

Coffey, C.E., Lucke, J.F., Saxton, J.A., Ratcliff, G., Unitas, L.J., Billig, B., & Bryan, R.N. (1998). Sex differences in brain aging: A quantitative magnetic resonance imaging study. *Archives of Neurology, 55,* 169–179.

Coffey, C.E., Wilkinson, W.E., Parashos, I.A., Soady, S.A., Sullivan, R.J., Patterson, L.J., Figiel, G.S., Webb, M.C., Spritzer, C.E., & Djang, W.T. (1992). Quantitative cerebral anatomy of the aging human brain: A cross-sectional study using magnetic resonance imaging. *Neurology, 42,* 527–536.

Cohen, G. (1996). Memory and learning in normal aging. In R.T. Woods (Ed.), *Handbook of the clinical psychology of ageing* (pp. 43–58). London: Wiley.

Cohen, G. (1998). The effects of aging on autobiographical memory. In P. Thompson & D.J. Herrmann (Eds.), *Autobiographical memory: Theoretical and applied perspectives* (pp. 105–123). Mahwah, NJ: Erlbaum.

Coleman, P.D., & Flood, D.G. (1987). Neuron numbers and dendritic extent in normal aging and Alzheimer's disease. *Neurobiology of Aging, 8,* 521–545.

Cowell, P.E., Turetsky, B.I., Gur, R.C., Grossman, R.I., Shtasel, D.L., & Gur, R.E. (1994). Sex differences in aging of the human frontal and temporal lobes. *Journal of Neuroscience, 14,* 4748–4755.

Craik, F.I.M. (1994). Memory changes in normal aging. *Current Directions in Psychological Science, 3,* 155–158.

Craik, F.I.M., & Jennings, J.M. (1992). Human memory. In F.I.M. Craik & T.A. Salthouse (Eds.), *The handbook of aging and cognition* (pp. 51–110). Hillsdale, NJ: Erlbaum.

Davies, D.F., & Shock, N.W. (1950). Age changes in glomerular filtration rate, effective renal plasma flow, and tubular excretory capacity in adult males. *Journal of Clinical Investigation, 29,* 496–507.

Dawson-Hughes, B., Harris, S.S., Krall, E.A., Dallal, G.E., Falconer, G., & Green, C.L. (1995). Rates of bone loss in postmenopausal women randomly assigned to one of two dosages of vitamin D. *American Journal of Clinical Nutrition, 61,* 1140–1145.

DeCarli, C., Murphy, D.G., Gillette, J.A., Haxby, J.V., Teichberg, D., Schapiro, M.B., & Horwitz, B. (1994). Lack of age-related differences in temporal lobe volume of very healthy adults. *American Journal of Neuroradiology, 15,* 689–696.

de Groot, C.P., Perdigao, A.L., & Deurenberg, P. (1996). Longitudinal changes in anthropometric characteristics of elderly Europeans. SENECA Investigators. *European Journal of Clinical Nutrition, 50,* 2954–3007.

de Leon, M.J., George, A.E., Golomb, J., Tarshish, C., Convit, A., Kluger, A., De Santi, S., McRae, T., Ferris, S.H., Reisberg, B., Ince, C., Rusinek, H., Bobinski, M., Quinn, B., Miller, D.C., & Wisniewski, H.M. (1997). Frequency of hippocampal formation atrophy in normal aging and Alzheimer's disease. *Neurobiology of Aging, 18,* 1–11.

de Lignieres, B. (1993). Transdermal dihydrotestosterone treatment of 'andropause'. *Annals of Medicine, 25,* 235–241.

Denti, L., Pasolini, G., Sanfelici, L., Ablondi, F., Freddi, M., Benedetti, R., & Valenti, G. (1997). Effects of aging on dehydroepiandrosterone sulfate in relation to fasting insulin levels and body composition assessed by bioimpedance analysis. *Metabolism: Clinical and Experimental, 46,* 826–832.

De Santi, S., de Leon, M.J., Convit, A., Tarshish, C., Rusinek, H., Tsui, W.H., Sinaiko, E., Wang, G.J., Bartlet, E., & Volkow, N. (1995). Age-related changes in brain: II. Positron emission tomography of frontal and temporal lobe glucose metabolism in normal subjects. *Psychiatric Quarterly, 66,* 357–370.

Diehl, M., Coyle, N., & Labouvie-Vief, G. (1996). Age and sex differences in coping and defense across the life span. *Psychology and Aging, 11,* 127–139.

Edelstein, S.L., & Barrett-Connor, E. (1993). Relation between body size and bone mineral density in elderly men and women. *American Journal of Epidemiology, 138,* 160–169.

Edwards, J.R., & Baglioni, A.J. (1991). Relationship between Type A behavior pattern and mental and physical symptoms: A comparison of global and component measures. *Journal of Applied Psychology, 76,* 276–290.

Einstein, G.O., McDaniel, M.A., Smith, R., & Shaw, P. (1998). Habitual prospective memory and aging: Remembering instructions and forgetting actions. *Psychological Science, 9,* 284–288.

Eisen, A., Entezari-Taher, M., & Stewart, H. (1996). Cortical projections to spinal motoneurons: Changes with aging and amyotrophic lateral sclerosis. *Neurology, 46,* 1396–1404.

Elias, M.F., Elias, P.K., D'Agostino, R.B., Silbershatz, H., & Wolf, P.A. (1997). Role of age, education, and gender on cognitive performance in the Framingham Heart Study: Community-based norms. *Experimental Aging Research, 23,* 201–235.

Epstein, M. (1996). Aging and the kidney. *Journal of the American Society of Nephrology, 7,* 1106–1122.

Farmer, K.C., & Naylor, M.F. (1996). Sun exposure, sunscreens, and skin cancer prevention: A year-round concern. *Annals of Pharmacotherapy, 30,* 662–673.

Ferrara, A., Barrett-Connor, E., & Shan, J. (1997). Total, LDL, and HDL cholesterol decrease with age in older men and women: The Rancho Bernardo Study 1984–1994. *Circulation, 96,* 37–43.

Field, A.E., Colditz, G.A., Willett, W.C., Longcope, C., & McKinlay, J.B. (1994). The relation of smoking, age, relative weight, and dietary intake to serum adrenal steroids, sex hormones, and sex hormone-binding globulin in middle-aged men. *Journal of Clinical Endocrinology and Metabolism, 79,* 1310–1316.

Fliser, D., Franek, E., Joest, M., Block, S., Mutschler, E., & Ritz, E. (1997). Renal function in the elderly: Impact of hypertension and cardiac function. *Kidney International, 51,* 1196–1204.

Frette, C., Barrett-Connor, E., & Clausen, J.L. (1996). Effect of active and passive smoking on ventilatory function in elderly men and women. *American Journal of Epidemiology, 143,* 757–765.

Friedman, H.S., Tucker, J.S., Schwartz, J.E., Martin, L.R., Tomlinson-Keasey, C., Wingard, D.L., & Criqui, M.H. (1995). Childhood conscientiousness and longevity: Health behaviors and cause of death. *Journal of Personality and Social Psychology, 68,* 696–703.

Friedman, M., & Rosenman, R.H. (1974). *Type A behavior and your heart.* New York: Knopf.

Garnero, P., Sornay Rendu, E., Chapuy, M.C., & Delmas, P.D. (1996). Increased bone turnover in late postmenopausal women is a major determinant of osteoporosis. *Journal of Bone and Mineral Research, 11,* 337–349.

Gold, D.P., Andres, D., Etezadi, J., Arbuckle, T., Schwartzman, A., & Chaikelson, J. (1995). Structural equation model of intellectual change and continuity and predictors of intelligence in older men. *Psychology and Aging, 10,* 294–303.

Golomb, J., Kluger, A., de Leon, M.J., Ferris, S.H., Mittelman, M., Cohen, J., & George, A.E. (1996). Hippocampal formation size predicts declining memory performance in normal aging. *Neurology, 47,* 810–813.

Gotthardt, U., Schweiger, U., Fahrenberg, J., Lauer, C.J., Holsboer, F., & Heuser, I. (1995). Cortisol, ACTH, and cardiovascular response to a cognitive challenge paradigm in aging and depression. *American Journal of Physiology, 268,* R865–R873.

Grimby, A., & Wiklund, I. (1994). Health-related quality of life in old age: A study among 76-year-old Swedish urban citizens. *Scandinavian Journal of Social Medicine, 22,* 7–14.

Hakkinen, K., & Pakarinen, A. (1995). Acute hormonal responses to heavy resistance exercise in men and women at different ages. *International Journal of Sports Medicine, 16,* 507–513.

Hasher, L., & Zacks, R.T. (1988). Working memory, comprehension, and aging: A review and a new view. In G.H. Bower (Ed.), *The psychology of learning and motivation* (Vol. 22, pp. 193–225). New York: Academic.

Henkel, L.A., Johnson, M.K., & De Leonardis, D.M. (1998). Aging and source monitoring: Cognitive processes and neuropsychological correlates. *Journal of Experimental Psychology: General, 127,* 251–268.

Huether, G. (1996). Melatonin as an antiaging drug: Between facts and fantasy. *Gerontology, 42,* 87–96.

Hurley, B.F. (1995). Age, gender, and muscular strength. *Journals of Gerontology. Series A, Biological Sciences and Medical Sciences, 50A,* 41–44.

Iida, I., & Noro, K. (1995). An analysis of the reduction of elasticity on the ageing of human skin and the recovering effect of a facial massage. *Ergonomics, 38,* 1921–1931.

Inoue, Y. (1996). Longitudinal effects of age on heat-activated sweat gland density and output in healthy active older men. *European Journal of Applied Physiology and Occupational Physiology, 74,* 72–77.

Inoue, Y., Nakao, M., Araki, T., & Ueda, H. (1992). Thermoregulatory responses of young and older men to cold exposure. *European Journal of Applied Physiology, 65,* 492–498.

Iqbal, P., & Castleden, C.M. (1997). Management of urinary incontinence in the elderly. *Gerontology, 43,* 151–157.

Isingrini, M., & Vazou, F. (1997). Relation between fluid intelligence and frontal lobe functioning in older adults. *International Journal of Aging and Human Development, 45,* 99–109.

James, K., Premchand, N., Skibinska, A., Skibinski, G., Nicol, M., & Mason, J.I. (1997). IL-6, DHEA and the ageing process. *Mechanisms of Ageing and Development, 93,* 15–24.

Kelly, K.S., Hayslip, B., Jr., & Servaty, H.L. (1996). Psychoneuroendocrinological indicators of stress and intellectual performance among older adults: An exploratory study. *Experimental Aging Research, 22,* 393–401.

Kern, W., Dodt, C., Born, J., & Fehm, H.L. (1996). Changes in cortisol and growth hormone secretion during nocturnal sleep in the course of aging. *Journal of Gerontology: Medical Sciences, 51A,* M3–M9.

Kidder, D.P., Park, D.C., Hertzog, C., & Morrell, R.W. (1997). Prospective memory and aging: The effects of working memory and prospective memory task load. *Aging Neuropsychology and Cognition, 4,* 93–112.

Kligman, A.M., Grove, G.L., & Balin, A.K. (1985). Aging of human skin. In C.E. Finch & E.L. Schneider (Eds.), *Handbook of the biology of aging* (2nd ed.). New York: Van Nostrand-Reinhold.

Krall, E.A., Dawson-Hughes, B., Hirst, K., Gallagher, J.C., Sherman, S.S., & Dalsky, G. (1997). Bone mineral density and biochemical markers of bone turnover in healthy elderly men and women. *Journals of Gerontology. Series A, Biological Sciences and Medical Sciences, 52,* M61–M67.

Lamberts, S.W.J., van den Beld, A.W., & van der Lely, A.-J. (1997). The endocrinology of aging. *Science, 278,* 419–424.

Laumann, E.O., Paik, A., & Rosen, R.C. (1999). Sexual dysfunction in the United States: Prevalence and predictors. *Journal of the American Medical Association, 281,* 537–544.

Launer, L.J., Masaki, K., Petrovitch, H., Foley, D., & Havlik, R.J. (1995). The association between midlife blood pressure levels and late-life cognitive function: The Honolulu-Asia Aging Study. *Journal of the American Medical Association, 274,* 1846–1851.

Lesourd, B.M. (1997). Nutrition and immunity in the elderly: Modification of immune responses with nutritional treatments. *American Journal of Clinical Nutrition, 66,* 478S–484S.

Lindenberger, U., & Baltes, P.B. (1997). Intellectual functioning in old and very old age: Cross-sectional results from the Berlin Aging Study. *Psychology and Aging, 12,* 410–432.

Lovat, L.B. (1996). Age related changes in gut physiology and nutritional status. *Gut, 38,* 306–309.

Lupien, S., Lecours, A.R., Lussier, I., Schwartz, G., Nair, N.P., & Meaney, M.J. (1994). Basal cortisol levels and cognitive deficits in human aging. *Journal of Neuroscience, 14,* 2893–2903.

Lupien, S., Lecours, A.R., Schwartz, G., Sharma, S., Hauger, R.L., Meaney, M.J., & Nair, N.P. (1996). Longitudinal study of basal cortisol levels in healthy elderly subjects: Evidence for subgroups. *Neurobiology of Aging, 17,* 95–105.

Maas, D., Jochen, A., & Lalande, B. (1997). Age-related changes in male gonadal function: Implications for therapy. *Drugs and Aging, 11,* 45–60.

Martin, L.R., Friedman, H.S., Tucker, J.S., Schwartz, J.E., Criqui, M.H., Wingard, D.L., & Tomlinson-Keasey, C. (1995). An archival prospective study of mental health and longevity. *Health Psychology, 5,* 381–387.

Matsumae, M., Kikinis, R., Morocz, I.A., Lorenzo, A.V., Sandor, T., Albert, M.S., Black, P.M., & Jolesz, F.A. (1996). Age-related changes in intracranial compartment volumes in normal adults assessed by magnetic resonance imaging. *Journal of Neurosurgery, 84,* 982–991.

May, H., Murphy, S., & Khaw, K.T. (1995). Bone mineral density and its relationship to skin colour in Caucasian females. *European Journal of Clinical Investigation, 25,* 85–89.

McCalden, R.W., McGeough, J.A., Barker, M.B., & Court-Brown, C.M. (1993). Age-related changes in the tensile properties of cortical bone: The relative importance of changes in porosity, mineralization, and microstructure. *Journal of Bone and Joint Surgery, 75*, 1193–1205.

McCalden, R.W., McGeough, J.A., & Court-Brown, C.M. (1997). Age-related changes in the compressive strength of cancellous bone: The relative importance of changes in density and trabecular architecture. *Journal of Bone and Joint Surgery American, 79*, 421–427.

McCartney, N., Hicks, A.L., Martin, J., & Webber, C.E. (1995). Long-term resistance training in the elderly: Effects on dynamic strength, exercise capacity, muscle, and bone. *Journals of Gerontology: Biological and Medical Sciences, 50*, B97–B104.

McCartney, N., Hicks, A.L., Martin, J., & Webber, C.E. (1996). A longitudinal trial of weight training in the elderly: Continued improvements in year 2. *Journals of Gerontology. Series A, Biological Sciences and Medical Sciences, 51*, B425–B433.

McCrae, R.R., & Costa, P.T.J. (1990). *Personality in adulthood.* New York: Guilford Press.

McEwen, B.S., Alves, S.E., Bulloch, K., & Weiland, N.G. (1997). Ovarian steroids and the brain: Implications for cognition and aging. *Neurology, 48*, S8–S15.

Miller, R.A. (1996). The aging immune system: Primer and prospectus. *Science, 273*, 70–74.

Miller, T.Q., Smith, T.W., Turner, C.W., Guijarro, M.L., & Hallet, A.J. (1996). Meta-analytic review of research on hostility and physical health. *Psychological Bulletin, 119*, 322–348.

Montgomery, S.A. (1990). Depression in the elderly: Pharmacokinetics of antidepressants and death from overdose. *International Clinical Psychopharmacology, 5*, 67–76.

Morley, J.E., Kaiser, F., Raum, W.J., Perry, H.M., III, Flood, J.F., Jensen, J., Silver, A.J., & Roberts, E. (1997). Potentially predictive and manipulable blood serum correlates of aging in the healthy human male: Progressive decreases in bioavailable testosterone, dehydroepiandrosterone sulfate, and the ratio of insulin-like growth factor 1 to growth hormone. *Proceedings of the National Academy of Sciences of the United States of America, 94*, 7537–7542.

Mroczek, D.K., & Kolarz, C.M. (1998). The effect of age on positive and negative affect: A developmental perspective on happiness. *Journal of Personality and Social Psychology, 75*, 1333–1349.

Murphy, D.G., DeCarli, C., McIntosh, A.R., Daly, E., Mentis, M.J., Pietrini, P., Szczepanik, J., Schapiro, M.B., Grady, C.L., Horwitz, B., & Rapoport, S.I. (1996). Sex differences in human brain morphometry and metabolism: An in vivo quantitative magnetic resonance imaging and positron emission tomography study on the effect of aging. *Archives of General Psychiatry, 53*, 585–594.

Murphy, S., Khaw, K.T., May, H., & Compston, J.E. (1994). Milk consumption and bone mineral density in middle aged and elderly women. *British Medical Journal, 308*, 939–941.

Nachbar, F., & Korting, H.C. (1995). The role of vitamin E in normal and damaged skin. *Journal of Molecular Medicine, 73*, 7–17.

National Center for Health Statistics. (1997). *Health, United States, 1996–97 and injury chartbook* (76-641496). Washington, DC: U.S. Government Printing Office.

Nicolson, N., Storms, C., Ponds, R., & Sulon, J. (1997). Salivary cortisol levels and stress reactivity in human aging. *Journals of Gerontology. Series A, Biological Sciences and Medical Sciences, 52*, M68–M75.

Nielsen Bohlman, L., & Knight, R.T. (1995). Prefrontal alterations during memory processing in aging. *Cerebral Cortex, 5*, 541–549.

O'Brien, J.T., Schweitzer, I., Ames, D., Tuckwell, V., & Mastwyk, M. (1994). Cortisol suppression by dexamethasone in the healthy elderly: Effects of age, dexamethasone levels, and cognitive function. *Biological Psychiatry, 36,* 389–394.

Park, D.C., Hertzog, C., Kidder, D.P., Morrell, R.W., & Mayhorn, C.B. (1997). Effect of age on event-based and time-based prospective memory. *Psychology and Aging, 12,* 314–327.

Perry, H.M., III, Horowitz, M., Morley, J.E., Fleming, S., Jensen, J., Caccione, P., Miller, D.K., Kaiser, F.E., & Sundarum, M. (1996). Aging and bone metabolism in African American and Caucasian women. *Journal of Clinical Endocrinology and Metabolism, 81,* 1108–1117.

Peskind, E.R., Raskind, M.A., Wingerson, D., Pascualy, M., Thal, L.J., Dobie, D.J., Veith, R.C., Dorsa, D.M., Murray, S., Sikkema, C., Galt, S.A., & Wilkinson, C.W. (1995). Enhanced hypothalamic-pituitary-adrenocortical axis responses to physostigmine in normal aging. *Journals of Gerontology. Series A, Biological and Medical Sciences, 50,* M114–M120.

Plassman, B.L., Welsh, K.A., Helms, M., Brandt, J., Page, W.F., & Breitner, J.C. (1995). Intelligence and education as predictors of cognitive state in late life: A 50-year follow-up. *Neurology, 45,* 1446–1450.

Prinz, P.N., Moe, K.E., Dulberg, E.M., Larsen, L.H., Vitiello, M.V., Toivola, B., & Merriam, G.R. (1995). Higher plasma IGF-1 levels are associated with increased delta sleep in healthy older men. *Journals of Gerontology. Series A, Biological Sciences and Medical Sciences, 50,* M222–M226.

Radvansky, G.A., Zacks, R.T., & Hasher, L. (1996). Fact retrieval in younger and older adults: The role of mental models. *Psychology and Aging, 11,* 258–271.

Ralphs, J.R., & Benjamin, M. (1994). The joint capsule: Structure, composition, ageing and disease. *Journal of Anatomy, 184,* 503–509.

Raz, N., Gunning-Dixon, F.M., Head, D., Dupuis, J.H., & Acker, J.D. (1998). Neuroanatomical correlates of cognitive aging: Evidence from structural magnetic resonance imaging. *Neuropsychology, 12,* 95–114.

Raz, N., Gunning, F.M., Head, D., Dupuis, J.H., McQuain, J., Briggs, S.D., Loken, W.J., Thornton, A.E., & Acker, J.D. (1997). Selective aging of the human cerebral cortex observed in vivo: Differential vulnerability of the prefrontal gray matter. *Cerebral Cortex, 7,* 268–282.

Resnick, S.M., Metter, E.J., & Zonderman, A.B. (1997). Estrogen replacement therapy and longitudinal decline in visual memory: A possible protective effect? *Neurology, 49,* 1491–1497.

Riedel, M., Brabant, G., Rieger, K., & von zur Muhlen, A. (1994). Growth hormone therapy in adults: Rationales, results, and perspectives. *Experimental and Clinical Endocrinology, 102,* 273–283.

Robbins, T.W., James, M., Owen, A.M., Sahakian, B.J., Lawrence, A.D., McInnes, L., & Rabbitt, P.M.A. (1998). A study of performance on tests from the CANTAB battery sensitive to frontal lobe dysfunction in a large sample of normal volunteers: Implications for theories of executive functioning and cognitive aging. *Journal of the International Neuropsychological Society, 4,* 474–490.

Ross, M.H., Yurgelun-Todd, D.A., Renshaw, P.F., Maas, L.C., Mendelson, J.H., Mello, N.K., Cohen, B.M., & Levin, J.M. (1997). Age-related reduction in functional MRI response to photic stimulation. *Neurology, 48,* 173–176.

Rossi, A., Ganassini, A., Tantucci, C., & Grassi, V. (1996). Aging and the respiratory system. *Aging, 8,* 143–161.

Salthouse, T.A. (1985). Speed of behavior and its implications for cognition. In J.E. Birren & K.W. Schaie (Eds.), *Handbook of the psychology of aging* (2nd ed., pp. 400–426). New York: Van Nostrand-Reinhold.

Salthouse, T.A. (1993). Speed and knowledge as determinants of adult age differences in verbal tasks. *Journal of Gerontology: Psychological Sciences, 48,* P29–P36.

Salthouse, T.A. (1996). The processing-speed theory of adult age differences in cognition. *Psychological Review, 103,* 403–428.

Schaie, K.W. (1983). The Seattle Longitudinal Study: A 21-year exploration of psychometric intelligence in adulthood. In K.W. Schaie (Ed.), *Longitudinal studies of adult psychological development* (pp. 64–135). New York: Guilford Press.

Schaie, K.W. (1996). Intellectual development in adulthood. In J.E. Birren, K.W. Schaie, R.P. Abeles, M. Gatz, & T.A. Salthouse (Eds.), *Handbook of the psychology of aging* (4th ed., pp. 266–286). San Diego, CA: Academic Press.

Schaie, K.W., Dutta, R., & Willis, S.L. (1991). Relationship between rigidity-flexibility and cognitive abilities in adulthood. *Psychology and Aging, 6,* 371–383.

Schugens, M.M., Daum, I., Spindler, M., & Birbaumer, N. (1997). Differential effects of aging on explicit and implicit memory. *Aging Neuropsychology and Cognition, 4,* 33–44.

Seaton, K. (1995). Cortisol: The aging hormone, the stupid hormone. *Journal of the National Medical Association, 87,* 667–683.

Seeman, T.E., McEwen, B.S., Singer, B.H., Albert, M.S., & Rowe, J.W. (1997). Increase in urinary cortisol excretion and memory declines: MacArthur studies of successful aging. *Journal of Clinical Endocrinology and Metabolism, 82,* 2458–2465.

Seeman, T.E., Singer, B., & Charpentier, P. (1995). Gender differences in patterns of HPA axis response to challenge: MacArthur studies of successful aging. *Psychoneuroendocrinology, 20,* 711–725.

Sherwin, B. (1996). Estrogen, the brain, and memory. *Menopause, 3,* 97–105.

Shinkai, S., Konishi, M., & Shephard, R.J. (1997). Aging, exercise, training, and the immune system. *Exercise Immunology Review, 3,* 68–95.

Silverman, H.G., & Mazzeo, R.S. (1996). Hormonal responses to maximal and submaximal exercise in trained and untrained men of various ages. *Journals of Gerontology. Series A, Biological Sciences and Medical Sciences, 51,* B30–B37.

Sinaki, M. (1996). Effect of physical activity on bone mass. *Current Opinions in Rheumatology, 8,* 376–383.

Smith, A.D. (1996). Memory. In J.E. Birren, K.W. Schaie, R.P. Abeles, M. Gatz, & T.A. Salthouse (Eds.), *Handbook of the psychology of aging* (4th ed., pp. 236–250). San Diego, CA: Academic Press.

Smits, C.H., Smit, J.H., van den Heuvel, N., & Jonker, C. (1997). Norms for an abbreviated Raven's Coloured Progressive Matrices in an older sample. *Journal of Clinical Psychology, 53,* 687–697.

Sone, Y. (1995). Age-associated problems in nutrition. *Applied Human Science, 14,* 201–210.

Spina, R.J., Miller, T.R., Bogenhagen, W.H., Schechtman, K.B., & Ehsani, A.A. (1996). Gender-related differences in left ventricular filling dynamics in older subjects after endurance exercise training. *Journals of Gerontology. Series A, Biological Sciences and Medical Sciences, 51,* B232–B237.

Squire, L.R. (1989). On the course of forgetting in very long term memory. *Journal of Experimental Psychology: Learning, Memory, and Cognition, 15,* 241–245.

Stampfer, M.J., Krauss, R.M., Ma, J., Blanche, P.J., Holl, L.G., Sacks, F.M., & Hennekens, C.H. (1996). A prospective study of triglyceride level, low-density lipoprotein particle diameter, and risk of myocardial infarction. *Journal of the American Medical Association, 276,* 882–888.

Steen, G., Berg, S., & Steen, B. (1998). Cognitive function in 70-year-old men and women: A 16-year cohort difference population study. *Aging, 10,* 120–126.

Suominen, H. (1997). Changes in physical characteristics and body composition during 5-year follow-up in 75- and 80-year-old men and women. *Scandinavian Journal of Social Medicine. Supplementum, 53,* 19–24.

Swick, D., & Knight, R.T. (1997). Event-related potentials differentiate the effects of aging on word and nonword repetition in explicit and implicit memory tasks. *Journal of Experimental Psychology: Learning, Memory, and Cognition, 23,* 123–142.

Taaffe, D.R., & Marcus, R. (1997). Dynamic muscle strength alterations to detraining and retraining in elderly men. *Clinical Physiology, 17,* 311–324.

Taaffe, D.R., Pruitt, L., Reim, J., Hintz, R.L., Butterfield, G., Hoffman, A.R., & Marcus, R. (1994). Effect of recombinant human growth hormone on the muscle strength response to resistance exercise in elderly men. *Journal of Clinical Endocrinology and Metabolism, 79,* 1361–1366.

Takema, Y., Yorimoto, Y., Ohsu, H., Osanai, O., & Kawai, M. (1997). Age-related discontinuous changes in the in vivo fluorescence of human facial skin. *Journal of Dermatological Science, 15,* 55–58.

Tankersley, C.G., Smolander, J., Kenney, W.L., & Fortney, S.M. (1991). Sweating and skin blood flow during exercise: Effects of age and maximal oxygen uptake. *Journal of Applied Physiology, 71,* 236–242.

Teramoto, S., Fukuchi, Y., Nagase, T., Matsuse, T., & Orimo, H. (1995). A comparison of ventilation components in young and elderly men during exercise. *Journal of Gerontology: Biological Sciences, 50A,* B34–B39.

Toogood, A.A., O' Neill, P., & Shalet, S.M. (1996). Beyond the somatopause: Growth hormone deficiency in adults over the age of 60 years. *Journal of Clinical Endocrinology and Metabolism, 81,* 460–465.

Trott, C.T., Friedman, D., Ritter, W., & Fabiani, M. (1997). Item and source memory: Differential age effects revealed by event-related potentials. *Neuroreport, 8,* 3373–3378.

van Boxtel, M.P., Paas, F.G., Houx, P.J., Adam, J.J., Teeken, J.C., & Jolles, J. (1997). Aerobic capacity and cognitive performance in a cross-sectional aging study. *Medicine and Science in Sports and Exercise, 29,* 1357–1365.

Van Cauter, E., Leproult, R., & Kupfer, D.J. (1996). Effects of gender and age on the levels and circadian rhythmicity of plasma cortisol. *Journal of Clinical Endocrinology and Metabolism, 81,* 2468–2473.

Vanhanen, M., Koivisto, K., Kuusisto, J., Mykkanen, L., Helkala, E.L., Hanninen, T., Riekkinen, P., Sr., Soininen, H., & Laakso, M. (1998). Cognitive function in an elderly population with persistent impaired glucose tolerance. *Diabetes Care, 21,* 398–402.

Venjatraman, J.T., & Fernandes, G. (1997). Exercise, immunity and aging. *Aging, 9,* 42–56.

Verhaeghen, P., Vandenbroucke, A., & Dierckx, V. (1998). Growing slower and less accurate: Adult age differences in time-accuracy functions for recall and recognition from episodic memory. *Experimental Aging Research, 24,* 3–19.

Villa, M.L., Marcus, R., Ramirez Delay, R., & Kelsey, J.L. (1995). Factors contributing to skeletal health of postmenopausal Mexican-American women. *Journal of Bone and Mineral Research, 10,* 1233–1242.

Vitiello, M.V., Wilkinson, C.W., Merriam, G.R., Moe, K.E., Prinz, P.N., Ralph, D.D., Colasurdo, E.A., & Schwartz, R.S. (1997). Successful 6-month endurance training does not alter insulin-like growth factor-1 in healthy older men and women. *Journals of Gerontology. Series A, Biological Sciences and Medical Sciences, 52,* M149–M154.

Wandersman, A., & Nation, M. (1998). Urban neighborhoods and mental health: Psychological contributions to understanding toxicity, resilience, and interventions. *American Psychologist, 53,* 647–656.

Welten, D.C., Kemper, H.C., Post, G.B., & van Staveren, W.A. (1995). A meta-analysis of the effect of calcium intake on bone mass in young and middle aged females and males. *Journal of Nutrition, 125,* 2802–2813.

West, S.K., Munoz, B., Rubin, G.S., Schein, O.D., Bandeen-Roche, K., Zeger, S., German, S., & Fried, L.P. (1997). Function and visual impairment in a population-based study of older adults: The SEE project Salisbury Eye Evaluation. *Investigative Ophthalmology and Visual Science, 38,* 72–82.

Whitbourne, S.K., & Collins, K.C. (1998). Identity and physical changes in later adulthood: Theoretical and clinical implications. *Psychotherapy, 35,* 519–530.

Wilkinson, C.W., Peskind, E.R., & Raskind, M.A. (1997). Decreased hypothalamic-pituitary-adrenal axis sensitivity to cortisol feedback inhibition in human aging. *Neuroendocrinology, 65,* 79–90.

Wilson, P.W., Anderson, K.M., Harris, T., Kannel, W.B., & Castelli, W.P. (1994). Determinants of change in total cholesterol and HDL-C with age: The Framingham Study. *Journal of Gerontology, 49,* M252–M257.

Wingfield, A., Lindfield, K.C., & Kahana, M.J. (1998). Adult age differences in the temporal characteristics of category free recall. *Psychology and Aging, 13,* 256–266.

Xu, S.Z., Huang, W.M., & Ren, J.Y. (1997). The new model of age-dependent changes in bone mineral density. *Growth, Development, and Aging, 61,* 19–26.

Yen, S.S., Morales, A.J., & Khorram, O. (1995). Replacement of DHEA in aging men and women: Potential remedial effects. *Annals of the New York Academy of Sciences, 774,* 128–142.

Young, A.J. (1991). Effects of aging on human cold tolerance. *Experimental Aging Research, 17,* 205–213.

Young, A.J., & Lee, D.T. (1997). Aging and human cold tolerance. *Experimental Aging Research, 23,* 45–67.

Zacks, R.T., Hasher, L., & Li, K.Z.H. (1998). Human memory. In F.I.M. Craik & T.A. Salthouse (Eds.), *Handbook of aging and cognition II.* Mahwah, NJ: Erlbaum.

Zelinski, E.M., & Burnight, K.P. (1997). Sixteen-year longitudinal and time lag changes in memory and cognition in older adults. *Psychology and Aging, 12,* 503–513.

Zioupos, P., & Currey, J.D. (1998). Changes in the stiffness, strength, and toughness of human cortical bone with age. *Bone, 22,* 57–66.

Zmuda, J.M., Cauley, J.A., Kriska, A., Glynn, N.W., Gutai, J.P., & Kuller, L.H. (1997). Longitudinal relation between endogenous testosterone and cardiovascular disease risk factors in middle-aged men: A 13-year follow-up of former Multiple Risk Factor Intervention Trial participants. *American Journal of Epidemiology, 146,* 609–617.

CHAPTER 3

Assessment of Older Adult Psychopathology

BARRY A. EDELSTEIN, RONALD R. MARTIN, AND
DEBORAH R. MCKEE

CASE STUDY

Mr. Toefert is a 76-year-old nursing home resident who was referred for psychological evaluation by the director of nursing. He is a retired university professor who was admitted two weeks ago with a broken hip that apparently resulted from a fall at his home. Since his admission to the nursing home, he frequently has refused to leave his room, has missed several meals, and has lost weight. Staff members have observed Mr. Toefert sobbing for periods of time in the mornings, but he has refused consoling attempts by the staff. Staff members also have attempted to coax Mr. Toefert out of his room to attend various activities and to interact with other residents. He has consistently refused, stating, "I don't want to leave my valuables unattended any longer than necessary. You know what's going on around here. I don't feel like doing anything anyway." The director of nursing is concerned that Mr. Toefert is having difficulty adjusting to the nursing home, that he might be depressed, and that the depression is compromising his health status.

The assessment of older adults invites the analogy and challenge of a complex puzzle with missing pieces, the pieces often comprising important elements of the older adult's presenting problem. When compared with the puzzle of a younger adult, the puzzle of an older adult includes a greater number and wider variety of pieces, frequently with more missing pieces. Older adults have longer histories of interactions with their environment, a greater probability of having experienced diseases, a greater number of prescription medications to address these diseases, a greater number of personal losses, and a greater likelihood of comorbid physical and mental disorders. All of these factors contribute to the complexity and challenge of assessing older adults.

In the following sections, we discuss the assessment of older adults, with particular emphasis on issues that are most relevant to this group. We begin with a discussion of multidimensional assessment, a prerequisite for the assessment of an aging individual, followed by discussions of multiple methods of assessment and the assessment process. As we mention various assessment instruments throughout the chapter, we briefly address their adequacy for use with older adults. Finally, we end with an application of material from the preceding sections in the assessment of Mr. Toefert.

MULTIDIMENSIONAL ASSESSMENT

The nature and complexity of mental and physical problems among older adults demands a multidimensional assessment, typically involving an interdisciplinary team of professionals (e.g., physicians, psychologists, social workers, nurses, physical therapists, activity therapists) (Zeiss & Steffen, 1996). The domains of functioning that are usually included in such an assessment are physical health, mental health, cognitive functioning, adaptive functioning, and social functioning (Edelstein & Kalish, 1999; Fry, 1986). The assessment of these multiple domains was recommended in the Omnibus Reconciliation Act (OBRA, 1987), which guides the care of older adults in facilities receiving reimbursement for these services through federal funds.

ASSESSMENT OF PHYSICAL HEALTH

Eighty percent of adults over the age of 65 experience at least one chronic illness (Health and Human Services Inspector General, 1989). The physical assessment of older adults is complicated by the interplay of illnesses and the multiple medications prescribed to address these illnesses. Moreover, physical illnesses can mask psychological problems, and psychological problems can mask physical illness (Morrison, 1997). For example, depression can mask hypothyroidism, and hypothyroidism can mask depression, as both can share overlapping symptoms. This can be especially complicating in the clinical presentation of older adults, who are less likely than younger adults to report depressed mood when experiencing major depression and more likely to report somatic complaints (Blazer, Bacher, & Hughes, 1987).

The assessment of physical functioning typically includes both a physical examination and laboratory tests (e.g., thyroid levels, vitamin B12 levels, folic acid levels, blood levels of medications). Examinations address both age-related changes (e.g., change in muscle strength, sensory changes) and those changes due to other factors (e.g., diseases, medications). The interested reader is referred to Whitbourne (1996) and Willott (1999) for thorough presentations of age-related biological changes.

ASSESSMENT OF COGNITIVE FUNCTIONING

Many people experience age-related changes in cognitive functioning; however, these changes are not experienced across all cognitive domains. Age-related declines may be observed in certain domains (e.g., working memory), whereas other domains may evidence stability or even improvement (e.g., semantic memory) (Babcock & Salthouse, 1990; Light, 1992).

Decline in cognitive functioning can be caused by a variety of factors beyond "aging" (e.g., cardiovascular disease, schizophrenia, dementia). Regardless of the source of these cognitive deficits, they can lead to declines in adaptive functioning (e.g., cooking, money management, dressing), social functioning, quality of life, and psychological functioning (e.g., depression, anxiety). Differentiating normal age-related changes from the changes due to these other factors is very important when assessing older adults.

A comprehensive assessment of cognitive functioning requires extensive neuropsychological assessment, a discussion of which is beyond the scope of this chapter. What is more common, and often the starting point for further cognitive assessment, is the use of a cognitive screening instrument. The interested reader is referred to Albert (1994) and MacNeil and Lichtenberg (1999) for discussions of various screening instruments.

The Mini-Mental State Examination (MMSE) is the most widely used cognitive screening instrument, requires little time to administer, and has extensive normative data available for various ages and education levels (see Crum, Anthony, Bassett, & Folstein, 1993). The MMSE is also reasonably good for following the dementing process, with declines of 3 to 4 points expected per year for Alzheimer's disease (Burns, Jacoby, & Levy, 1991). Moreover, most medical and mental health professionals are familiar with the MMSE and can relate aspects of functioning to MMSE scores. On the negative side, the MMSE is not particularly sensitive or specific for dementia and lacks a few elements that would be of value in assessing cognitive functioning (e.g., timed items, verbal fluency items, items sensitive to executive and subcortical functioning) (U.S. Department of Veterans Affairs, 1997).

ASSESSMENT OF PSYCHOLOGICAL FUNCTIONING

Psychological dysfunction is not a natural consequence of the aging process. Contrary to popular belief, older adults experience lower rates of some psychological disorders (e.g., depression) than younger adults (Blazer, 1994; Wolfe, Morrow, & Fredrickson, 1996). Of all the various mental disorders that are experienced by older adults, the three most diagnostically challenging are dementia, depression, and delirium. Moreover, the failure to accurately assess these disorders can lead to substantial long-term consequences for the older adult (Qualls, 1999). The symptoms of depression, delirium, and some dementias often can be decreased or eliminated with proper diagnosis and treatment. Adequate assessment of dementia, delirium, and depression typically includes medical and psychological evaluations and often more sophisticated neuropsychological assessment. As with many forms of psychopathology, the assessment of these disorders may begin with a broad, sensitive screening for a wide range of psychopathology, followed by a more focused assessment measure for the problem areas that become evident.

A variety of standardized assessment instruments have been used to assess psychopathology in older adults, but few have psychometric support for use with this population. Standardized tests have been developed for dementia, delirium, and depression, but a discussion of all of these disorders is beyond the scope of this chapter. The interested reader is directed to Broshek and Marcopulos (1999) for a thorough discussion of delirium assessment, and to LaRue (1992) and Riley (1999) for discussion of dementia assessment.

The assessment of depression often involves the administration of an individual test of depression. Though a variety of depression inventories exist, only two have demonstrated good psychometric properties with older adults: the Geriatric Depression Scale (GDS; Yesavage et al., 1983) and the Beck Depression Inventory (BDI; Beck, Ward, Mendelson, Mock, & Erbaugh, 1961). The GDS was specifically designed for older adults by excluding somatic items that might be more likely to be endorsed as a function of age and age-related factors (e.g., fatigue, sleep disturbance) and by using a dichotomous (yes/no) item format. The GDS has good sensitivity, specificity, reliability, and validity with a variety of older adult populations, such as medically ill outpatients (Norris, Gallagher, Wilson, & Winograd, 1987), noncognitively impaired nursing home residents (Lesher, 1986), and hospitalized older adults (Rapp, Parisi, Walsh, & Wallace, 1988). The BDI also has good psychometric properties with a variety of older adult populations, such as depressed outpatients (Olin, Schneider, Eaton, Zemansky, & Pollock, 1992) and medical outpatients (Norris et al., 1987). However, there is evidence that one must consider the influence of somatic complaints, particularly when assessing medical patients (see Rapp et al., 1988; Scogin, Hamblin, Beutler, & Corbishley, 1988). Moreover, the BDI employs a Guttman scale, which can be difficult for cognitively impaired older adults to complete.

ASSESSMENT OF ADAPTIVE FUNCTIONING

An individual's ability to perform activities of daily living (ADLs; eating, dressing, bathing) and instrumental activities of daily living (IADLs; meal preparation, money management) typically defines his or her level of adaptive functioning. The ability to care for oneself can be diminished severely by the presence of various forms of psychopathology, such as depression, dementia, substance abuse, and psychoses (LaRue, 1992).

Normal age-related changes also can have an impact on an older adult's level of adaptive functioning. For example, the age-related loss of bone density and muscle strength can limit the individual's ability to do yard work, such as mowing, weeding, and shoveling snow. Finally, disease processes (e.g., atherosclerosis, chronic obstructive pulmonary disease, diabetes, dementia) can impair significantly the older adult's level of adaptive functioning.

ADLs and IADLs can be assessed through self-report, direct observation, or report by others using standardized assessment instruments (e.g., the Katz Activities of Daily Living Scale; Hendrick, 1995; Katz, Downs, Cash, & Gratz, 1970). The Katz Activities of Daily Living Scale was designed to measure the independence in ADLs of chronically ill and older adults. The scale has shown high rates of interrater reliability (Kane & Kane, 1981), and scores on the ADL are related to scores on other measures of functional and cognitive abilities (Prineas et al., 1995). The advantage of the ADL is the ease of use by clinicians, caregivers, and clients. A limitation of the scale is that is does not address IADLs.

The Adult Functional Adaptive Behavior Scale (AFABS; Spirrison & Pierce, 1992) is a measure of both ADLs and IADLs. It was designed for use with older adults and measures levels of functioning in eating, ambulation, toileting, dressing, grooming, managing general personal needs, social interactions, orientation to environment, reality orientation, speech comprehension and expression, money management, memory, and health needs. A limitation of the AFABS is that the coverage of IADLs is limited and would not be adequate for a community-dwelling individual.

The Multidimensional Assessment Questionnaire (MFAQ; Duke University Center for the Study of Aging and Human Development, 1978; Fillenbaum, 1988) is a widely used measure that includes sections for the assessment of perceived mental health, perceived physical health, ADLs, and IADLs. The information is obtained by interviewing the client and/or a caregiver. Moderate to strong internal consistency coefficients have been reported for the MFAQ (George & Fillenbaum, 1985). Reliability and concurrent validity with other IADL and ADL measures has been well established (Whittle & Goldenberg 1996). The advantages of the MFAQ are the comprehensive nature of the information gathered on the client and the availability of normative data (McAuley, Arling, Nutty, & Bowling, 1980). The disadvantage is the amount of time needed to administer the MFAQ. Thus, some investigations have used only parts of the MFAQ, such as the section that assesses ADLs and IADLs.

ASSESSMENT OF SOCIAL FUNCTIONING

Social factors have been linked to mental (Burman & Margolin, 1992) and physical health (Thomas, Goodwin, & Goodwin, 1985) among older adults. Positive interactions have been shown to enhance physical and emotional functioning (Oxman & Berkman, 1990), and negative interactions have been associated with diminishing physical and emotional functioning (Rook, 1990).

Older adults will experience losses in their social networks (e.g., death or disease process in peers and family members) and encounter numerous relationship strains (e.g., illness of self or others, geographical distance from adult children). The size, construction, and complexity of an individual's social network will vary (Antonucci & Akiyama, 1987) across the life span. These changes require older adults to adapt and change to meet their continuing needs for positive social relationships, often by being more selective about these relationships (cf. Carstensen, 1991). That is, they cultivate their relationships with close friends and eliminate many acquaintance relationships to maximize the benefits (e.g., having a supportive listener) of their social networks and minimize the costs (e.g., energy expenditures). For reviews of relationships in old age, the reader is referred to Hanson and Carpenter (1994) and Lang and Carstensen (1998).

The assessment of social relationships and support can be an important element of a multidimensional assessment. The difficulty is in the selection of a suitable social support assessment instrument. Though numerous instruments have been used in the literature, each measures somewhat different aspects of social support, some are unreliable, some require considerable subjective judgment, and most are extremely time-consuming for both the interviewer and the participant (Kalish, 1997). Notwithstanding these shortcomings, these instruments can be helpful in examining facets of both negative and positive social interactions. A few representative instruments are the Social Support Structural Interview (Okun, Melichar, & Hill, 1990), the Arizona Social Support Interview Schedule (Barrera, Sandler, & Ramsay, 1981), and the Frequency of Interactions Inventory (Stephens, Kinney, Norris, & Ritchie, 1987).

MULTIMETHOD ASSESSMENT

Psychologists have employed a wide range of methods for assessing individuals (e.g., interview, direct observation, self-report inventory, report by others). No gold standard exists for assessment methods. Each method has strengths and weaknesses, and each delivers a different picture of the object of measure. These differences are typically attributed to method variance (cf. Campbell & Fisk, 1959). The relative strengths and weaknesses of each method often are minimized by combining methods in the assessment process. For example, an individual's suspected anxiety may be assessed through a combination of two or more of the following: structured interview, self-report instruments, reports by significant others, and heart rate, skin potential, and blood pressure responses to anxiety-arousing stimuli. Each method may contribute unique and corroborative information. The major advantages and disadvantages of the most common assessment methods are briefly reviewed as they pertain to older adults.

SELF-REPORT

The two most popular self-report instruments are the interview and the paper-and-pencil questionnaire or inventory. The clinical interview is the most commonly used clinical assessment instrument (Haynes & Jensen, 1979). All interviews offer the clinician an opportunity to observe directly various behavioral indicators of psychopathology (e.g., agitated behavior, depressed affect, motor retardation, inattention). This is a significant advantage over the self-report method.

Interviewing older adults is not unlike interviewing younger adults. The same general interviewing strategies that are effective with younger adults are effective with older adults (e.g., establishing rapport, active listening, careful questioning). Though similarities exist among the behaviors of different age groups, differences emerge as a function of the physiological and psychological considerations noted by Whitbourne in this volume. In contrast to younger adults, older adults have been found to refuse to participate in surveys at a higher rate (e.g., DeMaio, 1980; Herzog & Rodgers, 1988), to refuse to answer certain types of questions (e.g., Gergen & Back, 1966), and to respond "don't know" (Colsher & Wallace, 1989). Older adults also tend to be more cautious when responding (Okun, 1976) and give more acquiescent responses (Kogan, 1961). The length and complexity of the interview must be considered in light of the client's mental status and physical stamina. Some older adults may fatigue in a matter of minutes, whereas others may provide reliable information for hours. Several brief sessions may be required due to client fatigue or fluctuating cooperation.

Interviews vary in structure, ranging from structured and semistructured diagnostic interviews (e.g., Comprehensive Assessment and Referral Evaluation: Gurland et al., 1977; Geriatric Mental State Schedule: Copeland et al., 1976) to unstructured, free-flowing, nonstandardized clinical interviews. Overall, the structured interview offers unparalleled precision for arriving at reliable and valid diagnoses, although the trade-off for better psychometric characteristics is greater time consumption, more training required of interviewers, and reduced interviewer flexibility.

The unstructured interview is a very flexible and forgiving assessment instrument. It permits rephrasing of questions that appear unclear to the interviewee (e.g., offering various synonyms for depression, such as feeling blue, feeling down) and the exploration of topic areas that may be tangential but relevant to the presenting problems (Edelstein, Staats, Kalish, & Northrop, 1996). The interview also may enable one to determine which other assessment methods and instruments would be appropriate. For instance, the ability of the older adult to understand questions contained on a self-report questionnaire can be established. The interview also provides an opportunity to identify a significant other and/or care provider who can provide additional data on the client's current level of functioning. Moreover, the unstructured interview offers an opportunity to prompt and encourage responses and maintain the attention of the interviewee, who may be distracted easily and experience difficulty concentrating.

Paper-and-pencil self-report inventories and questionnaires also are used quite commonly with older adults, although the number of such instruments with good psychometric support for use with this group is limited. Among the advantages of inventories and questionnaires is the relatively small amount of professional staff time required to administer, score, and interpret them. They also are typically easy to administer, are more reliable than unstructured interviews, cover a wide range of information, and can provide access to privately held thoughts and beliefs.

Some of the disadvantages of self-report inventories are the requirements of good vision, adequate reading comprehension, and at least limited perceptual-motor skills. Problems in any of these domains can influence the reliability and validity of information obtained via questionnaires and inventories.

The self-report method, in general, is not without its shortcomings. The specific wording of questions, question format, and question context can influence the results (Schwarz, 1999). Dramatic demonstrations of such influence have appeared in the social psychological (e.g, Schwarz & Scheuring, 1988) and decision-making (e.g., Tversky & Kahneman, 1981) literatures. Moreover, both interviewers and self-report instruments may use words that are beyond the client's level of comprehension. Self-reporting can be particularly problematic with older adults who are experiencing communication-related cognitive deficits.

The evidence regarding the accuracy, reliability, and validity of older adult self-reports is mixed. Estimates of functional ability have been questioned by some researchers. For example, Rubenstein, Schairer, Wieland, and Kane (1984) found that geriatric patients overestimated their functional ability. Sager et al. (1992) found that older adults both under- and overestimated their ability to complete activities of daily living compared to performance-based measures. In addition to functional ability, some authors have reported that older adults' self-reports of memory impairment may not be accurate (e.g., Perlmutter, 1978; Rabbitt, 1982; A. Sunderland, Watts, Baddeley, & Harris, 1986; Zelinski, Gilewski, & Thompson, 1980).

The physical and mental health status of older adults can affect the accuracy of their reports. Responses can be altered by affective responses to acute illness, changes from previous levels of physical functioning occurring during hospitalization, and the presence of acute or chronic cognitive impairment (Sager et al., 1992). The cognitively impaired elderly pose a special challenge to clinicians. Typically, instruments are not validated for use with dementia patients. Some authors suggest that as levels of cognitive impairment increase, the validity of self-reports decreases (Sager et al.) Older adults with dementia who deny memory loss also tend to deny the presence of other symptoms (Feher, Larrabee, & Crook, 1992). Moreover, clients with severe dementia may not be able to comprehend the questions on the instruments or the nature of the information requested. Kiyak, Teri, and Borsom (1994) found that self-reports of functional health of demented individuals was consistently rated as poorer than reports by family members. Similarly, Kelly-Hayes, Jette, Wolf, D'Adostino, and Odell (1992) found low rates of agreement between self-reports of cognitively impaired individuals and performance-based measures.

On a more positive note, self-reported ADLs have been shown to correlate highly with performance measures in outpatient settings, where older adults perform ADLs daily and where a change in functioning is less likely (Sager et al., 1992). Similarly, older adults are no less accurate than younger adults in self-report, survey-type information (Rodgers & Herzog, 1987). Feher et al. (1992) also take a more positive view, suggesting that self-report instruments designed to measure mood may be utilized with older adults with mild to moderate dementia, arguing that accurate self-report of recent mood requires only minimal memory ability. Older adult self-reports of insomnia also have been quite accurate when compared against polysomnography (e.g., Reite, Buysse, Reynolds, & Mendelson, 1995), the gold standard for the assessment of sleep disorders.

Given these mixed results, broad generalizations regarding the accuracy of self reports by older adults should be avoided. The good news is that self-reports can be reliable under certain conditions. Consequently, it is important for clinicians and researchers to become knowledgeable of, and alert to, the factors that can influence self-report by older adults. Self-report measures remain an important source of data for geriatric assessment, especially for the relatively independent, well elderly (W.W. Morris & Boutelle, 1985). As with all age groups, self-reported information should be considered in light of its potential limitations and should be combined with other sources of information.

REPORT BY OTHERS

The report-by-other (e.g., spouse, caregiver, adult child) assessment method can provide valuable information on the history and course of symptoms, including unique and verifying data. Reports by others are particularly valuable when the older adult is incapable of conveying accurate information (e.g., when demented) and in institutional settings, where staff members observe residents throughout the day and night. In the latter case, nursing staff are often the principal source of information regarding day-to-day behaviors.

The disadvantages of report by others often depend on the relationship (Rubenstein et al., 1984) and proximity of the other to the client. Reports by others are susceptible to the same threats to reliability and validity as self-reports, with the added issue of bias by the reporter. For example, Zanetti, Geroldi, Frisoni, Bianchetti, and Trabucchi (1999) found that agreement between caregiver reports of patient ADLs and direct measures of ADLs of individuals with mild dementia was influenced by the caregiver's depressive symptoms and burden. Moreover, the correspondence between caregiver and performance-based ADL measures varied by activity. For example, the correspondence was high for motor performance (walking) but only moderate for telephone use, money use, and shopping.

In spite of its disadvantages, report by others is often a rich source of information, particularly with regard to the contextual factors related to the presenting problems. Reports by others can substitute for some self-report data when clients are unable (e.g., cognitively impaired) to provide needed information about their problem. Even when the ability to self-report is unimpaired, there may be reasons to seek reports by others. For example, there is considerable evidence that depressed individuals see the world somewhat differently from those who are not depressed (e.g., sometimes more accurately) and can distort and selectively attend to environmental information (Beck, Rush, Shaw, & Emery, 1979). As with each other source of information, report by others must be considered in the context of information gained from other methods.

Direct Observation

Direct observation of behavior can be one of the richest and most accurate assessment methods. Older adults may be observed in either natural settings or similar contrived situations. The information obtained can be utilized for a variety of purposes (e.g., needs assessment, planning of case management services, evaluation of functioning over time, admission planning for various living arrangements) (W.W. Morris & Boutelle, 1985).

There are several advantages to using direct observation. Direct observation can be useful when assessing older adults who are uncooperative, unavailable for self-report, or severely physically or mentally impaired (Goga & Hambacher, 1977). In addition, simple observational procedures can be taught easily to individuals with little or no previous experience. The data resulting from reliable observations can be incorporated into cost-effective institutionwide systems to identify goals, track behavior changes over time, and demonstrate facility patterns (Schnelle & Traughber, 1983). Finally, idiosyncratic patterns of impairment in ADLs caused by cognitive deficits can be noted with direct observations of performance on specific tasks (Kapust & Weintraub, 1988).

The clinician also can observe behaviors that may be clinically relevant but unreported. For the depressed older adult, observations might include speed of psychomotor behavior, social behavior (or lack thereof), agitated behavior, indicators of irritability, tearfulness, crying, and duration of attention. This method requires little on the part of the older adult, which is helpful when working with individuals experiencing moderate to severe cognitive impairment (Goga & Hambacher, 1977).

The potential disadvantages of direct observation methodology are both financial and practical. Third-party payers may not provide reimbursement for direct observation assessment (Kapust & Weintraub, 1988). More complex coding systems that provide richer sources of data may be too complicated or demand too much time for caregiver implementation. In addition, direct observations of ADLs, such as bathing and toileting, may be too intrusive and aversive to some older adults.

Overall, a combination of assessment methods can result in a more complete picture than that obtained by any single method. Moreover, such a combination can compensate for some of the limitations of the individual methods.

THE ASSESSMENT PROCESS

Specific Goals of the Assessment

Many specific goals may guide the assessment process, including (1) screening for various disorders (e.g., dementia); (2) evaluating capacity (e.g., in making medical decisions); (3) predicting adjustment to new environments (e.g., relocations to nursing homes); (4) evaluating functional skills (e.g., the ability to prepare meals); and (5) monitoring change over time (e.g., before and after surgery, pre- and poststroke, documenting memory loss). Beyond these specific goals, clinicians may have more general objectives. Two common, general goals of the assessment process are screening for psychopathology and diagnostic classification.

Goal: Screening Older Clients

Screening is carried out when clinicians want to cast a broad net designed to be maximally sensitive to any indicators of psychopathology. For example, clinicians may want to screen older clients for signs of dementia and, therefore, may select such instruments as the MMSE (Folstein, Folstein, & McHugh, 1975) or the Cognistat (Kiernan, Mueller, Langston, & Van Dyke, 1987). These instruments are designed broadly to assess for a variety of signs (e.g., memory and language disturbances) that may signal the presence of dementia. When scoring these instruments, one can use relatively low cutoff scores that have been demonstrated to maximize sensitivity. Clinicians also may screen for functional limitations by administering the ADL (Katz et al., 1970). Overall, the screening process is used when clinicians wish to adopt an economical yet comprehensive approach to the initial evaluation of older clients.

Goal: Classification/Diagnosis of Psychopathology among Older Clients

Another general goal of the assessment process may be to classify (i.e., diagnose) any psychopathology that may be present. Several alternatives exist regarding how clinicians may proceed (Hayes, Wilson, Gifford, Follette, & Strosahl, 1996). Syndromal classification identifies syndromes and classifies them. Syndromes are collections of signs (i.e., what is observed) and symptoms (i.e., the client's complaints) that often will lead to the diagnosis of various disorders. The syndromal classification approach is currently used by the majority of clinicians and is reflected in the organization and content of the widely used fourth edition of the *Diagnostic and Statistical Manual of Mental Disorders* (*DSM-IV*; American Psychiatric Association [APA], 1994).

Several criticisms have been raised regarding the strategy of syndromal classification. Hayes et al. (1996) argued that the descriptions of syndromes may be continually changed and refined, thus leading to an ever increasing number of diagnostic categories found within the *DSM* system. Another criticism is that clinicians will direct their efforts toward classification at the expense of investigating factors that may predict or etiologically explain various diseases (Follette & Houts, 1996). Criticisms such as these similarly have led others (e.g., Follette, 1996; McFall & Townsend, 1998) to reexamine the foundations of psychological assessment and call for viable alternatives to the dominant strategy of syndromal classification. Alternative approaches to syndromal classification may be especially desirable for clinicians who work with older clients, as the signs and symptoms of a given disorder may differ between younger and older clients. For example, the expression of depressive disorders among older adults may involve more somatic complaints and fewer complaints of depressed mood in comparison to younger adults (Scogin, 1994).

As an alternative to syndromal classification, Hayes et al. (1996) also discussed functional classification. Using this strategy, problematic behaviors are organized by the functional processes that are hypothesized to have produced and maintained them. Proponents of the strategy of functional classification may use a functional analysis (for the specific steps involved in a functional analysis, see Hayes & Follette, 1992; Martin & Pear, 1996). This type of analysis generally involves the observation of clients' problematic behaviors in their natural environments to arrive at hypotheses about how the problem behaviors are controlled and maintained by their antecedents and consequences. For example, a functional analysis may be utilized with an older client exhibiting constant yelling or occasional aggressive behavior. The initial occurrence or maintenance of these behaviors may be understood from a functional perspective; for example, these behaviors may produce attention from others. Overall, the utilization of functional analyses as a means of functional classification has been criticized on several grounds. For example, Hayes et al. (1996) have reported that functional analyses are sometimes vague, hard to replicate and test empirically, and strongly ideographic (i.e., not very generalizable).

As an alternative to the syndromal and functional classification strategies, Hayes et al. (1996) have proposed the utilization of functional diagnostic dimensions. For example, experiential avoidance involves an unwillingness to stay in contact with certain private experiences (e.g., thoughts, emotions, bodily sensations) and any subsequent actions that are taken to alter the frequency or form of these private experiences and the contexts that lead to them. The authors describe functional diagnostic dimensions such as experiential avoidance in the following way: "They are dimensional processes, not all-or-nothing categories that suggest psychological processes relevant to etiology, that make coherent many topographical forms under a single functional process, and that can be readily linked to treatment" (p. 1163). From this definition, it is evident that functional diagnostic dimensions address some of the weaknesses of syndromal and functional classification strategies. Hayes et al. also suggest the possibility of the future identification and exploration of other possible functional diagnostic dimensions, such as poor rule generation, inappropriate rule following, and socially impoverished repertoires.

In addition to the classification strategies outlined by Hayes et al. (1996), other approaches to classification have been described that may benefit older adults. For example, Nease, Volk, and Cass (1999) have suggested that symptom severity should be incorporated into classification strategies. These authors investigated a severity-based classification of mood and anxiety symptoms in primary care patients. In their research, the authors were able to identify valid clusters of symptom severity (e.g., low severity, high severity) and define relations between these clusters and other outcomes (e.g., health-related quality of life and frequency of *DSM* disorders). The adoption of a severity-based classification strategy may be especially beneficial when assessing older clients, because they often exhibit subclinical symptoms of certain disorders (i.e., they may fail to meet all of the diagnostic criteria for a given disorder that are sufficient to warrant clinical attention and intervention). For example, whereas the prevalence rates for major depressive disorder among older adults are low, the rates for depressive symptoms have been reported to be as high as 20% to 30% on average (Wolfe, Morrow, & Fredrickson, 1996). Because subclinical symptoms of depression may be somewhat common among older adults, an assessment strategy that focuses on the severity of these symptoms may be more suited for older populations.

POTENTIAL STRATEGIES FOR ASSESSING OLDER CLIENTS

When screening older clients, or attempting to arrive at diagnoses, clinicians may choose to implement different assessment strategies. Two such strategies are addressed in this section: symptom-based hypothesis testing and test battery approaches.

Symptom-Based Hypothesis Testing

This strategy involves following up on any symptom-based hypotheses that are formed as the assessment unfolds. For example, if an older client complained of fatigue, difficulty thinking or concentrating, and sleep disturbance, clinicians might administer a set of instruments designed to assess for disorders related to mood or anxiety. Further, if the clinician hypothesizes that various symptoms may signal the presence of a disorder, and diagnosis is the ultimate goal, then the diagnostic criteria for that disorder may be referenced from the *DSM-IV* (APA, 1994). An advantage of this symptom-based hypothesis strategy is that the clinician may make judicious use of the resources (i.e., time, effort, and money) that are available for the assessment process. A disadvantage is that clinicians may focus on a set of symptoms that is too narrow and miss other forms of psychopathology. This might occur if older clients leave out important information when describing their problems, or when clinicians fail to adequately investigate other areas of functioning and terminate the assessment process prematurely.

Test Battery Approaches

This strategy involves the administration of a diverse battery of assessment instruments that are designed to cover a broad spectrum of psychopathology. For example, a battery may consist of instruments designed to grossly assess cognitive functioning, mood, anxiety, psychotic symptoms, adaptive functioning, and so on. This strategy may be more commonly employed in settings where a basic set of information is required regarding the overall functioning of an older adult. For example, admissions to nursing homes often require the assembly of a Minimum Data Set (MDS; J.N. Morris et al., 1990) that involves the inclusion of a basic set of assessment instruments. However, the contents of the assessment battery also may be guided by any initial impressions that may have been formed during the screening process (e.g., the older client may have reported feelings of depression and anxiety, which may lead the clinician to utilize instruments designed to assess for both of these problems). The administration of a battery of assessment instruments also would be useful in situations where an identified problem exists but the wide-reaching effects of the problem are unknown (e.g., difficulties with the older client's memory have been identified, but it is unclear how it has affected his or her emotional, social, or adaptive functioning). A strong advantage of the strategy of using a comprehensive battery of assessment instruments is that clinicians are less likely to miss important information. A disadvantage of this strategy is that clinicians may utilize such a large number of assessment instruments that an unnecessary strain is placed on the older client and the resources that are available for the assessment process.

Some clinicians may prefer to carry out a hybrid of the assessment strategies mentioned above (i.e., a blend of the symptom-based hypothesis testing strategy and the use of assessment batteries). The use of a hybrid approach may help clinicians to maximize the advantages of the separate assessment strategies and minimize their disadvantages. The final selection of the appropriate assessment strategy depends on the setting in which the older adult is assessed (e.g., private practice, clinic, nursing home), as well as the unique features of each older client's case (e.g., the presence of sensory, cognitive, or physical limitations).

REVIEWING ASSESSMENT RESULTS

Sources of Discrepancies in Assessment Results

To begin integrating the results, clinicians should note any discrepancies observed among the various findings and attempt to resolve these through further inquiry and assessment. One source of discrepancies might include natural fluctuations over time in the phenomenon of interest (e.g., normal fluctuations in mood or anxiety). Discrepancies also may arise among multiple sources of information (e.g., self-reported information and reports by others). Further, discrepancies may occur when questionnaires designed to measure the same construct (e.g., depression) feature different wordings, formats, and contexts (Schwarz, 1999).

Discrepancies in the older client's assessment results also may be due to the influence of a chronic health problem. The older client's experience of such chronic health problems may change (i.e., improve or worsen) over the course of the assessment, thus altering the assessment results. For example, older adults with advanced cases of Chronic Obstructive Pulmonary disease (COPD) may experience declines in mental alertness and efficiency, memory, complex problem solving, motor coordination, and speed (Frazer, Leicht, & Baker, 1996). These declines may create discrepancies over the course of the assessment process.

Similarly, acute health problems may arise and affect the results of the assessment process. Consider the example of an older client who has a minor stroke or an undetected transient ischemic attack (TIA) between assessment sessions. The effects of the stroke or the TIA may be subtle (e.g., slight motor or cognitive disturbances), but they may be sufficient to produce contrasting assessment results over time.

Another source of discrepancies in assessment results may be the influence of medications. Schneider (1996) has documented a vast array of psychiatric symptoms (e.g., confusion, delusions, forgetfulness, depression, hallucinations) that may be produced by various drugs or classes of drugs. Further, given that older adults commonly take multiple medications, the likelihood of drug interactions increases, which in turn may increase the complexity of the assessment process.

Finally, the presence of certain cognitive disorders may produce discrepant assessment results. For example, individuals with disorders such as Alzheimer's disease may exhibit anosognosia (a denial or unawareness of one's deficits) and may report having no cognitive impairments, despite evidence to the contrary (Vasterling, Seltzer, Foss, & Vanderbrook, 1995).

Identifying Common Themes

Once any discrepancies have been resolved through further inquiry or assessment, clinicians then should focus on identifying any common themes that may emerge, both within and across assessment measures. These themes may relate to the older client's level of functioning (e.g., consistent performance that is above or below average) or to the older client's strengths or weaknesses in particular areas of functioning (e.g., memory performance, functional skills). The presence of consistent results and certain themes may begin to suggest the possibility of specific diagnoses (i.e., assuming that diagnosis is the clinician's goal).

PRACTICAL RECOMMENDATIONS

Prior to the Assessment

When scheduling an assessment, clinicians may wish to keep in mind several practical suggestions. First, clinicians may find it helpful to remind their older clients to bring any assistive devices they require to the evaluation (e.g., hearing aids, glasses with prescription lenses, special writing instruments for arthritis sufferers). Second, clinicians might benefit from inquiring about any sensory, motor, or cognitive difficulties the older client may have, as these difficulties may alter significantly the content of the assessment. This is especially important to clinicians who act as consultants on cases where limited information is available regarding the older client. Consider the example of a consulting clinician who has carefully assembled a battery of paper-and-pencil tests, only to find that the older client sitting in the waiting room is visually impaired, unable to write, and cognitively impaired. Third, clinicians may be wise to schedule more time when assessing older clients, as they may take longer than younger clients to complete assessment instruments. Along these lines, clinicians may find it necessary to schedule regular rest periods during the course of the assessment to prevent their older clients from becoming unnecessarily fatigued.

During the Assessment Process

Four additional, practical suggestions also may be offered with regard to the assessment process itself. First, when describing the instructions of assessment instruments, clinicians should use a level of vocabulary that is appropriate to the older client's level of education and understanding. Second, clinicians are well advised from practical and ethical standpoints to use assessment instruments that are psychometrically sound for older populations. Third, clinicians may find it beneficial to be aware of how the older client's performance may be adversely affected by potential age-related declines in sensory, cognitive, and motor domains. A discussion of these age-related declines is beyond the scope of this chapter; interested readers are referred to Edelstein, Martin, and Goodie (in press) and Whitbourne (this volume).

Given that certain age-related declines may be present, clinicians may wish to structure the assessment process to minimize their influence. To this end, several basic suggestions may be offered. To minimize the influence of potential age-related visual declines, clinicians may choose to: (1) use written materials that feature a large type size (i.e., a minimum of 14- to 16-point type); (2) use large visual stimuli with good contrast (e.g., black and white colors); and (3) use indirect lighting to reduce the impact of glare on visual materials. Potential age-related auditory declines may be managed by: (1) speaking loudly and clearly at an individually appropriate distance from the client; (2) allowing a clear view of the clinician's face to facilitate lip reading; and (3) presenting auditory information at a neutral or lower pitch. In an effort to accommodate potential age-related declines in cognition (e.g., declines in memory, mental processing speed, inhibition of irrelevant information, or attention), clinicians may choose to: (1) provide clients with verbal or written reminders of instructions in response to various declines in memory; (2) present information at a slower pace in response to slower mental processing speeds; (3) eliminate any tangential information from instructions or dialogue; and (4) neutralize any stimuli that may distract the older client's attention, such as noisy office equipment. It is important to keep in mind, however, that some of these suggestions may run counter to the standardized protocols of various assessment instruments. For example, clinicians may not be able to repeat instructions or alter the stimuli of certain assessment instruments without invalidating their standardization requirements.

Finally, clinicians should keep in mind that although it may be possible to obtain a great deal of information from their older clients, it may be necessary in some cases to solicit information from other sources. These sources may include past records (e.g., psychological or medical evaluations) or reports from proxies (i.e., prominent individuals in the older client's life, such as spouses or children). Input from these sources may be required if the older client is experiencing memory difficulties or any other cognitive, sensory, or motor impairments that would interfere with the delivery of accurate information.

ASSESSMENT OF MR. TOEFERT

The assessment of Mr. Toefert began with an interview. This took place in his room while he was seated in his wheelchair. He was cooperative, well kempt, and colorfully dressed in a Hawaiian shirt with contrasting purple trousers.

Mr. Toefert appeared his stated age, although his skin appeared very darkly tanned, excessively wrinkled, and leathery. His speech was slow, labored, and of low volume. Eye contact was brief and occurred only following questions from the interviewer; otherwise, his eyes were downcast. Mr. Toefert slouched in his wheelchair and occasionally winced when attempting to reposition himself, apparently from pain in his broken hip. He displayed depressed affect during most of the interview, evidencing occasional episodes of tearfulness. He reported feeling very sad for the past few months, particularly since his fall and broken hip. Mr. Toefert also reported symptoms of anxiety in regard to his memory problems, inability to walk, and prospects for the future. He said he had always been a chronic worrier, but his worrying had become more severe in recent weeks.

When asked about his appetite, Mr. Toefert stated, "Everything I eat tastes like cardboard!" He reported sometimes having difficulty falling asleep and often waking in the middle of the night or around 4:00 A.M. and not being able to return to sleep. He also reported having difficulty concentrating. For example, he said he was rarely able to watch a complete television program and was easily distracted. He also stated that he found it difficult to think, particularly about difficult issues or problems that require a great deal of concentration. When asked how he liked living in the nursing home, he replied that it was okay except for the fact that he had to conceal many of his personal belongings. A box of chocolate candy recently given to him by an old friend was missing, and Mr. Toefert blamed the loss on other residents who he claimed stole from him. He noted that the most effective way to ensure the safety of his belongings was to leave his room as little as possible, as other residents often wandered into his room without invitation. When asked why he didn't have the staff lock his valuable belongings in a cabinet, Mr. Toefert stated that he didn't trust the staff, some of whom he believed were "out to get" him. When asked how he determined that, Mr. Toefert replied, "They keep taking my eyeglasses and dentures, and hiding my coat."

Following the interview, Mr. Toefert's medical chart was reviewed. The chart contained his social history, previous evaluations by other professionals (e.g., physician, neurologist, orthopedic surgeon), and the results of laboratory tests (e.g., blood tests, neuroimaging, urinalysis). The review of Mr. Toefert's laboratory test results revealed no remarkable findings. Because of his symptoms of depression and anxiety, particular attention was paid to the results of his thyroid function tests. The laboratory tests yielded normal values of T_4, T_3, and TSH, thus ruling out hypothyroidism and hyperthyroidism as potential causes of the symptoms of anxiety and depression.

The nursing notes revealed that Mr. Toefert was refusing breakfast every morning, choosing instead to sleep until 10:00 A.M. He consumed very little food during lunch and dinner, and skipped at least one of these meals each day. The weight records added support to these reports, indicating that Mr. Toefert had lost 10 pounds in seven days and was nearing the bottom on his ideal weight range. Nurses also noticed that Mr. Toefert had been spending more and more time in bed. When asked why he did this, he reported that he was always tired and could not get enough rest. Nursing staff reported that Mr. Toefert's recent recall was sometimes poor. He occasionally forgot that he had just eaten a snack and would ask for another, usually something containing chocolate.

A review of the activities staff progress notes revealed that repeated attempts to coax Mr. Toefert out of his room to attend social activities and interactions were consistently met with refusals. When asked why he did not want to leave his room, Mr. Toefert despondently replied, "What's the difference? Just leave me alone."

An interview with Mr. Toefert's sister revealed that he previously had expressed distrust of some family members and believed that they were either taking or moving his personal possessions (e.g., eyeglasses, car keys). His family also reported that Mr. Toefert occasionally experienced difficulty driving, particularly in areas with which he was less familiar. On at least two occasions he had become lost and confused, experienced severe anxiety (described as panic), and had to seek assistance in becoming reoriented. Mr. Toefert's sister also indicated that his mood changed significantly following these incidents and after the fall in which his hip was broken.

The information obtained from Mr. Toefert's medical chart, interview of family members, and the initial interview of Mr. Toefert suggested several possible problem areas, including depression, anxiety, dementia, and delusions. Formal psychological testing began with a cognitive screening for possible dementia in light of his reported memory and attention deficits. His performance on the MMSE suggested possible mild cognitive impairment, which could be due to a variety of reasons, including inattention stemming from the depression.

A second screening instrument employed with Mr. Toefert was a clock drawing test (Freedman et al., 1994; Royall, Mulroy, Chiodo, & Polk, 1999; T. Sunderland et al., 1989). Various versions of this test have been developed (see Freedman et al., 1994). It is useful as a screening instrument because it is sensitive to deficits in various cognitive domains (e.g., planning, organization, perseveration, direction following, visual-motor skills). It is also quick to administer and is apparently uninfluenced by language or cultural factors (Schulman, Pushkar-Gold, Cohen, & Zucchero, 1993). Using the T. Sunderland et al. (1989) scoring criteria, Mr. Toefert achieved a score within the normal range of functioning.

In light of Mr. Toefert's reported sadness and other symptoms indicative of depression (e.g., fatigue, sleep disturbance, weight loss), a depression inventory was administered. Because he exhibited some symptoms that suggested the possibility of dementia, the GDS was chosen for its true/false format. He obtained a score indicative of moderate depression. In light of this score, the GDS was followed with administration of the Hamilton Rating Scale for Depression (HRSD; Hamilton, 1967), which provided additional detailed information on the severity of depression (Scogin, 1994) using another assessment method. The HRSD has sound psychometric properties with older adult medical patients and is superior to self-report instruments with regard to sensitivity and specificity using a cutoff score of 12 on the 17-item version of the HSRD (Rapp, Smith, & Britt, 1990). Mr. Toefert obtained a score in the depressed range, again suggesting depression.

Based on the interview, material gleaned from the medical record, reports by others, and the two depression assessment instruments, Mr. Toefert met the *DSM-IV* criteria for major depression. At this point, we considered the concurrent symptoms of depression, dementia, and anxiety: Mr. Toefert could be suffering from depression, generalized anxiety disorder, dementia, or all three. Common combinations include depression and anxiety; depression and dementia (dementia syndrome of depression, DSD); and dementia anxiety. The process of sorting out this diagnostic problem is complicated, and typically involves eliminating as many potentially reversible sources of presenting symptoms as possible (e.g., physical diseases, abnormal levels of hormones, vitamin B12, folate). For example, hypothyroidism could yield symptoms of depression, hyperthyroidism could yield symptoms of anxiety, and low levels of vitamin B12 could yield symptoms of a reversible dementia that could appear to be Alzheimer's disease. Hyperthyroidism, hypothyroidism, and vitamin B12 deficiency were ruled out with the laboratory tests. To differentiate Alzheimer's disease from DSD, Kaszniak and Christensen (1994) recommend contrasting symptoms of these two disorders with regard to the following measures: symptom duration at time of seeking medical attention (long for AD and short for DSD), previous psychiatric history (unusual for AD and usual for DSD), progression of symptoms (slow for AD and rapid for DSD), patient complaints of deficit (variable for AD and abundant for DSD), emotional reaction (variable for AD and marked distress for DSD), patient valuation of accomplishments (variable for AD and minimized for DSD), behavior congruent with cognitive deficits (usual with AD and unusual with DSD), delusions (mood-dependent in AD and mood-congruent in DSD), and mood disorder (environmentally responsive in AD and persistent in DSD).

After applying these criteria to Mr. Toefert, we concluded that his cognitive deficits were likely due to depression rather than dementia, or the combination of the two. To increase our confidence in our analysis, we recommended that Mr. Toefert receive a thorough neuropsychological evaluation. The results of this evaluation supported our hypothesis that he was not experiencing dementia.

Mr. Toefert's symptoms of anxiety were evaluated further through an administration of the Beck Anxiety Inventory (BAI; Beck & Steer, 1993). The BAI is a measure of general anxiety and is perhaps the only one for which we currently have positive psychometric support for use with older adults (Stanley & Beck, 1998). Mr. Toefert's score on the BAI and further interviewing regarding his symptoms of anxiety suggested that he had a longstanding problem with generalized anxiety. The problem was exacerbated by his brief disorientation episodes, and concerns about his memory and his inability to walk unassisted following the healing of his hip. Anxiety and fear following falls among older adults is not uncommon and can be quite debilitating, even after the physical consequences of falls have abated (see Edelstein & Drozdick, 1998).

Mr. Toefert's concern that people were "out to get" him and were hiding objects from him was determined, through observation and discussions with staff and family, to be a function of primary memory failures. Mr. Toefert would forget where he had placed objects, particularly when he did not place them in their "usual" location, and then blame others for their loss. The results of the neuropsychological evaluation supported this hypothesis, and Mr. Toefert's memory difficulties were diagnosed as benign senile forgetfulness.

In summary, we began with symptoms of delusions, anxiety, depression, and dementia, all of which may coexist. Only the symptoms of depression met diagnostic criteria, and their cause was attributed to Mr. Toefert's fall and concern about the possibility of developing dementia. Other possible causes were ruled out. The apparent delusions were ruled out as a function of poor memory. The anxiety was apparently a longstanding problem that was intensified by Mr. Toefert's failing memory, fear of dementia, and recent fall. The cognitive deficits considered as possible symptoms of dementia were attributed to age-related memory loss and depression.

CONCLUSION

The assessment of psychopathology in late life is complex and challenging. The interplay of biological, psychological, and social factors is profound and often perplexing. Moreover, the symptoms of psychopathology can be multiply determined, and even generated by treatments used to address other disorders. There also is evidence that subsyndromal forms of anxiety and depression among older adults can be quite debilitating and vexing. Thus, the clinical gerontologist may need to reconsider the exclusive use of our current diagnostic criteria when engaged in the assessment process.

Though our current assessment methods are tried and true, most of our assessment instruments have little empirical support for their use with older adults. In addition, there is some evidence that the manifestations of some forms of psychopathology among older adults may differ from those of younger adults. If this evidence is confirmed, then the content of many of our current psychological assessment instruments will have to be revisited with an eye to age-related differences in psychopathological presentation.

STUDY QUESTIONS

1. What is multidimensional assessment, and why is it so important for the assessment of older adults?
2. What domains of functioning are important to assess when working with older adults?
3. What are some potential causes of a decline in adaptive functioning?
4. Why might an older adult (70 years old) report having a smaller group of friends now than 15 years ago?
5. How does a biopsychosocial model guide the assessment process?
6. What is multimethod assessment, what are the various methods, and what are the strengths and weaknesses of each method?

7. What is screening, and what role does it play in the assessment process?
8. Describe syndromal classification as an assessment goal. What are some of the drawbacks of syndromal classification as it applies to older clients?
9. What are some alternatives to syndromal classification, and how might they be beneficial when dealing with older clients?
10. A clinician conducts an assessment of an older client who lives in a nursing home and observes significant discrepancies in the results. Describe some of the possible origins of these discrepancies.
11. In working with older clients, name several practical considerations that clinicians should be aware of prior to and during the assessment process.

SUGGESTED READINGS

Cavanaugh, J.C., & Whitbourne, S.K. (Eds.). (1999). *Gerontology: An interdisciplinary perspective.* New York: Oxford University Press.

Edelstein, B., Drozdick, L.W., & Kogan, J.N. (1998). Behavioral assessment of older adults. In A.S. Bellack & M. Hersen (Eds.), *Behavioral assessment: A practical handbook* (4th ed., pp. 378–406). Boston: Allyn & Bacon.

Edelstein, B., Kalish, K., Drozdick, L., & McKee, D. (1999). Assessment of depression and bereavement in older adults. In P.A. Lichtenberg (Ed.), *Handbook of geriatric assessment.* New York: Wiley.

Hansson, R.O., & Carpenter, B.N. (1994). *Relationships in old age: Coping with the challenge of transition.* New York: The Guilford Press.

Kogan, J., Edelstein, B., & McKee, D. (In press). Assessment of anxiety in older adults: Current status. *Journal of Anxiety Disorders.*

La Rue, A., & Watson, J. (1998). Psychological assessment of older adults. *Professional Psychology, 29,* 5–14.

Lichtenberg, P.A. (1999). *Handbook of assessment in clinical gerontology.* New York: Wiley.

Morrison, J. (1997). *When psychological problems mask medical disorders: A guide for psychologists.* New York: Guilford Press.

Storandt, M., & Vanden Bos, G.R. (1994). *Neuropsychological assessment of dementia and depression in older adults: A clinician's guide.* Washington, DC: American Psychological Association.

REFERENCES

Albert, M. (1994). Brief assessments of cognitive function in the elderly. In M.P. Lawton & J.A. Teresi (Eds.), *Annual review of gerontology and geriatrics: Focus on assessment techniques* (pp. 93–106). New York: Springer.

American Psychiatric Association. (1994). *Diagnostic and statistical manual of mental disorders* (4th ed.). Washington, DC: Author.

Antonucci, T., & Akiyama, H. (1987). Social networks in adult life and a preliminary examination of the convoy model. *Journal of Gerontology, 42,* 519–527.

Babcock, R.L., & Salthouse, T.A. (1990). Effects of increased processing demands on age differences in working memory. *Psychology and Aging, 5,* 421–428.

Barrera, M., Jr., Sandler, I.N., & Ramsay, T.B. (1981). Preliminary development of a scale of social support: Studies on college students. *American Journal of Community Psychology, 9,* 435–447.

Beck, A.T., Rush, A.J., Shaw, B.F., & Emery, G. (1979). *Cognitive therapy of depression.* New York: Guilford Press.

Beck, A.T., & Steer, R.A. (1993). *Beck Anxiety Inventory manual* (2nd ed.). San Antonio, TX: Psychological Corporation.

Beck, A.T., Ward, C.H., Mendelson, M., Mock, J., & Erbaugh, J. (1961). An inventory for measuring depression. *Archives of General Psychiatry, 4,* 561–571.

Blazer, D.G. (1994). Epidemiology of late life depression. In L.S. Schneider, C.F. Reynolds, B.D. Lebowitz, & A.J. Friedhoff (Eds.), *Diagnosis and treatment of depression in late life* (pp. 9–19). Washington, DC: American Psychiatric Association.

Blazer, D.G., Bacher, J., & Hughes, D.C. (1987). Major depression with melancholia: A comparison of middle-aged and elderly adults. *Journal of the American Geriatrics Society, 34,* 519–525.

Broshek, D.K., & Marcopulos, B.A. (1999). Delirium assessment in older adults. In P.A. Lichtenberg (Ed.), *Handbook of assessment in clinical gerontology* (pp. 167–204). New York: Wiley.

Burman, B., & Margolin, G. (1992). Analysis of the association between marital relationships and health problems: An interactional perspective. *Psychological Bulletin, 112,* 39–63.

Burns, A., Jacoby, R., & Levy, R. (1991). Progression of cognitive impairment in Alzheimer's disease. *Journal of the American Geriatrics Society, 39,* 39–45.

Campbell, D., & Fisk, D.W. (1959). Convergent and discriminant validation by the multitrait-multimethod matrix. *Psychological Bulletin, 56,* 81–105.

Carstensen, L.L. (1991). Selectivity theory: Social activity in life-span context. In K.W. Schaie (Ed.), *Annual review of gerontology and geriatrics* (pp. 195–217). New York: Springer.

Colsher, P., & Wallace, R.B. (1989). Data quality and age: Health and psychobehavioral correlates of item nonresponse and inconsistent responses. *Journal of Gerontology: Psychological Sciences, 44,* P45–P52.

Copeland, J.R.M., Kelleher, M.J., Kellett, J.M., Gourlay, A.J., Gurland, B.J., Fleiss, J.L., & Sharpe, L. (1976). A semi-structured clinical interview for the assessment of diagnostic and mental state in the elderly: The Geriatric and Mental State Schedule I. Development and reliability. *Psychological Medicine, 6,* 439–449.

Crum, R.M., Anthony, J.C., Bassett, S.S., & Folstein, M.F. (1993). Population-based norms for the MMSE by age and education level. *Journal of the American Medical Association, 269,* 2386–2391.

DeMaio, T. (1980). Refusals: Who, where and why. *Public Opinion Quarterly, 44,* 223–233.

Duke University Center for the Study of Aging and Human Development (1978). *Multidimensional functional assessment: The OARS Methodology* (2nd ed.). Durham, NC: Author.

Edelstein, B., & Drozdick, L. (1998). Falls among older adults. In B. Edelstein (Ed.), *Clinical geropsychology* (pp. 349–370). Oxford, England: Elsevier.

Edelstein, B., & Kalish, K. (1999). Clinical assessment of older adults. In J.C. Cavanaugh & S.K. Whitbourne (Eds.), *Gerontology: Interdisciplinary perspectives.* New York: Oxford University Press.

Edelstein, B.A., Martin, R.R., & Goodie, J. (in press). Physiological and behavioral concomitants of aging. In W.E. Craighead & C.B. Nemeroff (Eds.), *Encyclopedia of psychology and neuroscience.* New York: Wiley.

Edelstein, B., Staats, N., Kalish, K., & Northrop, L. (1996). Assessment of older adults. In M. Hersen & V. Van Hasselt (Eds.), *Psychological treatment of older adults: An introductory textbook.* New York: Plenum Press.

Feher, E.P., Larrabee, G.J., & Crook, T.J. (1992). Factors attenuating the validity of the Geriatric Depression Scale in a dementia population. *Journal of the American Geriatrics Society, 40,* 906–909.

Fillenbaum, G.G. (1988). *Multidimensional functional assessment of older adults.* Hillsdale, NJ: Erlbaum.

First, M.B., Spitzer, R.L., Gibbon, M., & Williams, J.B.W. (1995). *The Structured Clinical Interview for Axis I DSM-IV Disorders—Patient Edition* (SCID-I/P version 2.0). New York: New York State Psychiatric Institute, Biometrics Research Department.

Follette, W.C. (1996). Introduction to the special section on the development of theoretically coherent alternatives to the *DSM* system. *Journal of Consulting and Clinical Psychology, 64,* 1117–1119.

Follette, W.C., & Houts, A.C. (1996). Models of scientific progress and the role of theory in taxonomy development: A case study of the *DSM. Journal of Consulting and Clinical Psychology, 64,* 1120–1132.

Folstein, M.F., Folstein, S.E., & McHugh, P.R. (1975). "Mini-mental state": A practical method for grading the cognitive state of patients for the clinician. *Journal of Psychiatric Research, 12,* 189–198.

Frazer, D.W., Leicht, M.L., & Baker, M.D. (1996). Psychological manifestations of physical disease in the elderly. In L.L. Carstensen, B.A. Edelstein, & L. Dornbrand (Eds.), *The practical handbook of clinical gerontology* (pp. 217–235). Thousand Oaks, CA: Sage.

Freedman, M., Leach, L., Kaplan, E., Winocur, G., Shullman, K.I., & Delis, D.C. (1994). *Clock drawing: A neuropsychological analysis.* New York: Oxford University Press.

Fry, P.S. (1986). *Depression, stress, and adaptations in the elderly: Psychological assessment and intervention.* Rockville, MD: Aspen.

George, L.K., & Fillenbaum, G.G. (1985). The OARS methodology: A decade of experiences in geriatric assessment. *Journal of the American Geriatrics Society, 33,* 607–615.

Gergen, K.J., & Back, K.W. (1966). Communication in the interview and the disengaged respondent. *Public Opinion Quarterly, 30,* 385–398.

Goga, J.A., & Hambacher, W.O. (1977). Psychologic and behavioral assessment of geriatric patients: A review. *Journal of the American Geriatrics Society, 25*(5), 232–237.

Gurland, B.J., Kuriansky, J.B., Sharpe, L., Simon, R., Stiller, P., & Birkett, P. (1977). The Comprehensive Assessment and Referral and Evaluation (CARE): Rationale, development, and reliability. *International Journal of Aging and Human Development, 8,* 9–42.

Hamilton, M. (1967). Development of a rating scale for primary depressive illness. *British Journal of Social and Clinical Psychology, 6,* 278–296.

Hanson, R.O., & Carpenter, B.N. (1994). *Relationships in old age: Coping with the challenge of transition.* New York: Guilford Press.

Hayes, S.C., & Follette, W.C. (1992). Can functional analysis provide a substitute for syndromal classification? *Behavioral Assessment, 14,* 345–365.

Hayes, S.C., Wilson, K.G., Gifford, E.V., Follette, V.M., & Strosahl, K. (1996). Experiential avoidance and behavioral disorders: A functional dimensional approach to diagnosis and treatment. *Journal of Consulting and Clinical Psychology, 64,* 1152–1168.

Haynes, S., & Jensen, B.J. (1979). The interview as a behavioral assessment instrument. *Behavioral Assessment, 1,* 97–106.

Hendrick, S.C. (1995). Assessment of functional status: Activities of daily living. In L.Z. Rubenstein, D. Wieland, & R. Bernabei (Eds.), *Geriatric assessment technology: The state of the art.* Milan, Italy: Editrice Kurtis.

Herzog, A.R., & Rodgers, W.L. (1988). Age and response rates to interview sample surveys. *Journal of Gerontology: Social Sciences, 43,* S200–S205.

Kalish, K. (1997). *The relation between negative social interactions and health in older adults: A critical review of selected literature.* Unpublished manuscript, West Virginia University at Morgantown.

Kane, R.A., & Kane, R.L. (1981). *Assessing the elderly.* Lexington, MA: Lexington Books.

Kapust, L.R., & Weintraub, S. (1988). The home visit: Field assessment of mental status impairment in the elderly. *The Gerontologist, 28,* 112–115.

Kaszniak, A.W., & Christensen, G.D. (1994). Differential diagnosis of dementia and depression. In M. Storandt & G.R. VandenBos (Eds.), *Neuropsychological assessment of dementia and depression in older adults: A clinician's guide.* Washington, DC: American Psychological Association.

Katz, S., Downs, T.D., Cash, H.R., & Gratz, R.C. (1970). Progress in development of the index of ADL. *The Gerontologist, 10,* 20–30.

Kelly-Hayes, M., Jette, A.M., Wolf, P.A., D'Adostino, R.B., & Odell, P.M. (1992). Functional limitations and disability among elders in the Framingham study. *American Journal of Public Health, 82,* 841–845.

Kiernan, R.J., Mueller, J., Langston, J.W., & Van Dyke, C. (1987). The Neurobehavioral Cognitive Status Examination: A brief but quantitative approach to cognitive assessment. *Annals of Internal Medicine, 107,* 481–485.

Kiyak, H.A., Teri, L., & Borsom, S. (1994). Physical and functional health assessment in normal aging and Alzheimer's disease: Self-reports vs. family reports. *The Gerontologist, 34,* 324–330.

Kogan, N. (1961). Attitudes towards old people in an older sample. *Journal of Abnormal and Social Psychology, 62,* 616–622.

Lang, F., & Carstensen, L. (1998). Social relationships and adaptation in late life. In B. Edelstein (Ed.), *Comprehensive clinical psychology, Volume 7: Clinical geropsychology* (pp. 55–72). Oxford, England: Elsevier.

LaRue, A. (1992). *Aging and neuropsychological assessment.* New York: Plenum Press.

Lesher, E.L. (1986). Validation of the Geriatric Depression Scale among nursing home residents. *Clinical Gerontologist, 4,* 21–28.

Light, L.L. (1992). The organization of memory in old age (pp. 111–165). In F.I.M. Craik & T.A. Salthouse (Eds.), *Emergent theories of aging.* New York: Springer.

MacNeil, S., & Lichtenberg, P.A. (1999). Screening instruments and brief batteries for assessment of dementia. In P.A. Lichtenberg (Ed.), *Handbook of assessment in clinical gerontology* (pp. 417–441). New York: Wiley.

Martin, G., & Pear, J. (1996). *Behavior modification: What it is and how to do it* (5th ed.). Upper Saddle River, NJ: Prentice Hall.

McAuley, W.J., Arling, G., Nutty, C.L., & Bowling, C.A. (1980). *Final report of the statewide survey of older Virginians.* Richmond: Virginia Center on Aging.

McFall, R.M., & Townsend, J.T. (1998). Foundations of psychological assessment: Implications for cognitive assessment in clinical science. *Psychological Assessment, 10,* 316–330.

Mor-Barak, M.E., Miller, L.S., & Syme, L.S. (1991). Social networks, life events, and health of the poor, frail elderly: A longitudinal study of the buffering versus the direct effect. *Family and Community Health, 14,* 1–13.

Morris, J.N., Hawes, C., Fries, B.E., Phillips, C.D., Mor, V., Katz, S., Murphy, K., Drugovich, M.L., & Friedlot, A.S. (1990). Designing the national resident assessment instrument for nursing home facilities. *The Gerontologist, 30,* 293–307.

Morris, W.W., & Boutelle, S. (1985). Multidimensional functional assessment in two modes. *The Gerontologist, 25*(6), 638–643.

Morrison, J. (1997). *When psychological problems mask medical disorders: A guide for psychotherapists.* New York: Guilford Press.

Nease, D.E. Jr., Volk, R.J., & Cass, A.R. (1999). Investigation of a severity-based classification of mood and anxiety symptoms in primary care patients. *Journal of the American Board of Family Practice, 12,* 21–31.

Norris, J.T., Gallagher, D., Wilson, A., & Winograd, C.H. (1987). Assessment of depression in geriatric medical outpatients: The validity of two screening measures. *Journal of the American Geriatrics Society, 35,* 989–995.

Okun, M. (1976). Adult age and cautiousness in decision: A review of the literature. *Human Development, 19,* 220–233.

Okun, M., Melichar, J.F., & Hill, M.D. (1990). Negative daily events, positive and negative social ties, and psychological distress among older adults. *The Gerontologist, 224,* 193–199.

Olin, J.T., Schneider, L.S., Eaton, E.E., Zemansky, M.F., & Pollock, V.E. (1992). The Geriatric Depression Scale and the Beck Depression Inventory as screening instruments in an older adult outpatient population. *Psychological Assessment, 4,* 190–192.

Omnibus Budget Reconciliation Act of 1987, Pub. L. No. 100–203, Subtitle C: Nursing Home Reform (December 22, 1987).

Oxman, T.E., & Berkman, L.F. (1990). Assessments of social relationships in the elderly. *International Journal of Psychiatry in Medicine, 21,* 65–84.

Patterson, R.L., & Dupree, L.W. (1994). Older adults. In M. Hersen & S.M. Turner (Eds.), *Diagnostic interviewing* (2nd ed., pp. 373–397). New York: Plenum Press.

Perlmutter, M. (1978). What is memory aging the aging of? *Developmental Psychology, 14,* 330–345.

Prineas, R.J., Demirovic, J., Bean, J.A., Duara, R., Gomez Marin, O., Loewenstein, D., Sevush, S., Sitt, F., & Szapocznik, J. (1995). South Florida program on aging and health: Assessing the prevalence of Alzheimer's disease in three ethnic groups. *Journal of the Florida Medical Association, 82,* 805–810.

Qualls, S.H. (1999). Mental health and mental disorders in older adults. In J.C. Cavanaugh & S.K. Whitbourne (Eds.), *Gerontology: An interdisciplinary perspective* (pp. 305–328). New York: Oxford University Press.

Rabbitt, P. (1982). Development of methods to measure changes in activities of daily living in the elderly. In S. Corkin, K.L. Davis, J.H. Growdon, E. Usdin, & R.J. Wurtman (Eds.), *Alzheimer's disease: A report of progress.* New York: Raven Press.

Rapp, S.R., Parisi, S.A., Walsh, D.A., & Wallace, C.E. (1988). Detecting depression in elderly medical inpatients. *Journal of Consulting and Clinical Psychology, 56,* 509–513.

Rapp, S.R., Smith, S.S., & Britt, M. (1990). Identifying comorbid depression in elderly medical patients: Use of the extracted Hamilton Depression Rating Scale. *Psychological Assessment, 2,* 243–247.

Reiger, D.A., Boyd, J.H., Burke, J.K., Rae, D.S., Myers, J.K., Kramer, M., Robins, L.N., George, L.K., Karno, M., & Locke, B.Z. (1988). One-month prevalence of mental disorders in the U.S.: Based on five epidemiological catchment area sites. *Archives of General Psychiatry, 45,* 977–986.

Reiger, D.A., Farmer, M.E., Rae, D.S., Locke, B.Z., Keith, S.J., Judd, L.L., & Goodwin, F.K. (1990). Comorbidity of mental disorders with alcohol and other drug abuse. *Journal of the American Medical Association, 264,* 2511–2518.

Reite, M., Buysse, D., Reynolds, C., & Mendelson, W. (1995). The use of polysomnography in the evaluation of insomnia. *Sleep, 18,* 58–70.

Riley, K.P. (1999). Assessment of dementia in older adults. In P. Lichtenberg (Ed.), *Handbook of assessment in clinical gerontology* (pp. 134–166). New York: Wiley.

Rodgers, W.L., & Herzog, A.R. (1987). Interviewing older adults: The accuracy of factual information. *Journal of Gerontology, 42(4),* 387–394.

Rook, K.S. (1990). Stressful aspects of older adults' social relationships. In M.A.P. Stephens, J.H. Crowther, S.E. Hobfoll, & D.L. Tennenbaum (Eds.), *Stress and coping in later-life families* (pp. 173–192). New York: Hemisphere.

Rosin, A.J., & Glatt, M.M. (1971). Alcohol excess in the elderly. *Quarterly Journal of Studies in Alcoholism, 32,* 53–59.

Rosse, R., Giese, A.A., Deutsch, S.I., & Morihisa, J.M. (1989). *Concise guide to laboratory and diagnostic testing in psychiatry.* Washington, DC: American Psychiatric Press.

Royall, D.R., Mulroy, A.R., Chiodo, L.K., & Polk, M.J. (1999). Clock drawing is sensitive to executive control: A comparison of six methods. *Journal of Gerontology: Psychological Sciences, 54B,* P328–P333.

Rubenstein, L.Z., Schairer, C., Wieland, G.D., & Kane, R. (1984). Systematic biases in functional status assessment of elderly adults: Effects of different data sources. *Journal of Gerontology, 39*(6), 686–691.

Sager, M.A., Dunham, N.C., Schwantes, A., Mecum, L., Halverson, K., & Harlowe, D. (1992). Measurement of activities of daily living in hospitalized elderly: A comparison of self-report and performance-based methods. *Journal of the American Geriatrics Society, 40,* 457–462.

Schneider, J. (1996). Geriatric psychopharmacology. In L.L. Carstensen, B.A. Edelstein, & L. Dornbrand (Eds.), *The practical handbook of clinical gerontology* (pp. 481–542). Thousand Oaks, CA: Sage.

Schnelle, J.F., & Traughber, B. (1983). A behavioral assessment system applicable to geriatric nursing facility residents. *Behavioral Assessment, 5,* 231–243.

Schulman, K.l., Pushkar-Gold, D., Cohen, C.A., & Zucchero, C.A. (1993). Clock drawing and dementia in the community: A longitudinal study. *International Journal of Geriatric Psychiatry, 8,* 487–496.

Schwarz, N. (1999). Self-reports: How questions shape the answers. *American Psychologist, 54,* 93–105.

Schwarz, N., & Scheuring, B. (1988). Judgments of relationship satisfaction: Inter- and intraindividual comparison strategies as a function of questionnaire structure. *European Journal of Social Psychology, 18,* 485–496.

Scogin, F.R. (1994). Assessment of depression in older adults: A guide for practitioners. In M. Storandt & G.R. VandenBos (Eds.), *Neuropsychological assessment of dementia and depression* (pp. 61–80). Washington, DC: American Psychological Association.

Scogin, F.R., Hamblin, D., Beutler, L., & Corbishley, A. (1988). Reliability and validity of the short-form Beck Depression Inventory with older adults. *Journal of Clinical Psychology, 44,* 853–857.

Spirrison, C.L., & Pierce, P.S. (1992). Psychometric characteristics of the Adult Functional Adaptive Behavior Scale (AFABS). *The Gerontologist, 32,* 234–239.

Stanley, M.A., & Beck, J.G. (1998). Anxiety disorders. In B. Edelstein (Ed.), *Comprehensive clinical psychology, Volume 7: Clinical geropsychology* (pp. 171–192). Oxford, England: Elsevier.

Stephens, M.A.P., Kinney, J.M., Norris, V.K., Ritchie, S.W. (1987). Social networks as assets and liabilities in recovery from stroke by geriatric patients. *Psychology and Aging, 2,* 125–129.

Sunderland, A., Watts, K., Baddeley, A.D., & Harris, J.E. (1986). Subjective memory assessment and test performance in elderly adults. *Journal of Gerontology, 41*(3), 376–384.

Sunderland, T., Hill, J.L., Mellow, A.M., Lawlor, B.A., Gunderscheimere, J., Newhouse, P.A., & Grafman, J. (1989). Clock drawing in Alzheimer's disease: A novel measure of dementia severity. *Journal of the American Geriatrics Society, 37,* 725–729.

Thomas, P.D., Goodwin, J.M., & Goodwin, J.S. (1985). Effect of social support on stress-related changes in cholesterol level, uric acid, and immune function in an elderly sample. *American Journal of Psychiatry, 121,* 735–737.

Tversky, A., & Kahneman, D. (1981). The framing of decisions and the psychology of choice. *Science, 211,* 453–458.

U.S. Department of Veterans Affairs. (1997). *Dementia identification and assessment: Guidelines for primary care practitioner.* Washington, DC: Author.

Vasterling, J.J., Seltzer, B., Foss, J.W., & Vanderbrook, V. (1995). Unawareness of deficit in Alzheimer's disease: Domain-specific differences and disease correlates. *Neuropsychiatry, Neuropsychology, and Behavioral Neurology, 8,* 26–32.

Whitbourne, S.K. (1996). *The aging individual: Physical and psychological perspectives.* New York: Springer.

Whittle, H., & Goldenberg, D. (1996). Functional health status and instrumental activities of daily living: Performance in noninstitutionalized people. *Journal of Advanced Nursing, 23,* 220–227.

Willott, J.F. (1999). *Neurogerontology: Aging and the nervous system.* New York: Springer.

Wolfe, R., Morrow, J., & Fredrickson, B.L. (1996). Mood disorders in older adults. In L.L. Carstensen, B.A. Edelstein, & L. Dornbrand (Eds.), *The practical handbook of clinical gerontology* (pp. 274–303). Thousand Oaks, CA: Sage.

Yesavage, J.A., Brink, T.L., Rose, L.R., & Adey, M. (1983). The Geriatric Depression Rating Scale: Comparison with other self-report and psychiatric rating scales. In T. Crook, S. Ferris, & R. Bartus (Eds.), *Assessment in geriatric psychopharmacology* (pp. 153–167). New Canaan, CT: Mark Powley.

Yesavage, J.A., Brink, T.L., Rose, T.L., Lum, O., Huang, V., Adey, M., & Leirer V. (1983). Development and validation of a geriatric depression screening scale: A preliminary report. *Journal of Psychiatric Research, 17,* 37–49.

Zanetti, O., Geroldi, C., Frisoni, G.B., Bianchetti, A., & Trabucchi, M. (1999). Contrasting results between caregiver's report and direct assessment of activities of daily living in patients affected by mild and very mild dementia: The contribution of the caregiver's personal characteristics. *Journal of the American Geriatrics Society, 47,* 196–202.

Zeiss, A., & Steffen, A. (1996). Interdisciplinary health care teams: The basic unit of geriatric care. In L. Carstensen & B. Edelstein (Eds.), *The practical handbook of clinical gerontology* (pp. 423–450). Thousand Oaks, CA: Sage.

Zelinski, E.M., Gilewski, M.J., & Thompson, L.W. (1980). Do laboratory tests relate to self-assessment of memory ability in the young and old? In L.W. Poon, J.L. Fozard, L.S. Cermak, D. Arenberg, & L.W. Thompson (Eds.), *New directions in memory and aging: Proceedings of the George A. Talland memorial conference.* Hillsdale, NJ: Erlbaum.

CHAPTER 4

Personality Disorders

Daniel L. Segal, Frederick L. Coolidge, and
Erlene Rosowsky

In this chapter, we discuss personality disorders (PDs) in older adults. After presenting a case study, our focus shifts to the *Diagnostic and Statistical Manual of Mental Disorders* (*DSM-IV;* American Psychiatric Association [APA], 1994) category of personality disorders and a description of the disorders contained therein. Next, we provide epidemiological data, followed by a presentation of relevant theories and treatments for personality disorders among older persons. The chapter concludes with study questions and suggestions for additional readings.

CASE STUDY

Mr. E., a 76-year-old married man, was referred from a hospital-based headache clinic where he had been seen for diagnosis and treatment in excess of two years. It was determined that his headaches did not reflect an organic etiology. Mr. E. was diagnosed by both a psychiatrist and a clinical social worker as suffering from major depressive disorder (recurrent type, moderate severity) and generalized anxiety disorder. Treatment had been unsuccessful, other than to learn what did not work. The failed approaches included antidepressant medications (as no therapeutic dose could be tolerated) and psychodynamic psychotherapy provided at the headache clinic.

Mr. E.'s transfer to a new therapist was a potential setup for yet another treatment failure. An extended evaluation was done, including the gathering of collateral and informant data. The therapist needed to understand how this man made meaning of his world. How did he come to such a position of unhappiness and pain? The evaluation resulted in the same Axis I diagnoses noted earlier, as well as an Axis II diagnosis of personality disorder NOS (not otherwise specified). Specifically, Mr. E. met formal criteria for dependent and obsessive-compulsive PDs, and he also had significant avoidant PD features, all Cluster C PDs.

Cluster C embraces the anxious and fearful group, and Mr. E. demonstrated many of the dominant features of this Cluster. He consistently talked about how inadequate he felt and how concerned he was about making mistakes and being perceived by others in a multitude of situations as inept. He was hypersensitive to criticism and perceived rejection by others. He presented in a timid manner. He was fretful, wrung his hands, and kept his eyes cast downward. He had a difficult time making even the most simple decisions. He was indecisive about setting an appointment: he obsessed over possible contingencies that might interfere, and the like. He reported and demonstrated extensive worrying, much of it anticipatory. He sought excessive reassurance and comfort from others. He was unable to soothe himself or stop his incessant worrying.

CRITERIA AND DESCRIPTION OF *DSM-IV* PERSONALITY DISORDERS

DIAGNOSIS AND CATEGORIZATION

Most of us can describe ourselves according to our prominent personality *traits.* For example, some people are characteristically shy, quiet, and reserved; others are typically outgoing, boisterous, and loud. Other examples of personality traits include friendliness, caring, thoughtfulness, optimism, hostility, arrogance, ruthlessness, and impulsivity. Personality *disorders* are diagnosed when one's personality traits are rigid and maladaptive. According to the *DSM-IV*, a personality disorder is "an enduring pattern of inner experience and behavior that deviates markedly from the expectations of the individual's culture, is pervasive and inflexible, has an onset in adolescence or early adulthood, is stable over time, and leads to distress or impairment" (p. 629).

Historically, these conditions were called character disorders, suggesting that it is one's characteristic way of being that is dysfunctional. Millon (1981) cites the derivation of the word *character* as emanating from the Greek word for "engraving," and notes that it was originally used to "signify distinctive features that serve as the 'mark' of a person" (p. 7). Although anecdotal and literary descriptions of individuals who may have had PDs are thousands of years old, the official diagnosis of PDs as a unique and separate diagnostic entity did not appear until 1952 with the publication of the original *DSM* (APA, 1952). Notably, the diagnostic category of PDs has evolved and changed substantially over subsequent editions of the *DSM* (for full discussion, see Coolidge & Segal, 1998). The current manual, *DSM-IV*, officially categorizes 10 PDs. Younger and older adults alike can suffer from the full spectrum of these disorders, and they are often serious and debilitating.

Most clinicians probably agree that the PDs are interesting (and challenging) forms of psychiatric illness. This is partially because PDs are very different from the major clinical disorders (e.g., depression, schizophrenia) that are often perceived as true "sicknesses" that happen to people. In contrast, the PDs do not seem to be illnesses that come from "outside" the person, but rather, signify a pathological development of the self, of who one actually is at one's core. As such, a classic hallmark of the diagnosis has been that those who suffer from PDs typically lack insight or are unaware of having the disorder. In psychodynamic terms, the symptoms are often perceived as ego-syntonic (congruent with one's self-image) and not ego-dystonic. (Our case example demonstrated this quality of PDs.)

Comorbidity between major psychiatric disorders (coded on Axis I of *DSM-IV*) and PDs (coded on Axis II) among older and younger persons is common and provides considerable challenge to clinicians who treat elderly clients with multiple and complex disorders. It is also unusual in clinical practice or research to encounter an older person who presents with a single prototypical PD. Rather, older persons with one PD are also likely to present with significant signs and symptoms of a number of PDs. Occurrence of more than one PD appears to be the rule rather than the exception, and this is true across the life span. (This was also evident in our case example.)

The *DSM-IV* provides specific diagnostic criteria for each of the 10 PDs, with criteria reflecting mostly behavioral manifestations of the disorder. Diagnosis is based on a polythetic list of criteria (i.e., multiple criteria, none of which is the sine qua non). In addition, multiple symptoms are listed in order of diagnostic importance, and there is a required number of symptoms necessary to meet the threshold for diagnosis. Little reference to age is made in the features of PDs, with the exception that a PD requires onset no later than early adulthood. *DSM-IV* does, however, acknowledge that a person with a PD may not receive mental health services until old age.

In the *DSM-IV*, PDs are grouped into three clusters based on descriptive similarities. Cluster A groups the disorders in which individuals often appear odd or eccentric: paranoid, schizoid, and schizotypal PDs. Cluster B includes disorders in which individuals appear to be dramatic, emotional, or erratic: antisocial, borderline, histrionic, and narcissistic PDs. Cluster C denotes the disorders in which individuals often appear fearful or anxious: avoidant, dependent, and obsessive-compulsive PDs.

Although we will not replicate the explicit criteria presented in *DSM-IV* here, it will be helpful to describe the essential characteristics and present a clinical picture for each of the 10 PDs included in the *DSM-IV*, with one additional but often neglected feature: the clinical presentation seen in the older adult, which may differ markedly from that seen in younger persons.

DSM-IV PERSONALITY DISORDERS

Paranoid Personality Disorder

This disorder manifests itself as a pervasive pattern of distrust, suspicion, and vigilance without justification. Persons with the disorder tend not to confide in others or share personal information, and they maintain the suspicion that others may be out to do them harm. The pervasiveness of suspicion is such that even events that have nothing to do with them will be interpreted as personal attacks. In older adults, declines in hearing, vision, or cognitive abilities may incorrectly lead to thoughts that others are talking about them or threatening them in some way. Older people with paranoid PD are often experienced as distrustful, argumentative, and hostile. They may be highly isolated and reject needed social support.

Schizoid Personality Disorder

Hallmark features of this disorder are a complete detachment from social relationships and a restricted range of emotional expression. Such people are often perceived as aloof and cold, but most notably, they seem to have no desire for interpersonal relationships, to the point where they seem immune to criticism or praise. The schizoid's lack of relationships is a lifelong characteristic and is not simply a function of age-related losses. The older schizoid's arelational style is ego-syntonic and, therefore, may cause distress when the person must by necessity depend on relationships with others for their care.

Schizotypal Personality Disorder

Individuals with this disorder are often described as odd, bizarre, or eccentric. Such persons experience extreme discomfort with interpersonal relationships and tend to be socially withdrawn. Ideas of reference and magical thinking in the form of odd beliefs or possession of special powers (e.g., clairvoyance, telepathic thinking) are reported. Perceptual distortions exist but are not as extreme as those experienced by people with schizophrenia. In the absence of an organic condition such as dementia, an older adult who is unkempt, malodorous, suspicious, paranoid, bizarre, and has few friends might suffer from this PD.

Antisocial Personality Disorder

The hallmark feature of this disorder is a pattern of disregard for and failure to comply with societal norms. Rights of others are never a consideration, and when these rights are violated, persons with this disorder experience no remorse. Such people are often perceived as aggressive and ruthless; they take what they want, when they want it, with no regard for the impact their action will have on others. They lack empathy. Lying, cheating, and stealing appear to be part of their nature. Some persons with severe antisocial PD likely do not survive into old age due to a lifestyle of risky behaviors. Moreover, many behavioral descriptors of the disorder, such as aggressiveness, impulsiveness, lawlessness, and physical fighting clearly require physical strength and agility (Kroessler, 1990), and these behaviors may diminish as the person's stamina declines naturally with age. For many persons, however, even externally imposed limitations (e.g., jail) and age-related physical declines do not assure that the PD will remit because the underlying psychological processes remain constant.

Borderline Personality Disorder

This often severe disorder is highlighted by extreme instability of interpersonal relationships, self-image, and emotions. Marked impulsivity is also present, which usually results in the person's engaging in high-risk and dangerous behaviors, such as substance abuse, sexual promiscuity, self-mutilation, and/or suicide attempts (Widiger & Trull, 1993). People with this disorder often feel chronically bored or empty, and are perceived by others as manipulative, mercurial, and demanding. Due to emotional dysregulation, their moods shift rapidly.

They appraise the world and people in black-and-white terms (e.g., all good or all bad), and they can shift their perspective with alarming alacrity. There is considerable debate whether or not borderline PD declines with age. Although controlled studies suggest lower levels of borderline PD in older versus younger persons (Coolidge, Burns, Nathan, & Mull, 1992), other authorities suggest that the *DSM* criteria is inadequate in detecting signs of the disorder in older persons (Rosowsky & Gurian, 1991, 1992). It is possible that the lower prevalence rates of the disorder in older adults "reflects more the lack of fit of our existing diagnostic yardsticks than the lack of borderline personality disorder in old age" (Rosowsky & Gurian, 1991, p. 39). Excessive early mortality due to risky behaviors and suicide might also reduce rates of the disorder among older persons.

Histrionic Personality Disorder

People diagnosed with this disorder tend to engage in excessive emotional displays, with the primary goal of securing attention from others. They often become angry or upset when they are not the center of attention. They typically present themselves in an overstated, dramatic, and seductive manner, although their relationships are often superficial and one-sided. Older adults with this disorder are often described by their adult children as "acting like spoiled little children." They are intolerant of the physical changes that come with age (e.g., wrinkles, sagging body parts) because their self-worth is based largely on superficial characteristics such as physical appearance. They may be excessive users of plastic surgery and other anti-aging techniques. Many have poor adjustment to aging when their flirtatious and seductive style becomes less rewarded.

Narcissistic Personality Disorder

The main features of this disorder are an exaggerated sense of self-importance (grandiosity) and an illusion of specialness, leading to entitlement. Such persons also tend to be preoccupied with themselves, have a strong need to be admired by others, lack sensitivity and compassion for others, and express discomfort in situations in which they are not surrounded by people they perceive as being as special and privileged as they. People with this disorder tend to take advantage of others because they see their own needs as primary. Older adults with the disorder are experienced by others as demanding, insensitive, and self-centered. Alienation of family members is common due to a lifetime of perceived callous disregard for and purposeful manipulation of others in their family. With advancing age, persons with this disorder may suffer a "narcissistic injury" when they lose power and prestige (perhaps due to retirement and/or physical declines) and become aware of messages from society that devalue older persons.

Avoidant Personality Disorder

This disorder manifests itself as a pervasive pattern of social inhibition and low self-esteem, coupled with a longing for relationships. People with the disorder have an extreme sensitivity to the judgment of others and consequently avoid placing themselves in social situations wherein they might be rejected. In essence, they reject others to avoid being rejected themselves. Such people have strong feelings of inadequacy and believe that they cannot cope with the anxiety and fearfulness associated with social relationships. Older persons with this disorder might not apply for and receive needed social and supportive services due to their serious fears of being evaluated and found wanting. They may not try to meet new people or engage in new activities unless they are "guaranteed" to be successful. Such individuals are typically lonely, anxious, and frightened.

Dependent Personality Disorder

Individuals with this disorder are submissive and clinging and desperately seek being taken care of by others. They are reluctant to make even minor decisions, relinquishing this responsibility to others. As a result, people with the disorder are left with an overwhelming fear of being abandoned. Although often characterized as passive and indecisive, people with the disorder are not without their own opinions or beliefs, but will retreat if challenged to prevent abandonment. Problems often arise for the dependent older person when the spouse dies, leaving the person in the threatening position of having to depend on himself or herself. After such a loss, dependent older adults appear helpless, unable to perform the most mundane functions after decades of relying excessively on their partner. Feeling lost and vulnerable, these older adults often turn to their adult children to fill the void left by the deceased spouse on whom they depended. Older persons with the disorder may actively seek out and overly rely on supportive individuals and services, and they easily become burdensome.

Obsessive-Compulsive Personality Disorder

People with this disorder are so preoccupied with details that it interferes with the completion of important tasks. They are controlled and controlling, and manifest a pervasively rigid and moralistic style that often challenges close interpersonal relationships. Often described by others as "workaholics," those with this disorder forgo leisure activities for the sake of productivity. Ironically, their productivity suffers because the point of many an activity is lost among the rules, regulations, lists, and schedules to which they scrupulously and conscientiously adhere. Delegation of responsibility or work to others is unheard of, usually for fear that the task will not be completed in the "right way." This disorder is believed to increase with age, perhaps as the need for control and rigid organization becomes paramount in the face of losses of real control due to physical and social declines in some older persons.

EPIDEMIOLOGICAL DATA

There is a small but growing body of literature regarding epidemiology of PDs among older persons. Notably, there are fewer studies with older persons than with younger persons. Reported rates for these conditions are far more inconsistent and controversial than estimates for more widely studied disorders among older persons, such as schizophrenia, dementia, and major depression.

Such inconsistencies may highlight the difficulty clinicians and researchers have in accurately diagnosing PDs in the elderly. Prevalence estimates for PDs are also known to vary widely due to such factors as varying methodologies, sampling techniques, diagnostic measures, and diagnostic criteria.

Surveys conducted in the 1980s show prevalence rates for PDs in the older adult community to range from as low as 2.8% to as high as 11% (Cohen, 1990). Agronin (1994) presented a review of some early epidemiological studies in various European communities and found prevalence rates of 1.8% to 6%. However, he noted that many of the diagnoses would not conform to modern *DSM-IV* PD criteria. Weissman (1993) presented somewhat higher estimates of the total lifetime prevalence rates for PDs in the general population, ranging from 10% to 13%.

Ames and Molinari (1994) administered a structured interview (based on *DSM-III-R* criteria) to 200 community-living elderly (mean age 72 years) and found a 13% prevalence rate. Ames and Molinari also noted that, due to the nature of their sample (a senior center), dependent PD may have been overreported, whereas schizoid and avoidant PDs may have been underreported. When they compared these rates to a sample of 797 younger adults given the same structured interview, they found a prevalence rate of 17.9%. Cohen et al. (1994) used a semistructured psychiatric examination to study PDs in a community-dwelling sample of 810 people. They found that older adults (age 55 years and older) had a 10.5% PD prevalence rate, and younger people had a 6.6% rate. They also found antisocial and histrionic PDs were much less prevalent in the older than in the younger subjects. Segal et al. (1998) administered the self-report Personality Diagnostic Questionnaire–Revised (using *DSM-III-R* criteria) to 189 community-dwelling elderly (mean age 76 years) and found that 63% of the respondents received at least one PD diagnosis. Segal et al. proposed that their high prevalence rate may have been a function of the self-report measure and the fact that the sample participants were members of senior centers who may have been more likely to seek out this kind of social service because of existing personality and interpersonal dysfunction. Abrams and Horowitz (1996) have also noted that the elderly often self-report more Axis II symptoms when compared to clinicians' observations.

Prevalence figures have also been adduced in mental health settings. For example, in a retrospective chart review of a mixed sample of inpatient and outpatient older persons, Mezzich, Fabrega, Coffman, and Glavin (1987) found that 5.1% had a PD diagnosis. Casey and Schrodt (1989) reviewed charts of 100 consecutive admissions to a geriatric psychiatry unit and found that 7% received a diagnosis of PD as determined by psychiatrist rating. In a larger retrospective study, Fogel and Westlake (1990) ascertained prevalence of PDs in 2,332 older inpatients suffering from major depression. Again, diagnoses were assigned by attending psychiatrists, with results showing a 15.8% PD rate.

In other clinical studies, Kunik et al. (1993) evaluated depressed elderly inpatients and found that 37 of 154 (24%) met criteria for a PD based on consensus diagnosis among psychiatrists. Similarly, Thompson, Gallagher, and Czirr (1988) reported that 33% of depressed elderly clients participating in a psychotherapy outcome study were diagnosed with a PD. Molinari and Marmion (1995) used a structured PD scale to assess PDs in elderly patients with mood disorders, reporting a 63% prevalence rate. Similarly high prevalence rates were also found among older (58%) and younger (66%) adults suffering with a chronic mental illness (Coolidge, Segal, Pointer, et al., in press). In the only study we are aware of regarding PDs among clinically anxious older persons, Coolidge, Segal, Hook, and Stewart (in press) found that 61% met criteria for at least one PD.

Another epidemiological issue concerns differential rates for PDs among older males and females. According to the *DSM-IV*, borderline, dependent, and histrionic PDs are diagnosed more frequently in females, and antisocial and obsessive-compulsive PDs and, to a lesser extent, paranoid PD, are diagnosed more in males. However, it is unclear to what extent these differences apply to older individuals because most studies did not include older adults. At least one recent study of community-dwelling older persons (Segal et al., 1998) failed to find support for the claims in *DSM-IV* regarding gender differences for these specific PDs. Instead, results suggested that older females were more likely to be diagnosed with avoidant and schizoid PDs compared to older males (no differences for the remaining PD diagnoses).

Definitive data are also lacking about the stability or change in PD symptoms across the life span. In fact, there is some controversy in the geropsychological literature regarding whether or not PDs decline or "mellow" with advancing age (Coolidge et al., 1992; Molinari, Kunik, Snow-Turek, Deleon, & Williams, 1999; Segal & Coolidge, 1998; Segal, Hersen, Van Hasselt, Silberman, & Roth, 1996). The *DSM-IV* was the first version of the manual to include a specific section (along with cultural and gender topics) on the developmental issue of aging in the diagnosis of PDs. As noted earlier, *DSM-IV* describes a PD as a lifelong, stable pattern of thinking, feeling, and behaving. However, *DSM-IV* also suggests that some PDs (e.g., antisocial and borderline) tend to remit with age, whereas remission may be less likely for other PDs (e.g., obsessive-compulsive and schizotypal). In contrast, several researchers have suggested that some PDs (most notably borderline) may actually worsen with advanced age (Rose, Soares, & Joseph, 1993; Rosowsky & Gurian, 1991, 1992; Siegel & Small, 1986).

Tyrer (1988) suggested that "mature" forms of PD such as obsessive-compulsive, paranoid, schizoid, and schizotypal remain stable with age, whereas more "immature" or flamboyant disorders such as antisocial, borderline, histrionic, and narcissistic are likely to decrease with age. This observation certainly has some anecdotal support. For some elderly clients, their current personality and social functioning appears markedly improved compared to the interpersonal and occupational disasters characteristic of their earlier years. Conversely, some older adults show exacerbation of their personality styles.

In one of the few cross-sectional studies to date, Coolidge et al. (1992) directly compared PD rates in community-dwelling older adults ($n = 36$, M age = 69.4 years) and younger adults ($n = 573$, M age = 24 years). Results showed that the older adults were more schizoid and obsessive-compulsive than the younger adults, there were no age differences on the dependent and avoidant scales, and younger adults were higher on the remaining PD scales. Notably, these results of age-related elevations on obsessive-compulsive and schizoid PD scales were recently replicated with larger samples (Segal, Hook, & Coolidge, in press). In a recent and large cross-sectional study, Molinari et al. (1999) reported higher rates of compulsive and dependent PDs (as assessed by the Millon Clinical Multiaxial Inventory I, MCMI-I) in older versus younger inpatients.

A recent meta-analysis (Abrams & Horowitz, 1996) also evaluated this issue from a different statistical perspective. In the meta-analysis of 11 studies of prevalence in older adults (age 50 and above) from 1980 through 1994, a prevalence rate of 10% ranging from 6% to 33% was reported. Interestingly, in three of these studies that included under-50 age groups, the younger groups' overall prevalence was 21% with a range from 17% to 30%. However, in all three studies, there was no significant difference in the rate of PDs between younger and older adults. Abrams and Horowitz also found no gender differences in their older group and, contrary to their expectations, greater prevalence rates were found in outpatient or community settings than in inpatient settings. They also found consensus methods and chart reviews to yield higher rates of PDs compared to structured interviews. Despite the comprehensiveness and thoroughness of their meta-analytic approach, Abrams and Horowitz concluded that "the literature at this time appears to be inconclusive on the question of an age effect in personality disorder diagnosis" (p. 278).

If age changes are confirmed with further research, an intriguing question is: Why do some PDs decline with age and others intensify? Is it simply an artifact of activity level or sociability, or does it represent inadequate measurement of some PDs in the aged? Another possibility hints at a more complicated phenomenon: that is, to what extent do the abnormal behavioral changes associated with aging reflect underlying changes in neural substrate or chemical neurotransmitter functioning in the brain? It is apparent that systematic research is necessary to clarify clinical manifestations and develop clearer profiles of each PD in the aged. Longitudinal studies following personality-disordered individuals into later life are needed to assess changes over time in symptom patterns and personality characteristics of older individuals. Likely, some symptoms are robust, some appear in muted form in the aged, and some become irrelevant. As such, elder-specific diagnostic criteria may need to be developed. When evaluating and diagnosing PDs in the elderly, clinicians are encouraged to recognize and be sensitive to potential age biases in the *DSM-IV* system.

Establishing prevalence rates in older adults is not a simple task. It seems that the prevalence rates vary as a function of the mean age and age range of the sample, where the sample was gathered (e.g., community, inpatient psychiatric, outpatient psychiatric), the criteria used (e.g., *DSM, ICD-10*), the measurement device (e.g., self-report, structured interview, psychiatric examination), and statistical methodology (e.g., meta-analytic techniques). The National Institute of Mental Health Epidemiological Catchment Area (ECA) programs were successful at providing quality epidemiological data for many common mental disorders, but the PDs (with the exception of antisocial PD) were neglected in those surveys. Although these cross-sectional studies are intriguing, definitive research on the long-term course of individual PDs is lacking. Large-scale longitudinal studies that employ standardized, objective, and validated diagnostic instruments are warranted to investigate fully the prevalence of PD in the aged and to address in a rigorous manner the questions about age-related changes. Such studies will provide the clearest evidence about this issue, but unfortunately, are obviously time-consuming and expensive. However, information is sorely needed about this important clinical issue if we are to better understand and serve older adults.

THEORETICAL CONSIDERATIONS

It should be noted at the outset that there are no specific paradigmatic theories regarding the development of PDs in later life. It is likely that most cases of PDs in later life reflect the continuation of the same PD from earlier adulthood into old age. Other cases may appear to be new in later life, and these can perhaps be conceptualized as representing a deterioration of more adaptive personality traits in vulnerable older adults, likely due to an accumulation of stressors in old age. Several major theories of PDs are discussed next, followed by an analysis regarding how relevant they are to aging issues.

A THEORY OF TEMPERAMENTS, PERSONALITY, AND PERSONALITY DISORDERS

Rutter (1987) noted that temperaments are hypothesized to be biologically inherited predispositions for behaving in particular ways, and they emerge early in life. He specifically hypothesized, however, that temperaments were limited. According to Rutter, there are not a particularly large number of temperaments influencing behavior, and they are nonmotivational and noncognitive. The search for the core number of temperaments may parallel the search for the core number of personality traits or factors, with the number varying from as few as 3 to as many as 16. There is a fairly substantial body of empirical research in the developmental psychology literature in support of heritability of temperaments and their enduring influence on behavior (e.g., McGue, Bacon, & Lykken, 1993). Relatively undisputed is the hypothesis that the extraversion-introversion dimensional trait reflects a prominent temperament. Emotionality and activity levels have also received strong support as temperaments.

According to Rutter's theory, this limited number of temperaments helps to form what comes to be recognized as the person's unique personality, although personality is much broader than a simple collection of temperamental traits. Rutter further proposes that, as one interacts with one's family and society, these temperamental features may become reinforced by the social environment one experiences, thus producing the long-standing, enduring patterns of behavior that are characteristic of adult personalities. However, when particular temperamental features appear in the extreme or provoke unusual responses from the individual's environment, PDs may result. A PD's temperamental basis, along with its reinforcement history, therefore accounts for the enduring and inflexible nature of PDs.

Rutter's theory is confined to speculations about early childhood through adulthood, and there is little mention of issues related to later adulthood and the aged. His theory can be used, however, to generate a few hypotheses. Rutter argued that several longitudinal studies have shown "heterotypic" continuity, meaning that the phenotypic quality of the behavior changes over time, whereas individual differences remain stable. Thus, early childhood passivity is predictive of noncompetitiveness in later adult life (Kagan & Moss, 1962). With respect to PDs, therefore, it is possible that the elderly should perhaps be evaluated according to different criteria, or, at the least, the PD criteria should be examined for changes as a function of middle and later adulthood.

A Cognitive Theory of Personality Disorders

Pretzer and Beck (1996) have noted difficulties in the psychotherapeutic treatment of patients with PDs, and they argue that even cognitive-behavioral treatments may prove counterproductive or ineffective if the therapist fails to recognize the specific nature of the PD and fails to modify treatment accordingly. In terms of the etiology of PDs from a cognitive perspective, it is assumed that PDs develop phenomenologically, that is, through the person's view of his or her world. Thus, an individual's perception of stimuli interacts with his or her prior beliefs and assumptions. An individual may react consciously and logically, resulting in the observed emotional and behavioral responses to the perceived stimuli. However, prior misbeliefs and false assumptions about the world may lead to inappropriate or maladaptive emotional responses and behavior. An individual may also commit "systematic errors in reasoning," which Pretzer and Beck label "cognitive distortions," that result in inappropriate and maladaptive responses. They noted the prominence of at least 12 common cognitive distortions, such as viewing events in terms of mutually exclusive categories (dichotomous thinking) and focusing on one aspect of a complex situation to the exclusion of others (selective abstraction).

According to the theory, individuals are also likely to respond unconsciously or automatically to perceived stimuli. These ways of acting may once have been adaptive in an evolutionary sense. Beck (1992) has termed them "primeval strategies," and further, Pretzer and Beck (1996) propose that "human social change has outstripped physiological evolution [such that] we may well have also retained some biases in information processing that now tend to be maladaptive" (pp. 44–45). Thus, they argue, our inherited predispositions poorly fit some of the demands of modern society. For example, an earlier adaptive primeval strategy of predatory behavior may lead to the development of the antisocial PD, the earlier help-eliciting behavior may now result in the dependent PD, and earlier competitive behavior may now result in the narcissistic PD.

Nevertheless, Pretzer and Beck (1996) have argued that PD phenomena can be understood and treated without regard to inherited or inborn defects, and that inherited predispositions toward the development of PDs has not been clearly established. Moreover, their contribution does not appear to be simple and straightforward. Overall, cognitive theory tends to emphasize that interactions among predispositions, the environment, and significant life events shape development rather than predispositions alone, and it is not external events that shape the personality but an individual's perception of those events that forms his or her thinking and consequent behavior.

Although Pretzer and Beck's cognitive theory has a developmental perspective, it emphasizes early childhood influences on the adult personality. Even though they hypothesize that traumatic experiences, either singular or recurrent, may alter one's personality over time, they do not address the influence of traumatic experiences on the later adult personality. In fact, it could be easily hypothesized that 80 years of traumatic experiences should far outweigh a singular early traumatic experience. However, dramatic adult personality change is highly unlikely except for clear physiological reasons (e.g., brain disease, toxins). Thus, this aspect of their theory neglects personality issues of middle and late adulthood.

AN EVOLUTIONARY THEORY OF PERSONALITY DISORDERS

Millon and Davis (1996) have proposed a highly complex and sophisticated evolutionary theory of PDs that attempts to link both normal and abnormal behavior to both phylogenetic and ontogenetic processes. Their theory explains why early experiences play a more profound role in the development of the personality than do later experiences, drawing on diverse sources of evidence such as Freud's writings about the influence of early childhood on the later adult personality and ethologists' observations of critical imprinting periods in maturational development.

Central to Millon and Davis's (1996) evolutionary theory is the hypothesis that four evolutionarily based "bipolarities" interact with four stages of early neuropsychological development to produce stable and consistent patterns of behavior that can either be adaptive or maladaptive. These bipolarities are pain-pleasure, active-passive, self-other, and thinking-feeling. The four bipolarities also reflect the parallel evolutionary processes of existence, adaptation, replication, and abstraction, respectively. The four parallel neuropsychological stages are sensory-attachment, sensorimotor-autonomy, pubertal-gender identity, and intracortical-initiative, respectively. Although their theory is comprehensive and far-reaching, they do not address specifically the issue of PD in the elderly. In addition, despite the magnitude of their theory, it offers little heuristically for the differential waxing and waning of PDs in this population.

A BIOSOCIAL THEORY OF PERSONALITY DISORDERS

Cloninger (1987) has proposed a biosocial theory that asserts that phenotypic personality traits are the product of the interaction of genetically determined brain systems and environmental influences. He offers an operationalization of his theory in the Temperament and Character Inventory (TCI; Cloninger, Przybeck, Svrakic, & Wetzel, 1994). The TCI consists of seven major dimensions. There are four purportedly genetically independent trait dimensions: novelty seeking, harm avoidance, reward dependence, and persistence. The first three dimensions form the physiological component of the biosocial theory and are identified with three primary monoamine neurotransmitters: dopamine, serotonin, and norepinephrine. The first three traits are linked with these three neurotransmitters, respectively. Cloninger hypothesized that the three form neural temperaments that serve as discrete systems for the activation, inhibition, and maintenance of behavior in response to novelty, danger, and reward. The fourth character dimension, persistence, was not thought to be associated with a specific neurotransmitter. The decision to classify it as an autonomous factor in the model was based on empirical statistical factor analyses.

The TCI also assesses three character dimensions: self-directedness, cooperativeness, and self-transcendence. These dimensions became later additions to the TCI to account for behavior not otherwise described by the initial three physiological dimensions and to determine whether a PD was present or not. The four temperament dimensions were designed to delineate clinical subtypes of personality, but it appeared that they did not discriminate those individuals with PDs from those without PDs.

To account for PDs, Cloninger proposed that particular combinations of trait dimensions were predictive of various PDs. For example, he thought that the combination of high novelty seeking (high dopamine), low harm avoidance (low serotonin), and high reward dependence (high norepinephrine) was indicative of the histrionic PD, whereas the antisocial PD would be high on novelty seeking and low on both harm avoidance and reward dependence. Presumably, all of the PDs would be low on the three character dimensions of self-directedness, cooperativeness, and self-transcendence. Notably, a few studies have recently shown at least modest support for Cloninger's biosocial theory (e.g., Griego, Stewart, & Coolidge, 1999; Pfohl, Black, Noyes, Kelly, & Blum, 1990).

To date, Cloninger's biosocial theory makes no predictions about PDs as a function of the aging process. However, his theory is certainly fruitful for speculation. For example, there is substantial evidence (e.g., Morgan, May, & Finch, 1987) that there are normal age-related changes in the dopamine systems in humans and other mammals. There is an age-related, but not disease-related, loss in dopamine and its metabolites, a loss of dopaminergic neurons, and a decrease in particular types of dopamine receptors. Severe dopamine losses (greater than 75%) are characteristic of Parkinson's disease. Interestingly and anecdotally, these age-related losses of dopamine may, in part, account for the observation that some elderly persons do not typically engage in high novelty-seeking behaviors. It appears that there are little or no age-related changes in the serotonin systems in humans. Although there appears to be a modest reduction in particular serotonin receptor sites, serotonin levels appear to be stable across the life span. Major serotonin level declines and serotonin receptor site losses are, however, consistent with Alzheimer's disease. Evidence regarding age-associated decreases in norepinephrine is scant to date.

It appears that Cloninger's biosocial theory is provocative and capable of generating a plethora of hypotheses concerning both pathological (PDs and brain syndromes) and nonpathological behaviors in the elderly. However, neurotransmitter systems in the brain are extremely complex and interactive, and it is doubtful whether singular descriptions of human behavior (e.g., novelty seeking) are based on singular neurotransmitting systems. Furthermore, it is popularly suspected that many more neurotransmitters than have presently been discovered are yet to be discovered. In this latter light, Cloninger's theory, at least in regard to PDs, may be only speciously sophisticated.

RELEVANCE OF PERSONALITY DISORDER THEORIES TO OLDER ADULTS

Overall, many of the popular theories of PDs ignore issues related to aging and the elderly. Most of the theories, however, are useful in generating hypotheses about PDs in the elderly in terms of etiology, diagnosis, and treatment. For example, Rutter's (1987) hypothesis of heterotypic continuity in the life span is useful diagnostically, and it appears that comparisons of younger and older adults in terms of the *DSM* criteria for PDs may also be useful. Pretzer and Beck's (1996) cognitive theory is provocative in that it appears to minimize the influence of traumatic experiences in the elderly. It would be fruitful to examine how, why, and if traumatic experiences vary from childhood to later adulthood. Also, it might be useful to determine whether and to what extent traumatic experiences differentially affect older people; that is, what characteristics do individuals possess that make them vulnerable or invulnerable to traumatic experience? Are there ways of inoculating the vulnerable? Are the elderly, as a group, more or less vulnerable? Also, Pretzer and Beck's primeval strategies are fascinating as a basis for the development of differences among the various PDs.

Millon and Davis's (1996) evolutionary theory also does not address aging-related issues. However, the four bipolarities (pain-pleasure, active-passive, self-other, and thinking-feeling) should be examined with respect to aging. Are there differences between younger and older persons? Also, evolutionary theories, in general, tend to ignore the latter end of the life span. After adaptation and replication, are humans simply devoid of evolutionary purpose? Do dramatic behaviors such as memory loss in the elderly have evolutionary meaning? What evolutionary purpose does personality stability possess?

Cloninger's (1987) biosocial theory can also be used to generate hypotheses about personality stability and change and PDs in the elderly. To what extent do the chemical neurotransmitters in the brain affect behavior differentially in the elderly? How do declines in the neurotransmitter systems affect behavior in the elderly? Can classes of behaviors be directly linked to neurotransmitter systems in the elderly? If PDs are created by varying levels of neurotransmitters, can chemical interventions be developed to "cure" PDs?

This discussion of the etiology of PDs is far from an exhaustive review. However, a number of trends clearly emerge. The currently popular theories of PDs attempt to integrate the biological and evolutionary factors with environmental influences. Most of these theories virtually, if not totally, ignore issues related to aging. It appears, however, that one can generate a host of provocative hypotheses from the theories with regard to aging issues, and scientists should be encouraged to do so.

TREATMENT OF PERSONALITY DISORDERS IN OLDER ADULTS

GENERAL ISSUES AND STRATEGIES

PDs present great challenges to psychotherapy at any age, and perhaps especially in old age. The personality-disordered older adult is often ill-equipped to handle the challenges and changes associated with the normal aging process. A lifetime of social and occupational failures can also exacerbate the clinical picture and can increase the older person's sense of disappointment and hopelessness. As such, these individuals are often in need of psychotherapy and supportive services to reduce their frustrations and difficulties. As psychological researchers and clinicians, we are beginning to work toward a clearer understanding of the natural history of PDs as well as an understanding of how they respond to frequently occurring stressors of later life. Many models of psychotherapy have been applied to work with PDs, but there are scant empirical data to guide the choice among them. An appreciation of the "rules" of PDs, the utility of the countertransference, as well as what is known about treatment of PDs at younger ages and treatment of older adults with any psychological condition can be helpful in guiding the therapy.

The Route to Treatment

Older adults with PDs seldom seek mental health treatment. De facto, their personality, the self, feels syntonic (DeLeo, Scocco, & Meneghal, 1999). Interpersonal struggles can "feel like me," even as it is recognized that the pathology typically lies between the individual and another with whom the person is in an intimate relationship (Rosowsky, 1999). These patients come to treatment with problems resulting from an Axis II condition, because of a comorbid Axis I disorder, or both. Unfortunately, we know that therapy for any condition where a comorbid PD exists complicates the course and predicts a less positive outcome (Gradman, Thompson, & Gallagher-Thompson, 1999).

The following circumstances are often catalysts to problems requiring treatment:

1. When something occurs that compels the client to make an essential change, for example, when he or she is diagnosed with a health condition that requires a significant change in routine (dietary, medication, exercise) or lifestyle.
2. When what had been in place to limit the expression of pathology and the experience of distress is no longer available. This could develop through

the loss of significant others, or roles or tasks that had served to buffer the individual from stress, bolster his or her more adaptive strategies, or bind the more maladaptive ones.

3. When the exit is blocked for less pathological expression of intense affect. For example, when there is an organic brain disorder, especially involving the frontal lobe (resulting in disinhibition), or when there are real limitations to "escaping the field."

4. At the insistence of another on whom one perceives dependence, the so-called court order.

The "Rules" of Personality Disorders

1. The PD is ego-syntonic: It "feels like me."
2. The problem(s) is externalized: "I'm fine; the world is wrong."
3. The PD patient holds a closed versus open position to the possibility (and necessity) of change.
4. The PD patient embraces an "illusion of uniqueness" regarding his or her problem or circumstances, thereby denying the possibility of being understood and helped.

These rules typically conspire to discourage the formation of a therapeutic alliance. An alliance requires that therapist and patient be able to join together in an authentic relationship to be able to do the work of therapy (Greenson, 1965). The extent of impairment and distress reflects a quantification of the PD, called PDism. The greater the PDism, the more the therapy needs to be structured from the "outside in" rather than the "inside out." For severely compromised patients, the treatment is actually in the domain of environmental engineering, where change is affected through interventions at the level of the context, whether institutional or family.

Psychotherapy Requirements of the Older Adult

Older adults have expectations and requirements of any treatment, including psychotherapy. A major requirement is that treatment be clearly relevant. The older patient has come to address a specific problem or condition, and this needs to be addressed. The treatment must respect clients' resources of time, energy, and money. It must also appear "wise" and must be perceived as doable and moderately novel. If it is not novel enough, it is perceived as obvious, tried before, a preemptive failure. If it is appraised as too novel, it is experienced as threatening or "not for me." For PDs especially, any change prompted by treatment must feel reasonably effortless so it can come to "feel like me."

The Purpose and Focus of Therapy

The purpose of therapy is not the reconfiguration of one's character, but rather the reconfiguration of one's universe. This includes relief of symptoms, accommodation, adaptation, tolerance of interdependence, and the reinforcement of self (shoring up healthy narcissism). The focus of therapy, to meet the requirement of relevance and minimize the probability of resistance, can be guided by responses to three core questions:

1. Where is the distress coming from? As noted earlier, often with PDs, it is not "from within" but rather "from between" the individual and other(s) with whom the individual is in an intimate relationship. (This locus defines the "patient.")
2. Where in the "system" is it anticipated that the maximum change (movement toward the goal) can be achieved with the least resistance? (This identifies the point of entry.)
3. What does the patient need to have occur in treatment to appraise the therapy as successful? (This defines the assessment of outcome.)

The Stance versus Dance of the Therapist

In therapy with the older adult with a PD, the stance of the therapist needs to be active, protective, and flexible (DeLeo et al., 1999; Goldfarb, 1967). This is to counter the patient's stance of being stuck, vulnerable, and rigid. The frame of therapy needs to be consistent and reliable. The therapist needs to be experienced as able to "be there and stay with" the patient, neither threatening abandonment nor fusion, which defines the core conflict of the pathology (Westen, 1990). The therapist must avoid becoming inducted into the dance of the PD (DeLeo et al., 1999).

Special Utility of the Countertransference

Patients with PDs typically evoke strong feelings in their clinicians (Rosowsky, 1999). This response, the countertransference, of the "other" with whom the individual is in a close relationship (including the clinician) is pathognomonic of the pathology. The countertransference is not to be discounted or minimized, but rather to be used. It can offer a unique window into how the individual creates his or her universe, what the individual engenders in close relationship with others. If the treatment focus is in large part between the individual and his or her relationships, therapy offers an excellent living laboratory for diagnostic refinement as well as a medium for change. Although the diagnostic criteria for PD in old age remain less than precise, what appear as robust over the life course are the defensive structure and the problems these individuals historically have in close relationships (Rosowsky & Gurian, 1991).

TREATMENT OUTCOME: SUMMARY OF STUDIES

At all ages those with PDs being treated for Axis I disorders have a more complicated treatment course, a longer course, and poorer outcome than those with the same Axis I disorders without PDs. Overall, those with PDs develop the Axis I disorders earlier, have more symptoms, experience longer episodes, and relapse more frequently than those without PDs (Fava et al., 1996).

Pharmacological Treatment

There is no literature of which we are aware reporting data on the pharmacological treatment of PDs in older adults. Therefore, clinicians at this time are encouraged to use as guidelines what is extrapolated from what is known about psychopharmacological treatment of older adults in general and younger adults with PDs. Notably, there are psychobiologic models to serve as guidelines, and psychopharmacology can be invaluable for certain symptoms and maladaptive behaviors.

For example, in patients with Cluster A disorders, psychopharmacological agents can be useful for the transient psychotic and near-psychotic symptoms consistent with schizotypal PD. Neuroleptics (major tranquilizers) have been shown to be useful (DeLeo et al., 1999). For the more impulsive, acting-out behaviors consistent with Cluster B disorders, the serotonergic system has been implicated, and serotonergic enhancing agents have been shown to be helpful (Coccaro, 1993; DeLeo et al., 1999). The noradrenergic system has also been implicated in aggression and impulsivity (DeLeo et al., 1999).

Depressive symptoms are common among patients with PDs, especially for those in Clusters B and C. Pharmacological treatments are effective for depression in general, but appear to be less effective with the presence of PD. For anxiety, especially prevalent with Cluster C disorders, available data suggest that the selective serotonin reuptake inhibitors (SSRIs) may be the pharmacological treatment of choice for comorbid PD and anxiety (Sternbach, 1990).

It can be anticipated that, even following conservative psychopharmacology practice, the drug treatment of the PD older adult will be difficult. Compliance for older adults is often poor, as it is for PD patients; one can reasonably suspect a synergistic effect in a negative direction for this specific population (Agronin, 1999). Another complication is that older PD patients can act out by overtaking or undertaking their medications, prematurely aborting drug trials, or minimizing or exaggerating side effects. Such patients often have a poor relationship with their prescribing clinician (Agronin, 1999). This can be revealed through a number of manipulative and risky behaviors, including not disclosing multiple medications, taking but not reporting over-the-counter drugs, not revealing multiple prescribers, and being dishonest about alcohol practices. Especially with Cluster B disorders, there appear to be geriatric variants of risky and self-harming behaviors, acting out, in different ways, the same psychopathology as in younger life (Rosowsky & Gurian, 1991).

Psychotherapeutic Treatment

Psychotherapies, no matter what kind, are more difficult with patients with PDs: it is more difficult to structure a therapeutic alliance, these clients are less compliant, and they are more likely to terminate treatment prematurely (DeLeo et al., 1999; Krupnick et al., 1996). It is ironic that although this population has a high need for help, it has a low ability for engaging and accepting help.

Treatment outcome studies of patients of mixed ages with PDs and depression indicate poorer outcome with PD (Gradman et al., 1999). Cluster B clients may evidence selectively poor treatment outcome. Cluster C clients respond to treatment similarly to those without PD, but, as is true for all PDs, because they begin more symptomatic, even with an equal treatment response, they end being more symptomatic as well (Hardy et al., 1995). Within Cluster C, those with dependent and avoidant PDs may benefit more from treatment for depression than those with obsessive-compulsive and passive-aggressive PDs (Thompson et al., 1988).

There are scant outcome data reported for PDs and anxiety disorders. Reports on the efficacy of cognitive-behavioral therapy with diverse mixed-aged samples indicate that patients do benefit from therapy. However, as with depression, those with PD are more symptomatic, before and after treatment, than those without PD (Gradman et al., 1999; Mersch, Jansen, & Arntz, 1995).

No treatment outcome studies with older adults have been reported where PD has been the primary focus of treatment, except for single-case and anecdotal reports (Havens, 1999; Myers, 1999). For adults of mixed ages, most attention has been given to behavioral, cognitive-behavioral, and dialectical behavior therapy (Linehan, 1993).

THERAPY MODELS

Brief models appear to have some advantage in the treatment of older adults with PDs. This is because they offer what patients came to treatment for. Unlike the more analytically based long-term models, they do not directly tackle the underlying defensive structure, and they generally respect self resources. All treatment with the frail elderly is conducted against a backdrop of the inexorable running out of time. In addition, the medical model of doing a piece of work and being available for future work on an "as needed" basis (in other words, establishing the therapist as a member of the health care team) is an appropriate fit with the well-known "vicissitudes" of old age. Termination, which has unique meaning in old age, should, in its classical sense, be dispensed with in favor of the patient's taking comfort in knowing of the therapist's ongoing availability (DeLeo et al., 1999).

Psychodynamic Psychotherapy
This approach is generally not effective or appropriate as an exclusive model for older persons with PD because it has potential to violate several "rules." PD patients especially may not be able to tolerate the mainstay techniques of this model, such as confrontation and interpretation, and they are often maladept at self-reflection. These techniques are experienced as critical and threatening, can exacerbate anxiety or depression, can serve as catalysts for regression, and can lead to the premature abandonment of therapy. It is not wise at this life stage and with this population to dismantle defenses, especially at a time when there are many concurrent attacks on self-esteem and competing claimants for psychic energy, including the developmental tasks of review, reminiscence, and reconciliation (Solomon, Falette, & Stevens, 1982). This is

not because challenging and dismantling defenses cannot be accomplished, as intimated by Freud, but because it just may not be wise to do so.

Cognitive-Behavioral Therapy

This orientation appears to be a good choice in that it respects the rules of relevance and wisdom. It is also a good choice because it targets the symptoms (i.e., unhelpful thoughts and maladaptive behaviors) for treatment and does not target the psychic infrastructure (Goisman, 1999). This is especially relevant because, with PD, many of the symptoms *are* the infrastructure. It may not be a good choice, however, because it violates the rules of "no change" and energy conservation. Indeed, cognitive-behavioral therapy requires the patient to play an active role in the change process. Cognitive therapy also requires that the patient's cognitive abilities be adequately intact to support it. Further, it requires the patient's having the capacity for self-reflection and identification of self as the agent of change, and these abilities are weak with PDs and perhaps even more compromised in some older persons.

Interpersonal Therapy

This short-term model focuses on interpersonal relations and, as such, is intuitively a good fit with PDs. It helps the patient anticipate consequences of behaviors and interactions without threatening him or her with interpretations and probes for historical material. The focus is on present relationships and how to improve them. This approach uses structural, cognitive, and behavioral techniques to modify maladaptive relationship patterns while training and coaching more adaptive ones. It respects the rules of relevance, invisibility, and concreteness, and is typically perceived as doable and moderately novel.

Dialectical Behavior Therapy (DBT)

Although the efficacy of DBT with older adults awaits report, it has been shown to be effective for mixed ages in reducing hospitalizations and parasuicidal behaviors, particularly among patients with borderline PD. Notably, it has trained them to expand their response repertoire with more adaptive responses and likely will be shown to be a good fit with older adults with the more immature PDs as well. The model is based on an understanding of the pathology as an expression both of biologic dysregularities and social learning. The treatment can include medications where indicated, as well as direct modifications of the individual-environmental interactions (Linehan, 1993). The core of the DBT model includes individual therapy, skill training sessions, and telephone consultation, all with the goals of reducing maladaptive, especially self-harming, behaviors and improving adaptive coping behaviors (DeLeo et al., 1999).

Supportive Therapy and Environmental Engineering

This is the most appropriate approach with frail and cognitively compromised older adults with PD. This model meets the patient where the patient is; it does not challenge the patient by actively promoting personal change. Rather, the emphasis is to align with strengths that remain intact, are most available, and are relevant to the patient's reality. This is the "inside out" position, with the patient as subject and the context as object; the "outside in" position holds the context as subject and the patient as object. The therapy focuses on environmental changes that can be made to promote the patient's best adaptation while, reciprocally, inhibiting the more pathological responses.

RETURN TO THE CASE STUDY

Now, let's revisit our case study with the focus on treatment issues. Remember that Mr. E. was diagnosed with personality disorder NOS, he met full criteria for dependent and obsessive-compulsive PDs, and he also had significant avoidant PD features, all of which are classified as Cluster C PDs.

Questions to guide therapy with Cluster C patients include: What are the salient personality traits that need to be considered in the treatment plan? Which traits would you choose to strengthen/align with, and which would you select to diminish/not align with? How might you go about doing this? How would you expect the transference to manifest? What countertransference might you anticipate, and how might you use this? These questions helped direct the intervention with Mr. E.

The therapy plan for Mr. E. developed into six general segments:

1. The pharmacotherapy was split off from the psychotherapy. The purpose was to clear a space for therapeutic work that was not focused exclusively on somatic concerns, specifically the headache and medication side effects. He was referred to a geriatric psychopharmacologist, who introduced an anxiolytic along with an SSRI antidepressant, at the outset both at subtherapeutic doses. As the therapy progressed, the SSRI was increased gradually to a therapeutic dose, and ultimately the anxiolytic was discontinued.

2. The therapist "shaped" the content of the session, over time, away from the somatic focus. The therapist listened while the patient reported on his medications, but referred his questions and concerns to the psychopharmacologist. Mr. E. reported on his headaches using a 10-point SUDS (subjective units of distress scale) to quantify distress, but he was not encouraged to elaborate.

3. Dynamic and social material were reinforced through active listening and questions showing an interest in learning more. The therapist used few interpretations or probes to intentionally deepen the material out of concern that it would increase Mr. E.'s affect level beyond his ability to tolerate it. Sensitive issues became clearly marked at the patient's own pace. These included the great loss his retirement had meant (two years before the onset of the headaches) and the meaning of his not having had children (revisited now that he considered himself old). Also included was a review of his personality labels, the "feels like me" aspect of the PD that, because of the confluence of aging and age-related events, resulted

in a lessening of the ego-syntonic quality that subsequently led to his experience of subjective distress. Notably, Mr. E. had been labeled as a child as frail, weak, and vulnerable, someone needing the care and protection of others.

4. His obsessional tendencies were used as part of an overall plan to achieve better health and functioning. For example, Mr. E. was initially obsessionally stuck while considering a proposed walking regimen. He could not decide what footwear would be best, what route to take, and so on. He was assigned the task of doing a comparative analysis of footwear (suitable for serious walking for older men), and he extended his assignment to include an evaluation of elder-friendly sporting goods stores in the area. This use of his obsessional tendencies in the service of self-continuity and health promotion ultimately helped him secure a volunteer job, join a social group, and begin a gym program.

5. A large part of the therapy was psychoeducational. Topics discussed included the mind-body connection; biological, cognitive, and social learning contributions to depression; understanding personality and temperament (who he is, how he got to be that way, and how he might anticipate responding to age-related events); and understanding anxiety (reducing fear and worry by reframing his somatic preoccupation as "special sensitivity" to usual bodily sensations).

6. Adjunctive therapies were also tried, with variable success. Mr. E. did well with biofeedback, progressive relaxation, and visualization techniques. He was not able to tolerate hypnosis (due to the threat of perceived loss of control) or massage (due to the threat of too much body-related pleasure).

CONCLUSION

Older adults typically do not seek psychotherapy for PDs per se, yet these disorders greatly shape their quality of life, perhaps especially in older age. PDs are not readily diagnosed or considered in treatment plans for a number of reasons. Chief among these are the difficulty of making a clear clinical diagnosis and a paucity of reliable standardized test instruments specifically targeting and validated with older adults (Zweig & Hillman, 1999). In addition, there is often held an a priori opinion that PD, especially in old age, is immutable and therefore not an appropriate focus of clinical intervention. The available literature further supports the fact that when PD is comorbid with an Axis I condition, the treatment course is predictably more complicated and less effective. Patients with PDs have a high incidence of anxiety and depression; they have lifelong problems in dealing with others with whom they are, or need to be, in close relationship; they are limited and inflexible in their coping repertoire. Although this inflexibility is ego-syntonic ("feels like me") and may be a PD truism, another truism is that these individuals who come to clinical attention suffer enormous distress from the effect they have on others and their own inflexibility.

The purpose of therapy is clearly not to reconfigure the personality, but rather to relieve presenting symptoms and prevent additional ones. Effective therapy works both from the "outside in" and the "inside out." Psychotherapy needs to respect the rules of PD and also the requirements that older adults specifically have for treatment. The rules include ego-syntony, externalization, closed position, and illusion of uniqueness. The requirements of treatment include relevance, respect of self resources, wisdom, and novelty.

Certain therapy models intuitively, anecdotally, and with some empirical support offer guidelines for which psychotherapy might fit best with this population, and these have been addressed. A meld of therapies might be the best fit of all. This meld could include various combinations of dialectical behavior, cognitive-behavioral, interpersonal, psychoeducational, developmental (including guided life review), and brief psychodynamic therapies. The therapy offered would be relevant, focused, and not wasteful of self resources. Old age is not a time to tilt at windmills. The overarching purpose of therapy is to open up therapeutic space to enable change and relief by enhancing self-esteem and supporting healthy narcissism, effecting change from within and without. To this end, environmental engineering defines working mainly from the "outside in." It is probably most appropriate to those who are most deficient in the resources they can bring to the therapy. This group includes individuals with cognitive impairment to a degree that precludes other models of therapy, and those with such a degree of PD that it significantly compromises their ability to enter and maintain a therapeutic contract or to tolerate a self-as-object perspective.

STUDY QUESTIONS

1. In the case study, why do you think the earlier psychotherapy was not successful?
2. How do Axis II personality disorders differ from Axis I clinical disorders?
3. What special issues might aging be expected to present to the older person with a personality disorder?
4. Discuss the major variables that affect prevalence estimates of personality disorders in older adults.
5. How might an understanding of the theoretical models of personality disorders influence your treatment plan for an older person with a personality disorder?
6. Why is the treatment of the older adult with a personality disorder often focused on symptoms or on interpersonal problems in contrast to the psychic infrastructure?

SUGGESTED READINGS

Clarkin, J.F., & Lenzenweger, M.F. (Eds.). (1996). *Major theories of personality disorder.* New York: Guilford Press.

McCrae, R.R., & Costa, P.T., Jr. (1990). *Personality in adulthood.* New York: Guilford Press.

Millon, T. (1996). *Disorders of personality: DSM-IV and beyond* (2nd ed.). New York: Wiley.

Rosowsky, E., Abrams, R., & Zweig, R. (Eds.). (1999). *Personality disorders in older adults: Emerging issues in diagnosis and treatment.* Mahwah, NJ: Erlbaum.

Young, J.E. (1994). *Cognitive therapy for personality disorders: A schema-focused approach* (Rev. ed.). Sarasota, FL: Professional Resources Press.

REFERENCES

Abrams, R.C., & Horowitz, S.V. (1996). Personality disorders after age 50: A meta-analysis. *Journal of Personality Disorders, 10,* 271–281.

Agronin, M. (1994). Personality disorders in the elderly: An overview. *Journal of Geriatric Psychiatry, 27,* 151–191.

Agronin, M. (1999). Pharmacological treatment of personality disorders in late life. In E. Rosowsky, R. Abrams, & R. Zweig (Eds.), *Personality disorders in older adults: Emerging issues in diagnosis and treatment* (pp. 229–254). Mahwah, NJ: Erlbaum.

American Psychiatric Association. (1952). *Diagnostic and statistical manual of mental disorders.* Washington, DC: Author.

American Psychiatric Association. (1994). *Diagnostic and statistical manual of mental disorders* (4th ed.). Washington, DC: Author.

Ames, A., & Molinari, V. (1994). Prevalence of personality disorders in community-living elderly. *Journal of Geriatric Psychiatry and Neurology, 7,* 189–194.

Beck, A.T. (1992). Personality disorders (and their relationship to syndromal disorders). *Across-Species Comparisons and Psychiatry Newsletter, 5,* 3–13.

Casey, D.A., & Schrodt, C.J. (1989). Axis II diagnoses in geriatric inpatients. *Journal of Geriatric Psychiatry and Neurology, 2,* 87–88.

Cloninger, C.R. (1987). A systematic method for clinical description and classification of personality variants: A proposal. *Archives of General Psychiatry, 44,* 573–588.

Cloninger, C.R., Przybeck, T.R., Svrakic, D.M., & Wetzel, R.D. (1994). *The Temperament and Character Inventory (TCI): A guide to its development and use.* St. Louis, MO: Washington University, Center for the Psychobiology of Personality.

Coccaro, E. (1993). Psychopharmacologic studies in patients with personality disorder: Review and perspective. *Journal of Personality Disorder, 7,* 181–192.

Cohen, B.J., Nestadt, G., Samuels, J.F., Romanoski, A.J., McHugh, P.R., & Rabins, P.V. (1994). Personality disorder in later life: A community study. *British Journal of Psychiatry, 165,* 493–499.

Cohen, G.D. (1990). Psychopathology and mental health in the mature and elderly adult. In J.E. Birren & K.W. Schaie (Eds.), *Handbook of the psychology of aging* (3rd ed., pp. 359–371). San Diego, CA: Academic Press.

Coolidge, F.L., Burns, E.M., Nathan, J.H., & Mull, C.E. (1992). Personality disorders in the elderly. *Clinical Gerontologist, 12,* 41–55.

Coolidge, F.L., & Segal, D.L. (1998). Evolution of the personality disorder diagnosis in the *Diagnostic and Statistical Manual of Mental Disorders. Clinical Psychology Review, 18,* 585–599.

Coolidge, F.L., Segal, D.L., Hook, J.N., & Stewart, S. (in press). Personality disorders and coping among anxious older adults. *Journal of Anxiety Disorders.*

Coolidge, F.L., Segal, D.L., Pointer, J.C., Knaus, E.A., Yamazaki, T.G., & Silberman, C.S. (in press). Personality disorders in elderly inpatients with chronic mental illness. *Journal of Clinical Geropsychology.*

DeLeo, D., Scocco, P., & Meneghal, G. (1999). Pharmacological and psychotherapeutic treatment of personality disorders in the elderly. *International Psychogeriatrics, 11,* 191–206.

Fava, M., Alpert, J., Borus, J., Nirenberg, A., Pava, J., & Rosenbaum, J. (1996). Patterns of personality disorder comorbidity in early-onset versus late-onset major depression. *American Journal of Psychiatry, 153,* 1308–1312.

Fogel, B.S., & Westlake, R. (1990). Personality disorder diagnoses and age in inpatients with major depression. *Journal of Clinical Psychiatry, 51,* 232–235.

Goisman, R. (1999). Cognitive-behavioral therapy, personality disorders, and the elderly: Clinical and theoretical considerations. In E. Rosowsky, R. Abrams, & R. Zweig (Eds.), *Personality disorders in older adults: Emerging issues in diagnosis and treatment* (pp. 215–227). Mahwah, NJ: Erlbaum.

Goldfarb, A. (1967). Psychiatry in geriatrics. *Medical Clinics of North America, 51,* 1515–1552.

Gradman, T., Thompson, L., & Gallagher-Thompson, D. (1999). Personality disorders and treatment outcome. In E. Rosowsky, R. Abrams, & R. Zweig (Eds.), *Personality disorders in older adults: Emerging issues in diagnosis and treatment* (pp. 69–94). Mahwah, NJ: Erlbaum.

Greenson, R. (1965). The working alliance and the transference neurosis. *Psychoanalytic Quarterly, 34,* 155–181.

Griego, J.A., Stewart, S.E., & Coolidge, F.L. (1999). A convergent validity study of Cloninger's Temperament and Character Inventory with the Coolidge Axis II Inventory. *Journal of Personality Disorders, 13,* 256–267.

Hardy, G.E., Barkham, M., Shapiro, D.A., Stiles, W.B., Rees, A., & Reynolds, S. (1995). Impact of Cluster C personality disorders on outcomes of contrasting brief psychotherapies for depression. *Journal of Consulting and Clinical Psychology, 63,* 997–1004.

Havens, L, (1999). Personality and aging: A psychotherapist reflects late in his own life. In E. Rosowsky, R. Abrams, & R. Zweig (Eds.), *Personality disorders in older adults: Emerging issues in diagnosis and treatment* (pp. 17–28). Mahwah, NJ: Erlbaum.

Kagan, J., & Moss, H.A. (1962). *Birth to maturity.* New York: Wiley.

Kroessler, D. (1990). Personality disorder in the elderly. *Hospital and Community Psychiatry, 41,* 1325–1329.

Krupnick, J.L., Sotsky, S.M., Simmons, S., Moyer, J., Watkins, J., Elkin, I., & Pilkonis, P.A. (1996). The role of therapeutic alliance in psychotherapy and pharmacotherapy outcome: Findings in the National Institute of Mental Heath treatment of depression collaborative research program. *Journal of Consulting and Clinical Psychology, 64,* 532–539.

Kunik, M.E., Mulsant, B.H., Rifai, A.H., Sweet, R.A., Pasternak, R., Rosen, J., & Zubenko, G.S. (1993). Personality disorders in elderly inpatients with major depression. *American Journal of Geriatric Psychiatry, 1,* 38–45.

Linehan, M. (1993). *Cognitive-behavioral therapy of borderline personality disorder.* New York: Guilford Press.

McGue, M., Bacon, S., & Lykken, D.T. (1993). Personality stability and change in early adulthood: A behavioral genetic analysis. *Developmental Psychology, 29,* 96–109.

Mersch, P., Jansen, M., & Arntz, A. (1995). Social phobia and personality disorder: Severity of complaint and treatment effectiveness. *Journal of Personality Disorders, 9,* 143–159.

Mezzich, J.E., Fabrega, H., Coffman, G.A., & Glavin, Y. (1987). Comprehensively diagnosing geriatric patients. *Comprehensive Psychiatry, 28,* 68–76.

Millon, T. (1981). *Disorders of personality: DSM-III, Axis II.* New York: Wiley.

Millon, T., & Davis, R.D. (1996). An evolutionary theory of personality disorders. In J.F. Clarkin & M.F. Lenzenweger (Eds.), *Major theories of personality disorder* (pp. 221–346). New York: Guilford Press.

Molinari, V., Kunik, M.E., Snow-Turek, A.L., Deleon, H., & Williams, W. (1999). Age-related personality differences in inpatients with personality disorder: A cross-sectional study. *Journal of Clinical Geropsychology, 5,* 191–202.

Molinari, V., & Marmion, J. (1995). Relationship between affective disorders and Axis II diagnoses in geropsychiatric patients. *Journal of Geriatric Psychiatry and Neurology, 8,* 61–64.

Morgan, D.G., May, P.C., & Finch, C.E. (1987). Dopamine and serotonin systems in human and rodent brain: Effects of age and neurodegenerative disease. *Journal of the American Geriatric Society, 35,* 334–345.

Myers, W.A. (1999). Personality disorders in older adults: Some issues in psychodynamic treatment. In E. Rosowsky, R. Abrams, & R. Zweig (Eds.), *Personality disorders in older adults: Emerging issues in diagnosis and treatment* (pp. 205–214). Mahwah, NJ: Erlbaum.

Pfohl, B., Black, D.W., Noyes, R., Kelly, M., & Blum, N. (1990). A test of the tridimensional personality theory: Association with diagnosis and platelet imiprimine binding in obsessive-compulsive disorder. *Biological Psychiatry, 28,* 41–46.

Pretzer, J.L., & Beck, A.T. (1996). A cognitive theory of personality disorders. In J.F. Clarkin & M.F. Lenzenweger (Eds.), *Major theories of personality disorder* (pp. 36–105). New York: Guilford Press.

Rose, M.K., Soares, H.H., & Joseph, C. (1993). Frail elderly clients with personality disorders: A challenge for social work. *Journal of Gerontological Social Work, 19,* 153–165.

Rosowsky, E. (1999). The patient-therapist relationship and the psychotherapy of the older adult with personality disorder. In E. Rosowsky, R. Abrams, & R. Zweig (Eds.), *Personality disorders in older adults: Emerging issues in diagnosis and treatment* (pp. 153–174). Mahwah, NJ: Erlbaum.

Rosowsky, E., & Gurian, B. (1991). Borderline personality disorder in late life. *International Psychogeriatrics, 3,* 39–52.

Rosowsky, E., & Gurian, B. (1992). Impact of borderline personality disorder in late life on systems of care. *Hospital and Community Psychiatry, 43,* 386–389.

Rutter, M. (1987). Temperament, personality and personality disorder. *British Journal of Psychiatry, 150,* 443–458.

Segal, D.L., & Coolidge, F.L. (1998). Personality disorders. In A.S. Bellack & M. Hersen (Eds.), *Comprehensive clinical psychology: Vol. 7. Clinical geropsychology* (pp. 267–289). New York: Elsevier.

Segal, D.L., Hersen, M., Kabacoff, R.I., Falk, S.B., Van Hasselt, V.B., & Dorfman, K. (1998). Personality disorders and depression in community-dwelling older adults. *Journal of Mental Health and Aging, 4,* 171–182.

Segal, D.L., Hersen, M., Van Hasselt, V.B., Silberman, C.S., & Roth, L. (1996). Diagnosis and assessment of personality disorders in older adults: A critical review. *Journal of Personality Disorders, 10,* 384–399.

Segal, D.L., Hook, J.N., & Coolidge, F.L. (in press). Personality dysfunction, coping styles, and clinical symptoms in younger and older adults. *Journal of Clinical Geropsychology.*

Siegel, D.J., & Small, G.W. (1986). Borderline personality disorder in the elderly: A case study. *Canadian Journal of Psychiatry, 31,* 859–860.

Solomon, J., Falette, M., & Stevens, S. (1982). The psychologist as geriatric clinician. In T. Miller, C. Green, & R. Meagher (Eds.), *Handbook of clinical health psychology* (pp. 229–230). New York: Plenum Press.

Sternbach, H. (1990). Fluoxetine treatment of social phobia. *Journal of Clinical Psychopharmacology, 10,* 230.

Thompson, L.W., Gallagher, D., & Czirr, R. (1988). Personality disorder and outcome in the treatment of late-life depression. *Journal of Geriatric Psychiatry, 21,* 133–146.

Tyrer, P. (1988). *Personality disorders: Diagnosis, management, and course.* London: Wright/Butterworth.

Weissman, M.M. (1993). The epidemiology of personality disorders: A 1990 update. *Journal of Personality Disorders, 7,* 44–62.

Westen, D. (1990). Towards a revised theory of borderline object relations: Contributions of empirical research. *International Journal of Psychoanalysis, 71,* 661–693.

Widiger, T.A., & Trull, T.J. (1993). Personality and psychopathology: An application of the five-factor model. *Journal of Personality, 60,* 363–393.

Zweig, R., & Hillman, J. (1999). Personality disorders in adults: A review. In E. Rosowsky, R. Abrams, & R. Zweig (Eds.), *Personality disorders in older adults: Emerging issues in diagnosis and treatment* (pp. 31–53). Mahwah, NJ: Erlbaum.

CHAPTER 5

Anxiety in Older Adults

FORREST SCOGIN, MARK FLOYD, AND JENNIFER FORDE

Anxiety is one of the most prevalent disorders among older adults, yet it is one of the least researched, given much less attention than depression and the dementias. Recent surveys have found that up to 15% of the older population experience some type of anxiety disorder (Manela, Katona, & Livingson, 1996). It is important to focus on anxiety in older adults because it has been shown to reduce quality of life and is associated with increased mortality (Orrell & Bebbington, 1996). Encouragingly, several recent reviews of the topic (Acierno, Hersen, & Van Hasselt, 1996; Banazak, 1997; Sadavoy & LeClair, 1997; Sheikh & Salzman, 1995; Stanley & Beck, 1998) suggest increasing interest among basic and applied scientists. In our review of the topic, we discuss diagnostic issues, epidemiology, and treatment. Study questions and suggestions for further reading follow coverage of these content areas.

We begin with a case study presenting issues encountered in work with anxious older adults. This case is a composite of individuals we have seen in our clinical and research work.

CASE STUDY

Mrs. J. is a 71-year-old female who was referred by a family practice physician who works in a nearby town. Mrs. J. had become moderately depressed and extremely anxious following major orthopedic surgery, a total hip replacement. She was a retired office worker.

Mrs. J.'s physician contacted me to ask if I would be willing to see her for psychotherapy. She informed me that Mrs. J. had been on oxazepam, a benzodiazepine, for approximately six months. She was also taking an antidepressant. She had experienced a significant, but not total, remission of anxious and depressive symptoms. The referral for psychotherapy was to treat these remaining symptoms, particularly extreme worry. We agreed that continued pharmacotherapy was warranted and that we would stay in touch as to Mrs. J.'s progress, should she decide she wanted to try psychotherapy. The physician told me that Mrs. J. had agreed to psychotherapy when she brought it up.

I contacted Mrs. J. to set up our initial session. I was immediately struck by her general level of anxiety. For example, she expressed fears about her ability to get her husband to take her to an appointment and was concerned that she might not be the right type of person for psychological treatment. Her anxiety seemed to interfere with her ability to adequately attend to and process information. For example, she seemed to have difficulty getting down the directions to my office. I noted that assessment of cognitive functioning might be warranted during our early sessions. She stated that she was concerned about being able to find the building and that she would leave her house early in case she got lost.

Mrs. J. was early to her appointment. She looked distraught throughout the session. She wrung her hands, cried on a couple of occasions, and repeatedly stated "I don't want to be a burden." Her main concern was that due to her recent surgery, she might not be able to continue living in the home she and her husband had lived in most of her adult life. She was extremely afraid of having a fall and not being found for hours.

By the time we had discussed this issue in depth, I knew there would be no need for memory and cognitive testing. Mrs. J. evidenced good memory for recent events and had no problems in keeping up with the flow of our conversation. At one point in the session, I did ask her if she had any problems with memory, and she stated, "That's another thing! I definitely don't remember things as well as I did when I was working." I asked for specific examples, and she said she had to rely on notes to remember things now, whereas before, she did not need that kind of help. She was worried that she might be developing Alzheimer's disease.

To gain an appreciation of context, I also asked her about her history. "Tell me a little about your family, your work, your children if you have any, and so forth." Mr. and Mrs. J. had raised four children. She had two years of college credits but had to give up part-time higher education when her family grew. She worked in an office for a small business for most of her employed years. She was proud of herself for raising her children but expressed some regret that she continued to work when they were in their preschool years. She wondered if she had made the right decision.

I also asked about her history of anxiety and depression. She stated that when she was raising her children, she worried about their education and about money. Concerning depression, she stated that the only other time she had been really "blue" was when her husband and her sister were stricken with cancer in the same year 10 years ago. Her sister subsequently died.

Her children were living various distances away from her, so that their involvement, at least physically, was not an option. Mrs. J. indicated that she loved all her children but that she worried about two of them. Both had divorced and she was concerned about their well-being and that of her three grandchildren.

Toward the middle of the session, I began to assess Mrs. J.'s current level of anxious and depressive symptomatology. I used the *DSM-IV* criteria, asking for duration and intensity of symptoms. For example, I asked her, "How has your appetite been lately?" She reported not having the desire to eat because her stomach was "fluttery." I asked, "Do you find yourself worrying about things?", to which she responded, "Yes, a lot. I worry that I've begun to be a burden for my husband. I worry about my hip and I worry about not being able to get around. I guess I'm crazy because I worry about being worried so much." I assured her that she was not crazy, just anxious, which can oftentimes make you feel like you are crazy. Mrs. J. also indicated that she had feelings of guilt and had lost interest in previously enjoyable activities.

My initial diagnosis was that Mrs. J. suffered from generalized anxiety disorder with symptoms of major depression in partial remission. She did in fact engage in psychotherapy, and as our sessions continued, I realized that she had always been a particularly anxious person. She felt that this was just part of her personality. The change in her health made her worries more intense and began to interfere with her functioning.

Mrs. J. continued on anxiolytic and antidepressant medications, but gradually lowered the frequency and dosage on the benzodiazepine over the next year. She was intensely fearful of becoming addicted to this medication. In treatment, I used cognitive therapy to help combat her negative thinking patterns. She made steady progress, and after about 25 sessions, we terminated.

DSM CRITERIA FOR DIAGNOSIS

Anxiety, like many geriatric mental disorders, can be difficult to diagnose. A number of issues complicate diagnosis. Anxiety symptoms may also be produced by a variety of medical conditions. Many older adults presenting with anxiety symptoms have co-occuring medical conditions such as cancer or cardiovascular disease. These conditions can produce or exacerbate anxiety symptoms. Differential diagnosis can be challenging in such cases. Further, older adults themselves may be loath to report anxiety symptoms. They may minimize the impairment caused by anxiety or view it as a stable part of their personality. We have asked several older clients why they had not sought treatment for anxiety earlier in their life. They have responded with something to the effect of "I thought that was not a problem you went to a doctor about" and "I was afraid they would think I was crazy." We will have more to say on the topic of underreporting in the section on assessment. Also, many health providers are not accustomed to recognizing anxiety in older patients. Together, these factors lead not only to difficulties in diagnosis but, more important, to a problem in underdiagnosis. Underdiagnosis is understandable when one considers that the more common forms of anxiety problems, such as generalized anxiety disorder, have a very stable, traitlike quality and can lead to dispositional inferences, such as "That's just the way she is." This tendency toward underreporting and underdiagnosis is regrettable because anxiety disorders diminish quality of life. Fortunately, several treatments show promise in aiding anxious older adults.

SYMPTOMS AND CRITERIA

Anxiousness manifests itself in a variety of physical and emotional ways across the life span. In older adults, anxiety about loss of loved ones, mobility, status, or even fear of such losses can lead to some of the physical symptoms listed in Table 5.1.

Whether one likes it or not, the use of diagnostic criteria has become a standard aspect of clinical practice and clinical research. We present information on the *DSM-IV* (American Psychiatric Association [APA], 1994) criteria for anxiety disorders most often seen in older adults: generalized anxiety disorder (GAD),

Table 5.1 Symptoms of anxiety.

Anorexia	Backache	"Butterflies" in stomach
Chest discomfort	Diaphoresis	Diarrhea
Dizziness	Dyspnea	Dry mouth
Faintness	Fatigue	Restlessness
Headache	Hyperventilation	Sweating
Muscle tension	Pallor	Nausea
Palpitations	Paresthesis	Sexual dysfunction
Shortness of breath	Stomach pain	Tachycardia
Tremulousness	Urinary frequency	Vomiting
Insomnia	Body aches and pains	Facial flushing

Source: Small, 1997; Folks & Fuller, 1997.

panic disorder (PD), social phobia (SP), posttraumatic stress disorder (PTSD), acute stress disorder (ASD), and anxiety disorder due to a general medical condition (ADGMC). We also present information on a diagnosis under consideration for the next iteration of *DSM,* mixed anxiety-depression disorder (MADD; unfortunate acronym, we know). Adjustment disorders (ADJD) and dependent personality disorder (DPD), in which anxiety is prominent, are also overviewed.

Generalized Anxiety Disorder
GAD is considered one of the most prevalent of the anxiety disorders experienced by elders (Regier et al., 1988). The cardinal symptom of GAD is worry. According to the diagnostic criteria, the worry should be about a number of events and of at least six months duration, occurring more days than not. Additionally, persons should experience at least three of the following symptoms:

- Restlessness or feeling keyed up or on edge.
- Being easily fatigued.
- Difficulty concentrating or mind going blank.
- Irritability.
- Muscle tension.
- Sleep disturbance.

Furthermore, the worry or physical symptoms must cause significant distress or impairment. In our work, the distress/impairment clause has been readily fulfilled by the older clients meeting the above criteria.

Older and younger adults experiencing GAD tend to differ in the content of their worry. In a developmentally consistent fashion, older adults tend to worry more about their health, whereas younger adults are more likely to worry about finances (Person & Borkovec, 1995). Unfortunately, the predictability of these concerns may promote underdetection of the disruptive effects of excessive worry. We have had to catch ourselves from falling prey to the tendency to think, Who wouldn't be worried about their health? For example, an older client experiencing severe arthritis and cardiovascular disease understandably may be worried about his or her ability to maintain independent function. As clinicians, we are required to make a subjective decision about what constitutes realistic worry versus clinically significant worry. Judging the extent of impairment and distress resultant to the worry reduces but does not eliminate the diagnostic uncertainty.

GAD is a common anxiety disorder in older adults and has been shown primarily to begin early in life (Blazer, George, & Hughes, 1991). Some cases of GAD, however, do begin in later life. In most such cases, an anxious temperament is present but not an anxiety disorder, until stressful events aggravate an onset. Only then does anxiety begin to interfere with functioning. It appears that age of onset is an important factor in an individual's psychological profile. Those older adults with GAD who report early onset of anxiety tend to have more severe anxiety and are more likely to have depressive symptomology than those with late onset (see section on depression and anxiety). Older adults with GAD also have elevated levels of anxiety, worry, depression, and social fears, which are not present in a normal sample of older adults (Beck, Stanley, & Zebb, 1996). As noted previously, clinicians must be alert to the tendency to dismiss excessive worry in older adults as part of the natural aging process.

Panic Disorder

PD can occur in several forms, depending on the presence of agoraphobia. The basic criterion for PD is recurrent, unexpected panic attacks. Panic attacks, according to *DSM-IV*, comprise a discrete period of intense fear or discomfort in which four or more of the following symptoms occur:

- Palpitations.
- Sweating.
- Trembling or shaking.
- Shortness of breath.
- Feeling of choking.
- Chest pains.
- Nausea or abdominal distress.
- Dizziness.
- Derealization or depersonalization.
- Fears of losing control or going crazy.
- Fear of dying.
- Numbness or tingling sensations.
- Chills or hot flushes.

Further criteria for PD stipulate that one or more of the panic attacks be followed by at least one month of either anxiety about the potential for future attacks or the possible consequences of an attack or significant change in behavior related to the attacks. PD can occur with or without agoraphobia, which is the fear of being unable to escape a situation should a panic attack occur. Persons evidencing agoraphobia also tend to avoid situations that might lead to a panic attack. However, in PD, the situations that lead to an attack do not necessarily follow a pattern. Older adults may experience PD with agoraphobia in which outside activities such as shopping, church attendance, or socializing may be avoided due to fears of embarrassing panic attacks. Most surveys suggest that PD is a relatively rare anxiety disorder among older adults.

Agoraphobia is another common anxiety disorder in older adults. Whereas GAD tends to begin early in life, agoraphobia can develop at any time in life; in fact, it is common for this phobia to develop late in life (Lindesay, Briggs, & Murphy, 1989). Agoraphobia tends to appear in older adults after a physical illness or traumatic event (Lindesay, 1997). Medical conditions may also cause an older person to be fearful of leaving the house. For example, a senior may be afraid to be in large crowds due to bladder control problems, Parkinson-like tremors, or other potentially embarrassing symptoms of disease. It may be difficult to assess whether it is true agoraphobia that prevents elders from leaving their home or if their avoidant behavior is due to a medical condition (Fuentes & Cox, 1997). Thus, agoraphobia may be less related to panic attacks, which are often the critical precipitants to the development of agoraphobia in younger adults.

Social Phobia

SP develops from an extreme, persistent fear of situations where the individual may be exposed to unknown people or be scrutinized by others. Exposure to these types of events usually results in anxiety or even situationally bound panic attacks. This phobia results in avoidance of the feared situation to the detriment of overall functioning. Of particular importance for the elderly, this fear is not related to a medical condition (e.g., fear of shaking due to Parkinson's disease).

Post-Traumatic Stress Disorder and Acute Stress Disorder

Symptoms of PTSD and ASD are common in older adults, due in large part to grieving process sequelae (Rosenzweig, Prigerson, Miller, & Reynolds, 1997). PTSD is a complex disorder characterized by a traumatic event that is reexperienced in some manner. This leads to avoidance of certain stimuli and a decrease in responsiveness in the following manner:

- Efforts to avoid thoughts associated with the event.
- Efforts to avoid activities, people, or places that bring back memories of the event.
- Inability to recall important aspects of the trauma.
- Markedly diminished interest in activities.
- Feelings of detachment from others.
- Restricted range of affect.
- No sense of the future.

These symptoms occur for more than one month and can lead to insomnia, irritability, concentration difficulties, hypervigilance, and exaggerated startle responses. ASD is very similar to but shorter in duration than PTSD, lasting for less than one month. We are familiar with a client who evidenced acute stress disorder following an incorrect diagnosis of Alzheimer's disease and suggestions that her husband begin looking for a nursing home in which to place her. This was understandably a traumatic incident for the client and resulted in insomnia and diminished interest in activities.

PTSD is a common occurrence among combat veterans of all ages. Those who are veterans of World War II and the Korean War are presently in the older adult population, but in a few years, the first Vietnam veterans will begin to enter this age group. Presently, there are approximately one million elders with PTSD who served in either WWII or Korea (DVA, 1993). Because these veterans were raised in a time when discussing one's feelings was less accepted, these patients tend to emphasize their physical symptoms. Perhaps as a result of this phenomenon or as a result of the type of warfare utilized, WWII veterans tend to experience fewer and less dramatic psychological symptoms than the veterans of the Vietnam War (Davidson, Kudler, Saunders, & Smith, 1990). Several questions were developed to help physicians distinguish between physical illness and possible manifestations of PTSD (see Table 5.2; Snell & Padin-Rivera, 1997). Late-onset PTSD is also an increasing phenomenon in elderly combat veterans (Schnurr, Aldwin, Spiro, Stukel, & Keane, 1993). This is most likely due not to actual progression of the illness but to the Veterans Administration's acknowledgment of this disorder and the increasing acceptance of psychological treatment. This change in policy means that veterans can get treatment for their symptoms as well as disability benefits to attempt to compensate them for the potentially devastating effects of this illness on their interpersonal and work functioning.

Acute stress disorder is a new disorder, first introduced in *DSM-IV*, hence little research has been done involving the occurrence rates or symptomatology in elders. However, of relevance to ASD, evidence exists linking PTSD to the bereavement process (Bonanno & Kaltman, 1999; Prigerson et al., 1997). It has been suggested that some individuals may have extreme difficulty in dealing with the death of a loved one, particularly when this death was sudden,

Table 5.2   Senior veterans' PTSD screening instrument.

1. Are you bothered by unwanted memories about the war?
2. Is it hard for you to feel close to others, even family?
3. Are you angry or irritable much of the time?
4. Do you have nightmares about things that happened during the war?
5. Do you jump at noises when others do not?
6. Do you try to avoid thinking about what happened during the war?
7. Do you feel tense or on guard much of the time?
8. Have you repeatedly tried to remember important parts of the war but have not been able to do so?
9. Have you ever gotten upset when you saw or heard things that reminded you of the war?
10. Over the years, have you wanted to be alone rather than be with others?

Source: Snell & Padin–Rivera (1997).

and experience symptoms of traumatic stress. ASD is implicated by this research because the referenced data were typically collected after the end of the four week acute period and it is reasonable to assume the symptoms existed earlier in the bereavement process.

Anxiety Disorder Due to a General Medical Condition

This disorder is manifested by anxiety, panic attacks, and obsessions or compulsions related physiologically to a medical condition. According to *DSM-IV*, some of the medical conditions that can cause anxiety symptoms are endocrine conditions, cardiovascular conditions, respiratory conditions, metabolic conditions, and neurological conditions. This diagnosis is probably common among older adults due to their increased risk for many of these diseases. To our knowledge, no epidemiolgical data are available on ADGMC.

Table 5.3 lists clues for clinicians that there may be an underlying medical condition related to a patient's psychiatric symptoms, including anxiety.

Mixed Anxiety-Depression Disorder

MADD is a new classification for further research and possible inclusion in the next version of the *DSM* manual. This disorder combines anxiety and depression symptoms, as the name suggests, based on the observation that anxiety and depression are often co-occurring (Gallo, Rabins, & Iliffe, 1997). Individuals falling into this category have never met all of the criteria for major depressive disorder, dysthymic disorder, PD, or GAD. They have, however, experienced a persistent dysphoric mood for more than one month accompanied by four or more of the following symptoms:

- Difficulty concentrating.
- Sleep disturbance.
- Fatigue.
- Irritability.
- Worry.
- Crying easily.
- Hypervigilance.

Table 5.3   Clinical clues of an underlying medical condition related to psychiatric symptoms.

1. Atypical age of onset of symptoms.
2. Lack of family history of mental illness.
3. Lack of past personal history of mental illness.
4. Poor response to conventional treatments.
5. More severe symptoms than is typical.
6. The presence of abnormal cognitive functioning.

Source: Alessi & Cassel, 1996; Vickers, 1988.

- Anticipating the worst.
- Hopelessness.
- Low self-esteem or feelings of worthlessness.

The symptoms of this combined disorder cause significant impairment in important areas of functioning. We believe that this could become a common diagnosis among older adults, as often, symptoms of depression and anxiety occur together, though individually at a subsyndromal level. We discuss the comorbidity of depression and anxiety in a later section.

Adjustment Disorder with Anxious Features
This disorder occurs in response to an identifiable stressor and leads to emotional or behavioral symptoms within three months of the onset of the stressor. Symptoms should not meet criteria for another Axis I disorder such as PTSD or major depression. Behaviors are excessive distress and/or social or occupational impairment. This disorder can occur with anxiety symptoms or with mixed anxiety and depression symptoms. For example, we remember an older female client experiencing adjustment disorder with anxious features following the arrest of her oldest son on drug charges.

Dependent Personality Disorder
DPD is characterized by an excessive need to be taken care of, as seen in five or more of the following:

- Has difficulty making everyday decisions without advice from others.
- Needs others to assume responsibility for most major areas of life.
- Has difficulty expressing disagreement with others out of fear of disapproval.
- Has difficulty initiating projects or doing things on his or her own.
- Goes to excessive lengths to obtain support from others.
- Feels helpless when alone because of exaggerated fears of being unable to care for self.
- Urgently seeks new relationships when one ends.
- Is unrealistically preoccupied with fears of being left alone.

The clinician must carefully assess a person believed to have DPD, because several of the symptoms can appear to be GAD (e.g., fearfulness). The important distinguishing feature lies in the way the person relates to people. Persons with DPD seek new relationships because they fear being alone, and they will go to extremes to please their loved ones. Anxiety about being left alone could be a characteristic of GAD, but the extreme behavior regarding personal relationships is absent. DPD has been suggested as one of the more frequently occuring personality disorders among older adults. Losses in physical and cognitive functioning, as well as losses in significant relationships, can lead to diminished independence and provoke dependent reactions in those temperamentally disposed toward such behavior. Older adults with co-occurring personality disorders have been shown to have less successful outcomes in treatments for major depression (Gradman et al., 1999).

EPIDEMIOLOGY

As previously stated, anxiety is one of the most prevalent group of disorders among older adults (Stanley & Beck, 1998). Estimates range from 10% to 20% of older persons experiencing significant symptoms of anxiety (Banazak, 1997; Beekman et al., 1998). The most definitive source of information about mental disorders comes from the landmark Epidemiological Catchment Area (ECA) study. This study provides estimates of the prevalence of the major mental disorders by age and sex groupings. As was the case for other age groups, anxiety disorders were the most prevalent of the mental disorders (Regier et al., 1988). These authors report a one-month prevalence rate of 5.5% for the 65-years-and-older cohort. Phobias (4.8%), including agoraphobia, social phobia, and simple phobia (now termed specific phobia), were the most prevalent of the disorders. Obsessive-compulsive disorder (0.8%) and panic disorder (0.1%) were rarely observed. Similar figures were obtained in a companion survey (Weissman et al., 1985).

Notice that GAD, perhaps the prototypical anxiety disorder, is not included in the above prevalence estimates. This is because GAD was not a *DSM* diagnosis at the time of the initial ECA survey. Subsequent data collected by Blazer et al. (1991) revealed six-month GAD prevalence rates for older adults to be 1.9%. Lifetime prevalence of GAD was reported to be 4.6% for older adults.

As noted, the ECA is considered the gold standard in terms of the epidemiology of mental disorders generally and anxiety disorders in older adults specifically. However, several other surveys of anxiety disorders have been conducted. As reported by Flint (1994), prevalence estimates for phobic disorders ranged from 0 to 10%. Interestingly, agoraphobia, arguably the most serious of the phobic disorders, has been considered the most common of the phobias in older adults (Small, 1997). Although percentages vary by study, phobic disorder is the most common of the anxiety disorders in all age groups, including seniors (Beekman et al., 1998).

Anxiety disorders are consistently more prevalent in younger than in older cohorts, although they are certainly a significant problem among the elderly (Flint, 1994; Reiger et al., 1988). Anxiety disorders are more common in women in both age groups, as much as twice the rate of men (Beekman et al., 1998; Musil, 1998). Age of onset is not well researched in regard to geriatric anxiety. GAD has been observed to be approximately evenly distributed among earlier and late-onset cases. Blazer et al. (1991) found that 39% of community-surveyed elders had experienced GAD onset before late adulthood, whereas 50% had experienced duration of symptoms for five years or less.

The phenomenology of anxiety has also been a topic of some research attention. Particularly, studies have examined the nature of worry among older adults. Trends consistent with developmental challenges tend to emerge. For example, Powers, Wisocki, and Whitbourne (1992) found that older adults reported most worry about health, although the level of worry was similar to that reported by younger participants. Interestingly, Powers et al. found that worries occurred with relative infrequency among older participants. This investigation used the Worry Scale (Wisocki, 1988). These investigators also found that an external locus of control was associated with higher worry scores. Similarly, Person and Borkovec (1995) found that elders worried most about health and least about work. More recently, Diefenbach et al. (1999) compared worry content of 44 older adults diagnosed with GAD and 44 matched non-GAD participants. Worry topics were categorized as family/interpersonal, financial, work/school, illness/health/injury, and miscellaneous. GAD patients by definition reported more worries, but the content of the worries did not differ by diagnostic group. Both older adult groups indicated that family/interpersonal were the most frequent worries, followed by miscellaneous and illness/health/injury. The emergence of family/interpersonal themes is consistent with other observations (Miller & Silberman, 1996; Scogin, 2000).

Co-Occurrence and Overlap with Other Conditions

Anxiety and Depression

Anxiety and depression have been repeatedly shown to exist simultaneously, so much so that some question the independence of the two disorders. Alexopoulos (1990) reported that 38% of outpatients diagnosed with major depression were also diagnosed with an anxiety disorder. Studies with younger adults suggest that 60% to 90% of depressed patients experience at least some symptoms of anxiety (Stokes & Holtz, 1997). Anxiety may also be a significant indicator of depression in older adults. Of the specific anxiety disorders, GAD was found more often in correlation with depression than were the phobic types of anxiety (Manela et al., 1996). Lindesay et al.'s (1989) survey found that 91% of those older adults evidencing GAD and 39% of those evidencing a phobic disorder also met criteria for depression. Those with onset of depression early in life may show higher rates of anxiety than those with late-onset depression over the age of 59 (Baldwin & Tomenson, 1995). The converse is also true: those with early onset of anxiety disorders are more likely to experience comorbid depression (Beck et al., 1996). Of specific importance to the elderly, anxiety and depressive ideation have been found to impact negatively one's ability to carry out instrumental activities of daily living (Alexopoulos et al., 1996). Furthermore, those who experience anxious depression do not respond as well to antidepressant therapy and have poor compliance rates (Flint & Rifat, 1997). The unique experiences of individuals with comorbid anxiety and depression have prompted the authors of the *DSM-IV* (APA, 1994) to consider a new category termed mixed-anxiety and depression disorder.

The following is a list of symptoms common to depression and anxiety (Stokes & Holtz, 1997):

- High negative affect.
- Feelings of inferiority and rejection.
- Oversensitivity to criticism.
- Self-consciousness.
- Social distress.

Dementia and Anxiety

Among the many symptoms associated with dementia are cognitive decline, delusions, hallucinations, depression, and anxiety (Förstl, Satel, & Bahro, 1993). Anxiety, though commonly overlooked, may be present in one third of those with dementia. Some studies suggest that anxiety tends to appear more in the earlier stages of dementia (Wands et al., 1990), but others found no relation between cognitive decline and anxiety (Orrell & Bebbington, 1996). Forsell and Winblad (1997) found no significant differences between nondemented and demented elders as to prevalence of anxiety disorders. They go on to explain that in those patients they examined with moderate to severe dementia, little or no anxiety was present. Although this may be due in part to their method of assessment (severely demented patients could not respond to their questions), it does suggest that the beginning stages of dementia may be more anxiety-provoking, especially if the person is aware of his or her decline and fears that it may be due to Alzheimer's disease (Orrell & Bebbington, 1994).

Research using behavioral assessments has led to the belief that anxiety is present in the later stages of dementia as well; it simply manifests itself in different ways. Agitation is seen in 60% of the demented at some point during their illness (Eisdorfer et al., 1992). It has been hypothesized that agitation is the manifestation of GAD in those with late-stage dementia. According to this theory, agitation includes excessive worry, restlessness, irritability, fatigue, sleep difficulties, and unexplained verbal or motor activity, which can be seen as symptoms of GAD (Cohen-Mansfield, 1986; Mintzer & Brawman-Mintzer, 1996).

It has been suggested that the dynamics of social contact are associated with more anxiety among dementia patients (Orrell & Bebbington, 1996). Those with high levels of anxiety tended to be more dominant in their relationships prior to the development of dementia. Their anxiety may be due to their increasing dependence on others.

Pre-illness attachment style may also affect a demented person's anxiety levels. Magai and Cohen (1998) found that ambivalently attached patients had more anxiety than securely attached patients. Perhaps this finding can be explained, as before, by a growing dependence on others, to which the ambivalent person is not accustomed.

Illness and Anxiety

We have already discussed the *DSM* diagnosis of anxiety due to a general medical condition. Now we present further information on the link between various medical conditions and anxiety.

People of all ages commonly experience anxiety symptoms in response to thoughts about the possible implications of an illness (Small, 1997). For example, take an older man who fears that he may have prostate cancer. While waiting for the results of tests, he becomes anxious about the possible diagnosis, stories he has heard about painful treatments for cancer, the possibility of death, making sure his family is well cared for in case he should die, and so on. Evidence suggests that aging worriers (those who experience symptoms of anxiety but do not meet the criterion for diagnosis) are in poorer health and tend to experience more chronic illness (Wisocki, 1988). In addition, chronically ill patients with anxiety use health care services at a higher rate than nonanxious patients (Katon et al., 1990; Livingston, Manela, & Katona, 1997). Older adults who are anxious also tend to report more pain (Parmelee, Lawton, & Katz, 1998).

Penninx and colleagues (1996) found among older patients that the more diseases a person has, the more likely he or she will experience psychological dysfunction, including anxiety. Several studies have looked at specific illnesses and their relationship to anxiety (see Table 5.4 for illnesses with strong associations to anxiety). Of those afflicted with Parkinson's disease, 38% experience some type of anxiety disorder (Stein, Heuser, Juncos, & Uhde, 1990). Panic disorder is present in 8% of patient's with chronic obstructive pulmonary disease (Karajgi, Rifkin, Doddi, & Kolli, 1990); in our clinical experience, there is a much higher rate of anxiety in COPD. Castillo and associates (1993) studied stroke patients and found that 40% develop clinically significant anxiety, particularly GAD. In cases of early dementia, 38% experience anxiety to the extent of possible diagnosis (Wands et al., 1990).

A factor suggested to explain the differences in the prevalence of anxiety in different diseases is the extent of controllability of the particular disease. Diseases such as cancer that have an uncertain prognosis and are less controllable may be more anxiety-provoking than diseases like diabetes, which can be controlled with diet and medication (Cassileth et al., 1985; Felton, Revenson, & Hinrichson, 1984).

Table 5.4   Medical conditions with strong associations to anxiety.

Classification	Examples
Endocrine and metabolic disorders	Hypo- and Hyperthyroidism Hypoglycemia Cushing's Disease
Neurologic disorders	Dementia Stroke Parkinson's disease Central nervous system infections
Cardiovascular disorders	Arrhythmias Congestive heart failure
Respiratory disorders	Asthma Pneumonia Chronic obstructive lung disease

Source: Hocking & Koenig, 1995; Marsh, 1997.

MEASUREMENT

Data cited in the section on epidemiology suggested considerable range in the estimates of particular anxiety disorders. Undoubtedly, part of this can be attributed to the choice of assessment tools. Fuentes and Cox (1997) argue that many studies have used measures not validated with older persons or with vague definitions for anxiety disorders. Most inventories have been supported using data from college-age individuals, and research must examine their sensitivity to disorders in an older population. Here, we examine those instruments commonly used with aging adults.

INTERVIEW-BASED ASSESSMENT

The most frequently cited interview-based assessments of anxiety are the Hamilton Anxiety Rating Scale (HARS), the Structured Clinical Interview for *DSM* (SCID), and the Anxiety Disorders Interview Schedule (ADIS).

The HARS (Hamilton, 1959) is the sister instrument to the better-known Hamilton Rating Scale for Depression. The HARS is a measure of the severity of anxiety and is thus a useful tool for assessing change in anxiety over time. Beck et al. (1996) found good interrater agreement between two groups of older adults, one with independently diagnosed GAD and the other without. Further, total scores significantly differentiated the two groups. Thus, the HARS shows promise as a measure of anxiety symptom severity among older adults.

The SCID-IV (First, Spitzer, Gibbon, & Williams, 1997) is rapidly becoming the gold standard for interview-based assessment of mental disorders. The SCID, unlike the HARS, is not a measure of anxiety severity but instead provides information on the presence of diagnosable anxiety disorders. Using an earlier version (SCID-III-R), Segal, Hersen, Van Hasselt, Kabacoff, and Roth (1993) and Segal, Kabacoff, Hersen, Van Hasselt, and Ryan (1995) found good interrater diagnostic agreement for the anxiety disorders among older adults.

The ADIS (Brown, DiNardo, & Barlow, 1994) is a measure frequently used in clinical research. For example, Beck, Stanley, and colleagues have used the ADIS in their studies of geriatric anxiety (Beck, Stanley, & Zebb, 1995, 1996; Stanley, Beck, & Zebb, 1996). These investigators found excellent interrater agreement for the anxiety disorders, specifically GAD, social phobia, simple phobia, and panic disorder. These data suggest that the ADIS can be a useful tool for diagnosing anxiety disorders in elders.

SELF-REPORT MEASURES

The most commonly used self-report measure of anxiety across adulthood is the Speilberger State-Trait Anxiety Inventory (Speilberger, Gorsuch, & Lushene, 1970). Across several independent investigations, the State and Trait scales have been found to possess generally acceptable psychometric properties. Internal consistency and test-retest estimates were favorable; however, discriminant and convergent validity estimates have been less impressive (Stanley et al., 1996).

Other instruments appearing in the literature include the Worry Scale (Wisocki, Handen, & Morse, 1986), the Padua Inventory (Sanavio, 1988), the Penn State Worry Questionnaire (Meyer, Miller, Metzger, & Borkovec, 1990), the Fear Questionnaire (Marks & Matthews, 1979), and the Relaxation Inventory for Older Adults (Scogin, Floyd, & Rickard, 1998). Obviously, more work is needed to examine the psychometric properties of these and other measures of anxiety with older populations.

TREATMENTS

Among the first things to consider when examining treatments for mental health issues among older adults is that relatively few members of this cohort seek help for emotional problems. For example, Thompson and colleagues (1988) found that fewer than 1% of the older adults diagnosed with agoraphobia in the ECA study had seen a mental health professional in the preceding six-month period. Only about 2% of those evidencing a phobic disorder had seen a mental health professional.

Those older adults who do seek help tend to look to their family physician rather than to a mental health professional (Robinson, 1998). This fact may be related to the stigma associated with discussing feelings or being diagnosed with a mental disorder that pervades our culture and is even more predominant in contemporary older persons. It could also be related to the difficulty in obtaining sufficient coverage for behavioral health services from federal or private insurance.

Relatively few studies have been done involving the treatment of anxiety in older adults. Of those that have been done, most involve pharmacological treatments. In the following sections, we examine cognitive-behavioral therapies, relaxation therapy, and pharmacotherapy for anxiety disorders in the elderly.

COGNITIVE-BEHAVIORAL THERAPY (CBT)

CBT has received the most attention among the psychotherapies for geriatric anxiety. CBT is theorized to exert influence through helping patients identify and counteract negative thinking patterns that co-occur with anxiety. In this type of therapy, negative thoughts are challenged by pointing out types of thinking errors, such as all-or-nothing thinking, and identifying ways to modify these errors. The therapist may have patients view themselves from another perspective or explore their own unrealistic standards to appreciate how their thoughts are related to negative affect (Banazak, 1997).

A study by Stanley, Beck, and Glassco (1996) compared CBT to a supportive therapy control in older adults with GAD. They found few differences in efficacy between the two group therapies, which were given to 48 community-dwelling elders with an average symptom duration of 35 years. Although improvements were shown with both treatments, the interesting finding was that at six-month follow-up, only a few of the patients were functioning in the normal range. This finding suggests that additional or booster treatments may be necessary for full clinical response.

RELAXATION TRAINING

Relaxation training has been shown to be an effective form of treatment for anxiety symptoms. A study by DeBerry, Davis, and Reinhard (1989) showed that relaxation training reduced both state and trait anxiety as well as depression, whereas cognitive restructuring did not produce a change in state anxiety. Participants were 32 community-dwelling elders with anxious symptoms. Scogin, Rickard, Keith, Wilson, and McElreath (1992) examined the effects of progressive and imaginal relaxation training in elderly participants reporting tension and anxiety. The progressive and imaginal distinction is important because some older adults cannot participate in progressive relaxation, which involves tensing and relaxation of muscles. Persons with arthritic conditions find this procedure difficult. Imaginal relaxation is more appropriate for these individuals because it involves imagining the tensing and relaxation of muscles. We found that both types of treatment reduced state anxiety on the STAI and the SCL-90R anxiety subscale. At a one-year follow-up, patients had lower state and trait anxiety compared to their pretreatment scores (Rickard, Scogin, & Keith, 1994).

PHARMACOTHERAPY

As previously mentioned, treatment for mental disorders typically begins in the primary care setting. The predominant treatment provided in these settings is pharmacotherapy. Some have suggested that drug treatment should be considered a last resort only after other causes of anxiety have been ruled out, such as a medical condition or drug side effects, and after traditional types of psychotherapy have been ruled out (Smith, Sherrill, & Colenda, 1995). Drug treatment with older adults can be increasingly difficult due to age-related changes in drug absorption, distribution, metabolism, and sensitivity to side effects. Older adults typically are taking several prescription and over-the-counter medications that may have interaction effects with psychotropic medications (Salzman, 1991). All of these factors make dosing difficult for seniors. Some suggest starting at half the recommended dose to begin treatment (Banazak, 1997).

Benzodiazepines are the most prescribed anxiolytics for older adults, though few studies have been done to determine their efficacy with this population. Of these, oxazepam and lorazepam are preferred because of their shorter half-lives, which makes drug interactions less likely (Fernandez, Levy, Lachar, & Small, 1995). They also have a rapid response rate, making them particularly useful for acute anxiety. Studies have shown that elderly patients tend to use benzodiazepines much longer than indicated (Taylor, McCracken, Wilson, & Copeland, 1998). Further, older adults seem to use benzodiazepines more frequently than younger cohorts (Salzman, 1991). Unfortunately, these compounds are highly addictive and require higher and higher doses to maintain effect. Withdrawal can be so severe as to cause higher anxiety symptoms than before treatment. One study compared high and low doses of abecarnil to a placebo group and found that after discontinuation of treatment, the placebo group actually had fewer anxious symptoms than either of the treatment groups (Small & Bystritsky, 1997).

Several side effects could potentially be dangerous to seniors (Salzman, 1992):

- Potential for abuse.
- Unsteadiness (can lead to falls and bone fractures).
- Daytime sedation.
- Disinhibition.
- Impaired cognitive function.
- Sleep disorders.
- Cerebellar dysfunction.
- Slowed reaction time.

Buspirone has been used in the treatment of generalized anxiety disorder among older adults and has fewer side effects than the benzodiazepines. Whereas patients who discontinue use of benzodiazepines tend to experience an increase in symptoms after termination of drug treatment, the discontinuation of buspirone does not cause rebound symptoms (Pecknold, 1997). It has less potential for abuse because it does not cause withdrawal symptoms and is nonhabituating. It also has fewer drug interactions, so it is safer for patients with comorbid medical conditions (Cadieux, 1996). For those who are prone to falls, this drug is preferred because it causes less psychomotor slowing and unsteadiness. Very little research has examined buspirone use in the over-65 populations. Some side effects include gastrointestinal symptoms, dizziness, headache, sleep disturbance, nausea, uneasiness, and diarrhea (Palmer, Jeste, & Sheikh, 1997). However, it does not work well with acute anxiety symptoms, because it has a longer response time than some of the fast-acting benzodiazepines (Martin, Fleming, & Evans, 1995). Patients might be prone to discontinue treatment because it takes six to eight weeks for this drug to become effective, as opposed to the more immediate response time of the benzodiazepines (Banazak, 1997).

We found information on the efficacy of beta blockers in the treatment of anxiety in the elderly. Small doses have been suggested for treating anxiety in the general older population (Sadavoy & LeClair, 1997), consistent with the adage "Start low and go slow." In demented elders, higher doses of propranol may help control aggressive behavior (Sadavoy & LeClair, 1997). The main concern with a beta blocker use among older adults is the possibility of negative interactions with some medical illnesses. Those with COPD, diabetes mellitus, renal disease, vascular disease, and congestive heart failure should not use these drugs to treat anxiety, because they may lead to hypotension, cognitive impairment, confusion, and delirium (Schneider, 1996).

For those patients with anxiety and depression, selective serotonin reuptake inhibitors (SSRIs) have recently been shown to be effective and lack the sedating properties of previous treatments. Although little research has been done with older adults (Palmer et al., 1997), these medications have been effective with younger adults. When used in conjunction with buspirone, SSRIs can effectively treat patients with coexisting depression and anxiety (Cadieux, 1996). They are also effective in treating obsessive-compulsive disorder, panic disorder, and social phobias. Other antidepressants, such as tricyclics, tend to be useful in treating obsessive-compulsive and panic disorders. Again, very little research has been done with older adults (Palmer et al., 1997).

CONCLUSION

Although very little quantitative research has been done involving anxiety in the older population, it is clear that anxiety is a definite problem for some older adults. It is often undetected due to comorbidity with medical symptoms and the tendency of older adults to underreport their symptoms. Cultural factors also contribute, as there is a tendency to simply dismiss anxious symptoms as usual fears about getting older. Certainly, the potential for loss in late life makes elders susceptible to developing pathological reactions to life stressors. Fortunately, converging evidence suggests that many anxiety disorders experienced by older adults are treatable through psychological, pharmacological, or combination treatments. An important area of future investigation is how the course of anxiety may change in late life for those who have been afflicted for many years. Geriatric anxiety is a topic rich with clinical and scientific possibilities.

STUDY QUESTIONS

1. What area of research could lead to a new categorization of anxiety disorders in older adults? Why is this important?
2. What differences exist between those with early-onset and those with late-onset anxiety disorders?
3. Why is agoraphobia difficult to diagnose in older adults?
4. How does PTSD symptomology differ in older versus younger combat veterans?
5. Why is an aging person with anxiety and depression worse off than an elder with just an anxiety disorder?
6. What is the main difficulty in examining the comorbidity of dementia and anxiety disorders?
7. How are social relationships related to anxiety in the demented elderly?
8. Explain the negative cycle of anxiety due to a medical condition.

9. How does the issue of control factor into anxiety as it relates to a medical condition?
10. Why would CBT be inappropriate for the demented elder?
11. What is the main problem with traditional forms of relaxation therapy in the elderly population?
12. Why is drug treatment of anxiety difficult with seniors?
13. Which of the benzodiazepines are preferred for use in the elderly? Why?
14. What are some of the advantages of buspirone over the benzodiazepines? What are the disadvantages?
15. Why are beta blockers not the best choice for drug treatment of anxiety in the elderly?
16. How can antidepressants be used to treat anxiety disorders?

SUGGESTED READINGS

Beck, J.G., Stanley, M.A., & Zebb, B.J. (1996). Characteristics of generalized anxiety disorder in older adults: A descriptive study. *Behavior Research and Therapy, 34,* 225–234.
Orrell, M. & Bebbington, P. (1996). Psychosocial stress and anxiety in senile dementia. *Journal of Affective Disorders, 39,* 165–173.
Hocking, L.B. & Koenig, H.G. (1995). Anxiety in medically ill older patients: A review and update. *International Journal of Psychiatry in Medicine, 25,* 221–238.
Sheikh, J.I. & Salzman, C. (1995). Anxiety in the elderly: Course and treatment. *Psychiatric Clinics of North America, 18,* 871–883.

REFERENCES

Acierno, R., Hersen, M., & Van Hasselt, V.B. (1996). Anxiety-based disorders. In M. Hersen & V.B. Van Hasselt (Eds.), *Psychological treatment of older adults: An introductory text* (pp. 149–180). New York: Plenum Press.
Alessi, C.A., & Cassel, C.K. (1996). Medical evaluation and common medical problems. In J. Sadavoy, L.W. Lazarus, & L.F. Jarvik (Eds.), *Comprehensive review of geriatric psychiatry II* (2nd ed., pp. 251–285). Washington DC: American Psychiatric Press.
Alexopoulos, G.S. (1990). Anxiety-depression syndromes in old age. *International Journal of Geriatric Psychiatry, 5,* 351–353.
Alexopoulos, G.S., Vrontou, C., Kakuma, T., Meyers, B.S., Young, R.C., Klausner, E., & Clarkin, J. (1996). Disability in geriatric depression. *American Journal of Psychiatry, 153,* 877–885.
American Psychiatric Association. (1994). *Diagnostic and statistical manual of mental disorders* (4th ed.). Washington, DC: Author.
Baldwin, R.C., & Tomenson, B. (1995). Depression in later life: A comparison of symptoms and risk factors in early and late onset cases. *British Journal of Psychiatry, 167,* 649–652.
Banazak, D.A. (1997). Anxiety disorders in elderly patients. *Journal of the American Board of Family Practice, 10,* 280–289.
Beck, J.G., Stanley, M.A., & Zebb, B.J. (1995). Psychometric properties of the Penn State Worry Questionnaire in older adults. *Journal of Clinical Geropsychology, 1,* 33–42.

Beck, J.G., Stanley, M.A., & Zebb, B.J. (1996). Characteristics of generalized anxiety disorder in older adults: A descriptive study. *Behavior Research and Therapy, 34,* 225–234.

Beekman, A.T.F., Bremmer, M.A., Deeg, D.J.H., Van Balkom, A.J.L.M., Smit, J.H., De Beurs, E., Van Dyck, R., & Tilburg, W.V. (1998). Anxiety disorders in later life: A report from the longitudinal aging study, Amsterdam. *International Journal of Geriatric Psychiatry, 13,* 717–726.

Blazer, D., George, L.K., & Hughes, D. (1991). The epidemiology of anxiety disorders: An age comparison. In C. Salzman & B.D. Lebowitz (Eds.), *Anxiety in the elderly: Treatment and research* (pp. 17–30). Berlin, Germany: Springer.

Brown, T.A., DiNardo, P.A., & Barlow, D.H. (1994). *Anxiety Disorders Interview Schedule for DSM-IV.* Albany: State University of New York, Phobia and Anxiety Disorders Clinic Center for Stress and Anxiety.

Cadieux, R.J. (1996). Azapirones: An alternative to benzodiazepines for anxiety. *American Family Physician, 53,* 2349–2353.

Cassileth, B.R., Lusk, E.J., Strouse, T.B., Miller, D.S., Brown, L.L., & Cross, P.A. (1985). A psychological analysis of cancer patients and their next of kin. *Cancer, 55,* 72–76.

Castillo, C.S., Schultz, S.K., & Robinson, R.G. (1995). Clinical correlates of early-onset and late-onset poststroke generalized anxiety. *American Journal of Psychiatry, 152,* 1174–1179.

Cohen-Mansfield, J. (1986). Agitated behaviors in the elderly, II: Preliminary results in the cognitively deteriorated. *Journal of the American Geriatric Society, 34,* 722–727.

Davidson, J.R.T., Kudler, H.S., Saunders, W.B., & Smith, R.D. (1990). Symptom and comorbidity patterns in World War II and Vietnam veterans with post-traumatic stress disorder. *Comprehensive Psychiatry, 31,* 162–170.

DeBerry, S., Davis, S., & Reinhard, K.E. (1989). A comparison of meditation-relaxation and cognitive behavioral techniques for reducing anxiety and depression in a geriatric population. *Journal of Geriatric Psychiatry, 22,* 231–247.

Department of Veteran Affairs, Office of Public Affairs. (1993). Keeping track of the veteran population. *Vanguard, 15,* 6–7.

Diefenbach, G.J., Stanley, M.A., Beck, J.G., Novy, D., Averill, P.M., Bourland, S., & Shack, A. (1999, November). *Worry topics reported by older adults with generalized anxiety disorder.* Poster presented at the annual meeting of the Association for Advancement of Behavior Therapy, Toronto, Canada.

Eisdorfer, C., Cohen, D., Paveza, G.J., Ashford, J.W., Luchins, D.J., Gorelick, P.B., Hirschman, R.S., Freels, S.A., Levy, P.S., Semla, T.P., et al. (1992). An empirical evaluation of the Global Deterioration Scale for staging Alzheimer's disease. *American Journal of Psychiatry, 149,* 190–194.

Felton, B.J., Revenson, T.A., Hinrichsen, G.A. (1984). Stress and coping in the explanation of psychological adjustment among chronically ill adults. *Social Science Medicine, 18,* 889–898.

Fernandez, F., Levy, J.K., Lachar, B.L., & Small, G.W. (1995). The management of depression and anxiety in the elderly. *Journal of Clinical Psychiatry, 56,* 20–29.

First, M.B., Gibbon, M., Spitzer, R.L., & Williams, J.B.W. (1997). *Structured Clinical Interview for DSM-IV Axis I disorders.* New York: Biometrics Research Department.

Flint, A.J. (1994). Epidemiology and comorbidity of anxiety disorders in the elderly. *American Journal of Psychiatry, 151,* 640–649.

Flint, A.J., & Rifat, S.L. (1997). Anxious depression in elderly patients: Response to antidepressant treatment. *American Journal of Geriatric Psychiatry, 5,* 107–115.

Folks, D.G., & Fuller, W.C. (1997). Anxiety disorders and insomnia in geriatric patients. *Geriatric Psychiatry, 20,* 137–163.

Forsell, Y., & Winblad, B. (1997). Anxiety disorders in non-demented and demented elderly patients: Prevalence and correlates. *Journal of Neurology, Neurosurgery, and Psychiatry, 62,* 294–295.

Förstl, H., Satel, H., & Bahro, M. (1993). Clinical features of Alzheimer's disease. *International Review of Psychiatry, 5,* 327–349.

Fuentes, K., & Cox, B.J. (1997). Prevalence of anxiety disorders in elderly adults: A critical analysis. *Journal of Behavioral Therapy and Experimental Psychiatry, 28,* 269–279.

Gallo, J.J., Rabins, P.V., Iliffe, S. (1997). The "research magnificent" in late life: Psychiatric epidemiology and the primary health care of older adults. *International Journal of Psychiatry in Medicine, 27,* 185–204.

Gradman, T.J., Thompson, L.W., & Gallagher-Thompson, D. (1999). Personality disorders and treatment outcome. In E. Rosowsky, R.C. Abrams, & R.A. Zweig (Eds.), *Personality disorders in older adults: Emerging issues in diagnosis and treatment* (pp. 69–94). Mahwah, NJ: Erlbaum.

Hamilton, M. (1959). The assessment of anxiety states by rating. *British Journal of Medical Psychology, 32,* 50–55.

Hocking, L.B., & Koenig, H.G. (1995). Anxiety in medically ill older patients: A review and update. *International Journal of Psychiatry in Medicine, 25,* 221–238.

Karajgi, B., Rifkin, A., Doddi, S., & Kolli, R. (1990). The prevalence of anxiety disorders in patients with chronic obstructive pulmonary disease. *American Journal of Psychiatry, 147,* 200–201.

Katon, W., Von Korff, M., Lin, E., Lipscomb, P., Russo, J., Wagner, E., & Polk, E. (1990). Distressed high utilizers of medical care, *DSM-III-R* diagnoses and treatment needs. *General Hospital Psychiatry, 12,* 355–362.

Knauper, B., & Wittchen, H.U. (1994). Diagnosing major depression in the elderly: Evidence for response bias in standardized diagnostic interviews? *Journal of Psychiatric Research, 28,* 147–164.

Lindesay, J. (1997). Phobic disorders and fear of crime in the elderly. *Aging and Mental Health, 1,* 81–86.

Lindesay, J., Briggs, K., & Murphy, E. (1989). The Guy's Age Concern Survey: Prevalence rates of cognitive impairment, depression, and anxiety in an urban elderly community. *British Journal of Psychiatry, 155,* 317–329.

Livingston, G., Manela, M., & Katona, C. (1997). Cost of community care for older people. *British Journal of Psychiatry, 171,* 56–69.

Magai, C., & Cohen, C.I. (1998). Attachment style and emotion regulation in dementia patients and their relation to caregiver burden. *Journal of Gerontology: Psychological Sciences, 53,* 147–154.

Manela, M., Katona, C., Livingston, G. (1996). How common are the anxiety disorders in old age? *International Journal of Geriatric Psychiatry, 11,* 65–70.

Marks, I.M., & Matthews, A.M. (1979). Brief standard self-rating for phobic patients. *Behavior Research and Therapy, 17,* 263–267.

Marsh, C.M. (1997). Psychiatric presentations of medical illness. *Geriatric Psychiatry, 20,* 181–204.

Martin, L.M., Fleming, K.C., & Evans, J.M. (1995). Recognition and management of anxiety and depression in elderly patients. *Mayo Clinic Proceedings, 70,* 999–1006.

McNally, R.J. (1994). *Panic disorder: A critical analysis.* New York: Guilford Press.

Menza, M.A., & Liberatore, B.J. (1998). Psychiatry in the geriatric neurology practice. *The Neurology of Aging, 16,* 611–633.

Meyer, T.J., Miller, M.L., Metzger, R.L., & Borkovec, T.D. (1990). Development and validation of the Penn State Worry Questionnaire. *Behavior Research and Therapy, 28,* 487–495.

Miller, M.D., & Silberman, R.L. (1996). Using interpersonal therapy with depressed elders. In S.H. Zarit & B.G. Knight (Eds.), *A guide to psychotherapy and aging* (pp. 83–99). Washington, DC: American Psychological Association.

Mintzer, J.E., & Brawman-Mintzer, O. (1996). Agitation as a possible expression of generalized anxiety disorder in demented elderly patients: Toward treatment approach. *Journal of Clinical Psychiatry, 57,* 55–63.

Musil, C.M. (1998). Gender differences in health and health actions among community dwelling elders. *Journal of Gerontological Nursing, 24,* 30–38.

Orrell, M., & Bebbington, P. (1996). Psychosocial stress and anxiety in senile dementia. *Journal of Affective Disorders, 39,* 165–173.

Palmer, B.W., Jeste, D.V., & Sheikh, J.I. (1997). Anxiety disorders in the elderly: DSM-IV and other barriers to diagnosis and treatment. *Journal of Affective Disorders, 46,* 183–190.

Parmelee, P.A., Lawton, M.P., & Katz, I.R. (1998). The structure of depression among elderly institution residents: Affective and somatic correlates of physical frailty. *Journal of Gerontology: Psychological Sciences, 53,* 155–162.

Patterson, R.L., O'Sullivan, M.J., & Speilberger, C.D. (1980). Measurement of state and trait anxiety in elderly mental health clients. *Journal of Behavioral Assessment, 2,* 89–97.

Pecknold, J.C. (1997). A risk-benefit assessment of buspirone in the treatment of anxiety disorders. *Drug Safety, 16,* 118–132.

Penninx, B., Beekman, A., Ormel, J., Kriegsman, D., Boeke, A., Van Eijk, J., & Deeg, D. (1996). Psychological status among elderly people with chronic disease: Does type of disease play a part? *Journal of Psychosomatic Research, 40,* 521–534.

Person, D.C., & Borkovec, T.D. (1995). *Anxiety disorders among the elderly: Patterns and issues.* Paper presented at the 103rd annual convention of the American Psychological Association, New York.

Powers, C.P., Wisocki, P.A., & Whitbourne, S.K. (1992). Age differences and correlates of worrying in young and elderly adults. *Gerontologist, 32,* 82–88.

Regier, D.A., Boyd, J.H., Burke, I.D., Rae, D.S., Myes, J.K., Kramer, M., Robins, L.N., George, L.K., Karno, M., & Locke, B.Z. (1988). One-month prevalence of mental disorders in the United States: Based on five epidemiologic catchment area sites. *Archives of General Psychiatry, 45,* 977–986.

Rickard, H.C., Scogin, F., & Keith, S. (1994). A one-year follow-up of relaxation training for elders with subjective anxiety. *Gerontologist, 34,* 121–122.

Robins, L.N., Heizer, J.E., Croughan, J., & Ratcliff, K.S. (1981). National Institute of Mental Health Diagnostic Interview Schedule: Its history, characteristics, and validity. *Archives of General Psychiatry, 38,* 381–389.

Robinson, P. (1998). Behavioral health services in primary care: A new perspective for treating depression. *Clinical Psychology: Science and Practice, 5,* 77–89.

Rosenzweig, A., Prigerson, H., Miller, M.D., & Reynolds, C.F. (1997). Bereavement and late-life depression: Grief and its complications in the elderly. *Annual Review of Medicine, 48,* 421–428.

Sadavoy, J., & LeClair, J.K. (1997). Treatment of anxiety disorders in late life. *Canadian Journal of Psychiatry, 42,* 28–34.

Salzman, C. (1991). Pharmacologic treatment of the anxious elderly patient. In C. Salzman & B.D. Lebowitz. (Eds.), *Anxiety in the elderly: Treatment and research* (pp. 149–173). New York: Springer.

Salzman, C. (1992). *Clinical geriatric psychopharmacology* (2nd ed.). Baltimore: Williams & Wilkins.

Sanavio, E. (1988). Obsessions and compulsions: The Padua Inventory. *Behavior Research and Therapy, 26,* 169–177.

Schneider, L.S. (1996). Overview of generalized anxiety disorder in the elderly. *Journal of Clinical Psychiatry, 57,* 34–45.

Schnurr, P.P., Aldwin, C.M., Spiro, A., III, Stukel, T., & Keane, T. (1993). *A longitudinal study of PTSD symptoms in older veterans.* Paper presented at the American Psychological Association Conference, Toronto, Canada.

Scogin, F. (2000). *The first session with seniors.* San Francisco: Jossey-Bass.

Scogin, F., Floyd, M., & Richard, H.C. (1998). The Relaxation Inventory: Reliability, validity, and factor structure with older adults. *Journal of Clinical Geropsychology, 4,* 235–240.

Scogin, F., Rickard, H.C., Keith, S., Wilson, J., & McElreath, L. (1992). Progressive and imaginal relaxation training for elderly persons with subjective anxiety. *Psychology and Aging, 7,* 418–424.

Segal, D.L., Hersen, M., Van Hasselt, V.B., Kabacoff, R.I., & Roth, L. (1993). Reliability of diagnosis in older psychiatric patients using the Structured Clinical Interview for *DSM-III-R. Journal of Psychopathology and Behavioral Assessment, 15,* 347–356.

Segal, D.L., Kabacoff, R.I., Hersen, M., Van Hasselt, V.B., & Ryan, C.F. (1995). Update on the reliability of diagnosis in older psychiatric outpatients using the Structured Clinical Interview for *DSM-III-R. Journal of Clinical Geropsychology, 1,* 313–321.

Sheikh, J.I., & Salzman, C. (1995). Anxiety in the elderly: Course and treatment. *Psychiatric Clinics of North America, 18,* 871–883.

Small, G.W. (1997). Recognizing and treating anxiety in the elderly. *Journal of Clinical Psychiatry, 58,* 41–47.

Small, G.W., & Bystritsky, A. (1997). Double-blind placebo controlled trial of two doses of abecarnil for geriatric anxiety. *Journal of Clinical Psychiatry, 58,* 24–29.

Smith, S.L., Sherrill, K.A., & Colenda, C.C. (1995). Assessing and treating anxiety in elderly persons. *Psychiatric Services, 46,* 36–42.

Snell, F.I., & Padin-Rivera, E. (1997). Post-traumatic stress disorder and the elderly combat veteran. *Journal of Gerontological Nursing, 23,* 13–19.

Speilberger, C.D., Gorsuch, R.C., & Lushene, R.E. (1970). *Manual for the State-Trait Anxiety Inventory.* Palo Alto, CA: Consulting Psychologists Press.

Stanley, M.A., & Beck, J.G. (1998). Anxiety disorders. In M. Hersen & V.B. Van Hasselt (Eds.), *Handbook of clinical geropsychology* (pp. 217–238). New York: Plenum Press.

Stanley, M.A., Beck, J.G., & Glassco, J.D. (1996). Treatment of generalized anxiety in older adults: A preliminary comparison of cognitive-behavioral and supportive approaches. *Behavior Therapy, 27,* 565–581.

Stanley, M.A., Beck, J.G., & Zebb, B.J. (1996). Psychometric properties of four anxiety measures in older adults. *Behaviour Research and Therapy: Behavior Assessment, 34,* 827–838.

Stein, M.B., Heuser, J.L., Juncos, J.L., Uhde, T.W. (1990). Anxiety disorders in patients with Parkinson's disease. *American Journal of Psychiatry, 147,* 217–220.

Stokes, P.E., & Holtz, A. (1997). Fluoxetine tenth anniversary update: The progress continues. *Clinical Therapeutics, 19,* 1135–1250.

Taylor, S., McCracken, C.F.M., Wilson, K.C.M., & Copeland, J.R.M. (1998). Extent and appropriateness of benzodiazepine use. *British Journal of Psychiatry, 173,* 433–438.

Thompson, J.W., Burns, B.J., Bartko, J., Boyd, J.H., Taube, C.A., & Bourdon, K.H. (1988). The use of ambulatory services by persons with and without phobia. *Medical Care, 26,* 183–198.

Vickers, R. (1988). Medical aspects of aging. In L. Lazarus (Ed.), *Essentials of geriatric psychiatry* (pp. 65–101). New York: Springer.

Wands, K., Merskey, H., Hashinsky, V.C., Fisman, M., Fox, H., Bonifero, M. (1990). A questionnaire investigation of anxiety and depression in early dementia. *Journal of the American Geriatrics Society, 39,* 535–538.

Weissman, M.M., Myers, J.K., Tischler, G.L., Holzer, C.E., Leaf, P.J., Orvaschel, H., & Brody, J.A. (1985). Psychiatric disorders *(DSM-III)* and cognitive impairment among the elderly in a U.S. urban community. *Acta Psychiatrica Scandinavica, 71,* 366–379.

Wisocki, P.A. (1988). Worry as a phenomenon relevant to the elderly. *Behavior Therapy, 19,* 369–379.

Wisocki, P.A., Handen, B., & Morse, C.K. (1986). The Worry Scale as a measure of anxiety among homebound and community active elderly. *Behavior Therapist, 5,* 91–95.

CHAPTER 6

Mood Disorders in Older Adults

DEBORAH A. KING AND HOWARD E. MARKUS

CASE STUDY

Mrs. S. was a 76-year-old widowed mother of three children who came to the Clinic for Older Adults, an ambulatory psychiatric clinic for seniors, at the behest of her oldest son, Roger. When first greeted in the waiting room, Mrs. S. was sitting on the edge of her seat wringing her hands, looking anxiously from one corner of the room to another. Roger was sitting next to his mother, slumped in his chair and visibly irritated. Once she was alone with the interviewer, Mrs. S. explained that she was terribly upset because her bowel was no longer working. She had been constipated for five days and took this as evidence that her bowel had "died" and that she would likely be dead within a matter of days. She further stated that she had been to see her primary care physician repeatedly for the problem and got only false reassurances that she was basically healthy, but needed to adjust her diet and take a daily fiber supplement. She then tearfully related how "fed up" her children were with her and her bowel problems, and fervently asked the interviewer not to tell Roger that she had been talking about her problems again. She hinted that her children would be better off without her because "they just don't understand what I'm going through and are too busy with their own lives to worry about me." When asked if she had other difficulties, Mrs. S. stated only that she was quite lonely and wished her children would visit more frequently.

In response to specific questions about depressive signs and symptoms, Mrs. S. stated that her sleep had been quite interrupted for the past several months and that she woke typically around 5 A.M. with abdominal cramping and fears about dying. She estimated that in the past six months she had lost about 20 pounds, in part because she had lost her appetite and in part because she was afraid to eat and "clog up" her body. The interviewer then attempted to establish the point in time that most of the current difficulties began, but Mrs. S. was unable to offer any specific time line. When asked if there was anything she enjoyed, she replied that it was impossible for her to enjoy anything because of her medical problems. Although she had been an avid reader in the past, she now found it difficult to focus or concentrate on anything other than her bowel. She also stated that she was unable to go to church or other activities because of pain and cramping in her abdomen. When asked if her problems had gotten so bad that she thought about dying or

141

hurting herself, her eyes welled with tears and she admitted that she asked the Lord each night to take her and put her out of her misery. The interviewer asked Mrs. S. if she had had any unusual experiences that would be difficult to understand or explain to others, such as seeing things that others could not see or hearing voices or other sounds that others could not hear. Mrs. S. looked surprised at this question, saying, "You must really think I'm crazy . . . I guess everyone does!" The interviewer reassured her that this was not the case, but that she needed to ask a range of questions about experiences that people sometimes have when they have been through a very difficult time in terms of medical or emotional stress. At that point, she acknowledged that there were times at night, just before drifting off to sleep, when she felt the presence of her late husband. She denied hearing or seeing him, but felt that at times he came to be near her to offer comfort.

At this point, the interviewer asked if Mrs. S. would give permission for Roger to join the interview to add his perspective to her description of her problems. Roger joined the interview, stating angrily that his mother's "physical obsessions" were totally false and that she needed to "get a grip" on herself. At one point, he began to vehemently remind his mother that they had "been to all the doctors" and they had denied that she had any malignancy or other life-threatening illness. He then turned back to the psychologist and explained that he used to have his mother stay at home with him and his wife every other weekend, but had stopped inviting her over because her "obsessions" were driving him and his wife crazy. He further reported that his younger brother, Harry, was no longer speaking to Mrs. S. because she seemed so "down" and "self-absorbed." Similarly, his younger sister, Peggy, limited her interactions with Mrs. S. to a 10-minute "check-in" phone call each Wednesday night. When asked about friends or social supports for Mrs. S. outside of the family, Roger related that his mother had derived much satisfaction from her local church and from volunteer work at a local nursing home until recent months, when she began isolating herself in her apartment. Outside of these activities, she had few social contacts except for one surviving sibling, who was failing in a nursing home, and her children. The interviewer then asked Roger if he had a sense of when his mother began to have her current difficulties. He reported that she had been "an anxious worrier" all her life but that things had gotten much worse five or six months ago, when her older sister Harriet died unexpectedly from a stroke.

When asked how she was coping with this loss, Mrs. S. initially turned away and then wept bitterly. She began to describe how Harriet had been her close companion throughout life and especially since Mrs. S.'s husband died 10 years earlier of a protracted cardiac illness. After this brief release of sorrow, she then abruptly asked that the interview be terminated because she could not imagine how any of this could help her with her "real" problem.

DSM-IV CRITERIA FOR THE MAJOR MOOD DISORDERS FOUND IN OLDER ADULTS

Broadly speaking, mood disorders are diagnostic categories in which disturbance in mood is the central psychiatric feature. Mood disorders encompass affective, physiological, and cognitive symptoms. According to the fourth edition of the *Diagnostic and Statistical Manual of Mental Disorders* (American Psychiatric Association [APA], 1994), mood disorders can be divided into four general clusters depressive disorders (i.e., major depression, dysthymic disorder, and depressive disorder not otherwise specified), bipolar disorders (i.e., bipolar I, bipolar II, cyclothymic disorder, and bipolar disorder not otherwise specified), mood disorders due to a general medical condition, and substance-induced mood disorders. Mood disorders are distinguished from each other by means of specific diagnostic criteria, symptom severity, longevity, etiology, and personal history. We will focus on depressive disorders, as these are the most prevalent and most concerning mood disorder found in older adults. Although the other disorders are addressed, this chapter emphasizes the etiology, diagnosis, and treatment of unipolar major depression in older persons. The case of Mrs. S. is used throughout the chapter to highlight key factors and symptoms that facilitate a differential diagnosis of her mood disorder.

DEPRESSIVE DISORDERS

Depressive disorders are the most frequently occurring mood disorders found in old age. These disorders must be distinguished from normal fluctuation in mood and periods of sadness, demoralization, or bereavement. A clinical disorder reflects a severity and disruption in overall functioning that is significant, distressful, enduring, and in marked contrast to preepisodic status. When assessing elderly patients, clinicians must be mindful not to overlook or discount relevant symptoms and change in functioning due to a biased expectation that depression is a normal and inevitable result of the aging process or a normal response to a medical illness.

Major Depression

To meet *DSM-IV* diagnostic criteria for major depression, individuals must evidence depressed mood and/or a loss of interest in pleasurable activities nearly all day and every day for at least two weeks. In addition, they must experience at least three or more of the following symptoms, for a total of at least five depressive symptoms: significant weight change (i.e., a 5% weight change within a one-month period), sleep disturbance (i.e., insomnia or hypersomnia), psychomotor agitation or retardation, low energy, poor concentration, feelings of worthlessness or guilt, poor concentration, and recurrent thoughts of death or suicide. Cognitive impairments such as diminished decision-making ability, poor concentration, and slowed processing speed often become manifest in older depressed persons. Learning and memory deficits also are likely to become prominent with age. *DSM-IV* criteria allow clinicians to specify the nature of several depressive features. *Depression with psychotic features* (i.e., hallucinations or delusions) is more common in older cohorts than in their younger counterparts (Blazer, 1999). Another specification is *major depression with melancholic features*. Melancholia is an intense, intractable form of depression characterized by loss of interest or pleasure in all or almost all activities, worsening of mood in the morning, early morning awakening, psychomotor retardation or agitation, significant weight loss, or excessive guilt. The identification of psychotic features and melancholic features is important for determining the most appropriate treatment regimen.

Dysthymic Disorder

Dysthymic disorder is a chronic, enduring, yet less severe form of depression in which the individual experiences depressed mood and at least two additional symptoms of appetite disturbance, sleep dysregulation, fatigue, low self-esteem, poor concentration, and a sense of hopelessness for a period of at least two years (APA, 1994). Older persons with a dysthymic disorder may also demonstrate increased social isolation and tearfulness (Butler, Lewis, & Sunderland, 1998). Although dysthymic disorder and major depressive disorder share many similar symptoms, they are different in intensity and duration of symptoms. Individuals with dysthymic disorder may develop major depression. The course of such "double depression" may involve recurrent episodes of major depression separated by episodes of dysthymia.

Major Depression Due to a General Medical Condition

There are many medical illnesses that are associated with symptoms of depression. This diagnosis is reserved for conditions in which the disrupted mood is the direct physiological result of a specific medical condition. Common medical conditions whose symptoms mimic depression include multiple sclerosis, Cushing's disease, Parkinson's disease, Huntington's disease, Addison's disease, cerebrovascular disease, hypothyroidism, and chronic obstructive pulmonary disease. There are also nutritional problems, such as B12 deficiency, that cause lethargy and fatigue such as that associated with depression. Accordingly, a laboratory diagnostic workup and physical examination should be routinely completed to rule out physical illness as the cause of depressive symptoms. It should be noted, however, that some have questioned the utility of making a dichotomous distinction between major depression and major depression due to a general medical condition within the older adult population (Caine, Lyness, King, & Conners, 1994). Mood disorder is actually a *final common pathway* for the expression of a wide variety of pathological processes that become more predominant with age. Thus, the line between "functional" and "organic" becomes increasingly difficult to define as age increases.

A Diagnostic Caveat

One must be mindful that the syndromic diagnostic criteria set forth in the *DSM-IV* may not adequately capture the various ways in which depressive disorders are expressed by older adults. Older patients are less likely to report depressed mood, guilt, low self-esteem, and suicidal ideation (Baker, 1996; Blazer, 1994; Caine, Lyness, & King, 1993; Lyness et al., 1995; Marin, 1990), but more likely to present with somatic complaints (e.g., constipation, abdominal cramps, weight loss, aches), feelings of anxiety, psychomotor abnormalities, cognitive dysfunction, suicidal behavior, and delusions of a somatic or persecutory nature (Alexopoulos, 1996; Baker, 1996; Blazer, 1999; Butler et al., 1998; Caine et al., 1993). Thus, clinicians and researchers alike must be aware of the vast clinical and etiological heterogeneity of depressive disorders in late life.

Bipolar Disorders

The *DSM-IV* diagnostic criteria for bipolar disorders include a disturbance in mood characterized by one or more episodes of elevated or irritable mood and the presence of inflated self-esteem, decreased need for sleep, pressured speech, distractibility, flight of ideas, psychomotor agitation, increased goal-directed activity, and excessive involvement in goal-directed or pleasurable activities (APA, 1994). Elevated or irritable mood must be accompanied by at least two of the additional criteria in order for a diagnosis of a bipolar illness to be made.

Four categories of bipolar disorders exist: bipolar I disorder, bipolar II disorder, cyclothymic disorder, and bipolar disorder not otherwise specified. These disorders are distinguished by the severity and intensity of the experienced manic symptoms as well as the presence or absence of a major depressive episode.

Individuals with a bipolar I disorder have experienced one or more manic or mixed episodes as well as one or more episodes of major depression. People who have a bipolar II disorder have experienced one or more major depressive episodes and at least one hypomanic episode (i.e., a less severe manic episode) and no manic episodes. Cyclothymic disorder is characterized by a chronic fluctuation in mood that never achieves a full manic or major depressive episode as far as intensity and duration.

There is a relative deficiency in the amount of information known about bipolar illnesses in the older adult population. As in the depressive disorders, older individuals who suffer from a bipolar illness often present in a manner that differs from the criteria set forth in the *DSM-IV*. At present, there is no consensus on the similarities and differences in clinical features that may exist when comparing younger and older cohorts. However, older individuals may demonstrate increased agitation, irritability, hostility, and paranoia as well as mixed episodes of dysphoria, mania, and hypomania (Blazer, 1999; Koenig, 1997). Cognitive dysfunction such as attention deficits, memory problems, and delirium during manic episodes is also common in the older population (Chen, Altshuler, & Spar, 1998). Koenig notes that euphoria is less common and impaired cognitive functioning is more likely in late-life bipolar disorders. Chen et al. summarize the existing literature and conclude that older adults may experience more frequent mood cycles and longer duration of manic episodes and have a greater likelihood of relapse into a depressive episode following mania. Some studies have found that there is a greater latency period between an initial depressive episode and first onset of mania in this population, averaging approximately 15 years (Broadhead & Jacoby, 1990; Tohen, Shulman, & Satlin, 1994).

The likelihood of an individual's experiencing a manic episode for the first time in old age is relatively low. The onset of a bipolar illness typically occurs in late adolescence or early adulthood. Manic episodes in older adults are more likely the result of a general medical condition, tumors, cerebrovascular disease, a neurological disorder, closed head trauma, or the direct result of a psychoactive substance (Alexopoulos, 1996; Butler et al., 1998; Chen et al., 1998; Shulman, 1996). These episodes, often referred to as secondary mania, occur in the absence of any previous mood disorder history.

SUBSTANCE-INDUCED MOOD DISORDERS

The use of narcotics and alcohol, medication, and/or exposure to an environmental toxin may foster the occurrence of a mood disorder. Sedatives, hypnotics, and anxiolytic use and/or dependence are not uncommon in the older adult population. A range of medications commonly used to treat medical conditions in the elderly, such as cardiovascular drugs, antihypertensives, sedatives, central nervous system drugs, and cancer treatments, are associated with mood disturbances (Koenig, 1997). Both depressive and manic episodes may result from exposure to these substances.

DIFFERENTIAL DIAGNOSIS

Psychologists are often called on to assist in the differentiation of appropriate diagnoses. This task is complicated when working with elderly individuals due to the frequency of comorbid psychological and medical disorders. Common differential diagnosis questions include distinguishing between depression and bereavement and differentiating the presence of a true mood disorder versus an adjustment disorder with depressed mood or disturbed conduct. Clinicians must also be able to account for the comorbid symptoms of depression with anxiety, and discriminate between the expected cognitive decline due to the normal aging process as opposed to cognitive deficits due to either a mood disorder or dementia.

Grief and bereavement are time-limited emotional disturbances that result from the loss of an emotionally meaningful relationship or a cherished possession. The experience of bereavement is often characteristic of a major depressive episode in which an individual may report a subjective sense of sadness, irritability, fatigue, and anxiety as well as vegetative symptoms such as insomnia, decreased appetite, and weight loss. Although reactions to loss are far from universal, empirical evidence enables distinctions between normal and abnormal grief reactions (Stroebe, van den Bout, & Schut, 1994). In general, a diagnosis of major depressive disorder is not indicated unless the symptoms of bereavement go unattenuated for two or more months beyond the loss. In addition, the presence of profound guilt, thoughts that one would be better off dead, morbid preoccupation with own worthlessness, decreased psychomotor activity, prolonged functional impairment, and hallucinations (that go beyond the common "hearing" or transient images of the deceased) are suggestive of a mood disorder rather than bereavement alone (APA, 1994).

It is not uncommon for older adults to experience anxiety and agitation during an episode of a mood disorder. Older individuals who appear anxious may be suffering from an underlying depression. Accordingly, it becomes important to be able to distinguish between an "agitated depression" and a concurrent anxiety disorder. This distinction is made through careful assessment for other diagnostic features of depression as well as the presence or history of manic symptoms. Depressed mood, nervousness, and disturbed behavior that occur within three months of a clear psychosocial stressor may reflect an adjustment disorder and not a depressive episode. Accordingly, it is important to determine if there has been a clear precipitating event to the noted change in functional status.

It is often difficult to distinguish between deficits in cognitive and behavioral functioning that are due to a mood disorder from those caused by dementia. This is further complicated by the fact that depression and dementia may, in fact, exist comorbidly. The tendency for many depressed elderly individuals to present with cognitive dysfunction (e.g., decreased concentration, impaired memory) led to the classification of a depressive syndrome known as the *dementia syndrome of depression* or *pseudodementia*. The symptoms of pseudodementia were once thought to be transient and reversible. There is, however, a growing body of research that suggests that the distinct alterations in cerebral functioning that occur in depression do not always improve and increase the risk for future irreversible dementia (King & Caine, 1996). Differentiating between depression and dementia is difficult and is best accomplished through interdisciplinary collaboration and the use of neuropsychological tests, patient self-report, and caregiver report. There are some noteworthy distinctions between the presentation of depression and that of dementia in older adults. Depressive symptoms may be common to both, yet individuals with a mood disorder typically present with more severe symptoms of depression and less severe cognitive deficits (Kaszniak & Christenson DiTraglia, 1994). Depressed elderly patients are more likely to complain of memory problems than are their counterparts with dementia, and older adults with dementia are more likely to overestimate their memory ability despite evidence to the contrary. Depressed individuals often show compromised "free recall" but adequate memory recognition, whereas those who suffer from dementia demonstrate impaired recall and recognition memory skills. Last, depressed patients are more likely to report an abrupt onset of symptoms and demonstrate variability in their mental status.

DIAGNOSTIC IMPRESSION OF MRS. S.

Mrs. S. clearly met the syndromic criteria for a melancholic major depressive episode. Since the death of her sister, approximately six months prior to her clinic presentation, she had been experiencing depressed mood, anhedonia (i.e., having lost interest and pleasure in her volunteer work and other previously pleasurable activities), and significant weight loss, as well as worsening of mood in the morning. Additionally, her sleep was described as "quite interrupted" with early morning wakenings. Concentration and ability to maintain cognitive focus were impaired. Mrs. S. also noted feelings of worthlessness and guilt about being a burden to her grown children. Last, she reported having re-current thoughts of death and praying to die. Mrs. S. did not report a history of or recent hypomanic or manic symptoms. It is important to note that Mrs. S. herself did not describe *feeling* depressed but instead focused on somatic (i.e., "vegetative") symptoms. It was her son who provided the observations about depressed mood.

According to her primary care physician, Mrs. S.'s symptoms were not due to the direct physiological effects of either medication or a general medical condition. Furthermore, there was no evidence of alcohol or other substance use. Although Mrs. S. denied experiencing auditory or visual hallucinations, she seemed initially to be experiencing a persistent, false belief about her body (i.e., that her bowel had "died") that was in direct contradiction to her primary care physician's assessment. To assess the possible existence of depression with psychotic features or a delusional disorder, psychotic type, the inter-viewer asked further questions to clarify the nature and intensity of Mrs. S.'s beliefs about her intestinal malady. In response to several questions about how someone's bowel or intestine could actually "die," she acknowledged that this probably was impossible but that something was indeed terribly wrong inside her lower abdomen. When asked how to make sense of her doctor's report that she was basically healthy, she stated that the physician had good intentions and was trying to shield her from bad news. From this discussion, it was de-cided that there was not conclusive evidence of psychosis and that the patient demonstrated grossly intact reality testing (i.e., she was aware that it was not truly possible for one's bowel to die). Although it was clear that her thinking needed to be monitored regularly, her intestinal complaint and focus on her GI system appeared to be a persistent, somatic rumination that had not yet reached psychotic proportions.

EPIDEMIOLOGICAL DATA

Estimates of the prevalence of mood disorders in the older adult population vary according to research method. Large-scale studies, such as the Epidemio-logic Catchment Area survey (ECA) and the Established Populations for Epi-demiologic Studies of the Elderly (EPESE) have sought to quantify the rates of psychiatric disorders among the adult and aged populations. Yet caution must be used when interpreting the results of wide-scale epidemiologic investiga-tions due to multiple methodological and conceptual shortcomings (Blazer, 1994; Caine, Lyness, King, & Conners, 1994; Nussbaum, 1997; Roberts, Kaplan, Shema, & Strawbridge, 1997).

Epidemiological studies have been faulted for being overly rigid in applying inclusion criteria, inconsistent in the method used to assess the presence of a mood disorder (i.e., diagnostic criteria vs. symptom checklists), variable in their findings secondary to method of assessment (e.g., self-report vs. diagnos-tic interview; cross-sectional vs. longitudinal design), and biased by sampling technique. Snowdon (1990), for example, indicates that prevalence surveys of depression in older persons can be divided into *low-prevalence conclusions* and *high-prevalence conclusions* based on the employed research methods. Caine et al. (1994) note that there is a great deal of heterogeneity in the presentation of mood disorders in older adults, as well as comorbid medical illnesses, that are artificially excluded from clinical research and may lead to underdetection of psychopathology. Older adults demonstrate a tendency to underreport the presence and severity of depressive symptoms, making studies that rely on self-report suspect (Lyness et al., 1995). Diagnostic categories are dichotomous, whereas symptom checklists provide clinical data on a continuum. Accordingly, Gatz, Kasl-Godley, and Karel (1997) caution that an individual can attain a high score on a symptom checklist while not meeting the diagnostic criteria for a particular disorder.

Clearly, mood disorders in late life may be more difficult to detect and current research shortcomings limit the conclusions that can be made. Nevertheless, the aggregate data suggest that the prevalence of mood disorders is less common in the older adult population. Some evidence suggests that a curvilinear relationship between age and depression exists across the lifespan. Early adulthood and late adulthood (over the age of 75) appear to be the ages in which depression is most prevalent (Gatz et al., 1997). Older adults who have experienced a previous depression are more likely to experience a recurrence of their illness. In particular, those who are 70 years and older are significantly more likely to experience a relapse of their clinical symptoms (Reynolds, Frank, Dew, et al., 1999). Similarly, older adults who receive maintenance treatment during the first year are still significantly more likely to experience a recurrence of major depression (Reynolds, Frank, Perel, et al., 1999). There is growing evidence of a cohort effect in which the prevalence and relapse rates of depression are increasing and the age of initial onset is decreasing for successive generations. Accordingly, future generations of older adults will likely experience greater rates of depressive disorders (Blazer, 1994; Gatz et al., 1997). Although the overall rates of depressive disorders may be lower in older populations, the risk of suicide is greater (Conwell, 1994).

Most studies delineate between elderly who live in the community and those who reside in an institutionalized setting (e.g., nursing home, hospital) or seek care at an outpatient clinic. Although estimates vary across studies, the prevalence of major depression in individuals 65 years old and above who live in the community is between 1% and 3% (Blazer, 1999; Butler et al., 1998). Major depression is significantly more common in acute care or chronic care settings, with prevalence rates ranging from 12% to 20% (Blazer, 1999). Approximately 2% of the community-dwelling older adult population meet the diagnostic criteria for a dysthymic disorder (Blazer, 1994). Females are more likely to experience major depression or dysthymia than their male counterparts (Blazer, 1999). Few differences in prevalence rates cross-culturally have been documented; however, little is known about cultural and racial variability.

An even more striking picture emerges when the prevalence of clinically significant symptoms of depression that do not meet the full diagnostic criteria for major depression are assessed. Estimates suggest that approximately 8% to

15% of the community-living elderly experience depressive symptoms that are disruptive to their daily living (Blazer, 1999; Marin, 1990). Alexopoulos (1996) reports that up to 27% of older adults who live in the community report clinically significant depressive symptoms. The incidence of institutionalized elderly with clinically significant, functionally impairing symptoms of depression ranges from approximately 25% to 30% (Alexopoulos, 1996; Koenig, 1997).

Bipolar disorders in the elderly occur less frequently than in younger adults. Approximately 0.1% of the community-dwelling older adult population (as compared to 1.4% of younger adults) meet the diagnostic criteria for a bipolar illness (Alexopoulos, 1996). Again, concurrent medical conditions may overlap and misdiagnosis may confound epidemiologic findings (Koenig, 1997).

THEORIES OF DEPRESSION IN OLDER ADULTS

Mental health problems result from a complex blend of factors at the biological, psychological, and social levels of organization (Engel, 1980), the particular combination of which varies greatly across individuals. Many of the risk factors for depression in older adults are similar to those of young adulthood, for example, female gender, stressful life events, and lack of a supportive social network, but there are also some differences. It has been noted that genetic factors play a lesser role in the depression of older adults, whereas other biological factors such as medical illness and age-associated changes in the central nervous system play a greater role (Caine et al., 1993). Likewise, older adults experience normative changes in thinking and cognition, as well as altered or lost social roles and relationships, all of which may contribute to the onset of depression.

One useful model for understanding how biological and psychosocial factors combine to cause depression is the *diathesis stress* model. According to this model, an individual has a biological vulnerability to depression, which then becomes manifest when triggered by psychosocial factors, such as stressful life events. Here we review a variety of biological, psychological, and social theories of depression that have been applied specifically to older adults.

BIOLOGICAL THEORIES

Aging leads to changes in several neurobiological systems that have been implicated in the pathogenesis of depression. Age-associated changes in brain structure and chemistry, sleep architecture, and neuroendocrine systems are among the most prominent systems featured in theories of late-life depression.

Neuroanatomical Changes and Depression

Computed tomography (CT) and magnetic resonance imaging (MRI) are methods for obtaining static images of the brain. These techniques have revealed an increase in brain abnormalities of older depressed adults compared to nondepressed individuals of similar age (Coffey, Figiel, Djang, & Weiner, 1990; Nussbaum, 1994; Robinson, Morris, & Federoff, 1990). Although a vast heterogeneity of methods hampers interpretation of findings, there is some evidence of a relationship among age, changes in both white and gray matter of the brain, and depression. Specifically, older depressed patients have both central and cortical atrophy on CT scans (Jacoby & Levy, 1980; Morris & Rapoport, 1990), as well as an increased number of diffuse high-signal subcortical hyperintensities on T2-weighted MRI images (Rabins, Pearlson, & Aylward, 1991; Zubenko, Sullivan, & Nelson, 1990). These neuroimaging abnormalities have been associated with neuropsychological impairment (Lesser et al., 1991; Nussbaum, Kazniak, & Allender, 1991; Pearlson, Rabins, & Kim, 1989), suggesting that the well-documented cognitive impairments of older depressives may constitute a marker for subtle cerebral changes that influence the course of depression in the elderly (King, Caine, Conwell, & Cox, 1991; King, Cox, Lyness, & Caine, 1995; Nussbaum, Kaszniak, Allender, & Rapcsak, 1995). Alternatively, these impairments may be early indicators of brain disease such as Alzheimer's or other forms of dementia (Alexopoulus, 1996; Nussbaum, 1997).

Studies of stroke patients revealed an association between lesions in subcortical (especially the left basal ganglia) and frontal (especially left frontal) brain regions and depression (Robinson & Starkstein, 1991; Starkstein et al., 1991). Similar findings have emerged from functional neuroimaging methods (e.g., positron-emission tomography, PET, and single photon emission computed tomography, SPECT) that allow the examination of regional brain function by demonstrating regional metabolic rate or perfusion. Carefully conducted studies of younger depressives revealed decreased activity in frontal (especially left frontal) and subcortical (basal ganglia) brain regions (Baxter, Schwartz, & Phelps, 1989; Delvenne, Delecluse, & Hubain, 1990; Martinot, Hardy, & Feline, 1990). Combined with neuropsychological test findings of a similar pattern of cognitive dysfunction in depressed patients and patients with subcortically based diseases, such as Huntington's disease (Massman, Delis, Butters, Dupont, & Gillin, 1992), these studies suggest that depression is caused or mediated by subcortical brain changes or by disruption of the pathways bridging frontal and subcortical regions. However, in contrast to these investigations of younger patients, functional neuroimaging studies of older depressives have revealed widespread regional dysfunction (Sackheim, Prohovnik, & Moeller, 1990; Upadhyaya, Abou-Saleh, & Wilson, 1990), consistent with neuropsychological studies indicating a range of cognitive impairments in older depressives (King et al., 1995) or impairments that go beyond the typical subcortical pattern (Speedie, Rabins, & Pearlson, 1990). Rather than pointing to frontal and subcortical dysfunction, these latter studies suggest instead that late-life depression is associated with more diffuse cortical involvement. Further investigations are needed that follow early- and late-onset older depressives over time, combining careful diagnostic procedures with functional imaging techniques. Such longitudinal studies will provide a more thorough understanding of the relationship among neuroanatomical changes, cognitive dysfunction, and depression, while at the same time helping to clarify whether late-onset depression has a distinct etiologic basis.

Neurochemical Changes and Depression

Depression has been associated with medications that reduce the supply of certain brain neurotransmitters known as catecholamines and indoleamines (Goodwin & Bunney, 1973; Post, 1996), whereas improvement in depression has been associated with medications that increase the functional level of these neurotransmitters (Post, 1996; Schildkraut, 1973). These empirical findings, many of which were serendipitous, led to the biogenic amine hypothesis of depression, which maintains that depression results from a depletion of neurotransmitters, especially norepinephrine (NE) and serotonin, and that mania results from an increase in these neurotransmitters.

Controlled studies comparing the levels of biogenic amines or their metabolites in the cerebrospinal fluid or blood of depressed individuals have yielded mixed results (Akiskal, 1996; Post, 1996). However, there is some evidence that levels of monoamine oxidase (MAO), an enzyme that breaks down NE in the brain, increases markedly with age, supporting the notion that late-life depression results from depleted brain catecholamine. Although the amine hypothesis of depression (and late-life depression) has not received unequivocal support, it has provided meaningful links to psychopharmacologic interventions proven effective in treating depression.

Other Biological Theories

Compared to younger adults, older adults sleep less, experience more interrupted sleep, and experience decreased latency in the onset of rapid eye movement (REM) after falling asleep. Depressed individuals of all ages exhibit these same characteristic changes in sleep, especially the decreased REM latency. These findings led to the notion that disruption of circadian rhythms may be involved in the etiology of late-life depression (Blazer, 1999). Indeed, abnormalities in sleep architecture are noted to be among the most robust biological findings associated with depression and may represent a marker for underlying brain dysfunction that causes or mediates depressive illness.

Another biological theory of depression involves the neuroendocrine system, specifically the hypothalamic-pituitary-adrenal (HPA) axis. Hyperactivity of the HPA axis, resulting in relative hypersecretion of cortisol by the adrenal cortex, is evidenced by elevated cortisol levels at baseline or lack of suppression of cortisol when exogenous glucocorticoids are administered. It is commonly recognized that depressed individuals have elevated levels of cortisol, a finding that led to the development of the dexamethasone suppression test (DST) as a potential marker for treatment-responsive depression. There is evidence of increased cortisol secretion with age and even one report of an interactive effect of age, depressed state, and hypercortisolemia on neuropsychological deficits (Rubinow, Post, & Savard, 1984). However, depressed older adults are no more likely to demonstrate abnormal cortisol levels than younger depressed persons. Although

HPA axis abnormalities continue to be a focus of inquiry among some depression researchers, the DST has not proven to be a useful tool for the diagnosis of major depression because of its limited specificity.

Biological Treatment of Mood Disorders in Late Life

Pharmacotherapy has been proven effective for treatment of major depression in older adults at all levels of severity, with effectiveness rates from clinical trials ranging from 50% to 70% (Gerson, Plotkin, & Jarvik, 1988; Niederehe & Schneider, 1998). There are several classes of antidepressants with demonstrated usefulness in older adults, including selective serotonin reuptake inhibitors (SSRIs; fluoxetine, paroxetine, and sertraline) and related medications (including nefazodone, venlafaxine, buproprion, and trazodone); tricyclic antidepressants (TCAs, such as nortriptyline, desipramine, and doxepin), and monoamine oxidase inhibitors (MAOIs, such as phenelzine, tranylcypromine, and isocarboxazid). The SSRIs are relatively free of cardiovascular and other side effects associated with TCAs and MAOIs, making these preparations especially useful with older adults (Blazer, 1999). Pharmacotherapy is especially indicated for the treatment of depression with psychotic or melancholic features, as psychosocial treatments alone generally have been found to be ineffective when these features are present. Research indicates that the combination of psychotherapy and pharmacotherapy is the most effective treatment for major depression (Reynolds, Frank, Perel, et al., 1999; Thompson et al., 1991), perhaps because the two forms of treatment may target different types of symptoms or because psychotherapy may begin to reduce symptoms while antidepressant medication is yet to take effect. All medications have potential contraindications and side effects, to which older adults are especially vulnerable. Therefore, careful medical evaluation is conducted prior to the use of antidepressant medication, and, depending on the preparation used, laboratory, cardiovascular, or other medical studies may be indicated at regular intervals.

Patients with bipolar illness are treated with different medications, such as lithium carbonate, valproic acid, or carbamazapine. Like the antidepressant medications used to treat unipolar disorders, these medications are used only after careful medical evaluation and require ongoing clinical and laboratory follow-up to rule out contraindications and guard against toxic reactions.

Electroconvulsive therapy (ECT) is a safe and effective treatment for depression in older adults (Blazer, 1999; Mulsant & Sweeney, 1997). It is typically the treatment of choice for older adults with severe depressions that have not responded to pharmacotherapy or for those whose medical conditions, such as cardiovascular disease, prevent the use of antidepressant medication. Treatment usually involves a course of 6 to 12 sessions, followed by a course of antidepressant medication or maintenance ECT delivered at relatively less frequent intervals. Despite adverse publicity to the contrary, ECT is relatively lacking in side effects, except for transient memory loss or more permanent loss of memory for the events surrounding the period of treatment. However, because administration of ECT does temporarily increase intracranial pressure, it is contraindicated or used with great caution when individuals have certain medical conditions, including space-occupying cerebral tumors, retinal detachment, recent stroke or heart attacks, and cerebral aneurysms.

PSYCHOLOGICAL THEORIES

There are a variety of psychological approaches to the understanding and treatment of late-life depression. Here we focus on several major theories, representing psychodynamic, cognitive, and behavioral viewpoints, that have given rise to treatments specifically adapted to the needs of older adults. Where applicable, the case of Mrs. S. is used to highlight how theory helps to inform treatment.

Psychodynamic Approaches

In his classic work, *Mourning and Melancholia* (1975), Freud postulated that vulnerability to depression was caused by major disappointment in a significant interpersonal relationship early in life. According to this view, the early loss or disruption led to a lifelong pattern of relating to others with marked ambivalence, as well as a tendency to respond to actual or threatened interpersonal loss with self-destructive feelings and impulses. Depression was viewed as the result of unexpressed rage toward the lost love object that is turned inward on the self. Freud also noted the profound loss of self-esteem and self-reproach and guilt associated with melancholia.

Whereas classical psychoanalytic formulations of psychopathology focused predominately on intrapsychic conflict resulting from internal drive states, such as sex and aggression, post-Freudian developments in psychodynamic theory focused on the fundamental need for human attachment and the dynamic development of the self in relation to others (cf. Bowlby, 1977; Kohut, 1971). Here we focus on two specific approaches, self psychology and interpersonal psychology, because these have been applied most extensively to the understanding and treatment of psychopathology in older adults.

Self Psychology.   Self psychology views depression and other mental illnesses as resulting from a defect in the overall structure of the self that is derived from disturbances in "self/self object" relationships early in life. In developmental terms, the self object is the early caregiver who is consistently available to actively reflect, validate, and differentiate the emotions and needs of the young child. The self object provides a consistent "mirroring" presence that supports the development of basic trust in one's caregiver and forms the basis for a positive, stable sense of one's identity and worth. A child deprived of any such early, formative self/self object bond fails to develop the internal capacity for self-soothing during times of distress or crisis and becomes excessively reliant on others for this function. Thus, an adult who never developed adequate endogenous "supplies" of self-worth may compensate for such a deficit by maintaining one or more close, mirroring relationships that perform the supportive, self object function. If faced with the loss of such a significant relationship or its mirroring function because of death or serious illness, this vulnerable individual is prone to self-fragmentation resulting in agitation, despair, depression, or even suicidal impulses. Consistent with this view, there is considerable evidence of an association between early loss of a parent and later depression and/or suicidal behavior in young and middle-aged adults (Kaslow et al., 1998; Oakley Brown, Joyce, Wells, Bushnell, & Hornblow, 1995). Although older adults may be expected to experience the loss of a loved one relatively frequently and these losses may precipitate a depressive response, there has been little research addressing whether depression in older adults is associated with early childhood loss (Kivela, Luukinen, Koski, Viramo, & Pahkala, 1998).

Older adults experience more frequent threats to the self, as the aging process brings irrevocable changes in physical health, appearance, and social relationships. Loss of vitality and previous capabilities represent enormous assaults to the ability to maintain a stable sense of one's identity and worth, especially for those whose self-esteem was previously associated with mastery and leadership roles. Kohut's concept of the "bipolar self" provides a useful heuristic for understanding the necessary self-transformations precipitated by the physical, cognitive, and social changes of aging (Muslin, 1992). The pole of values, representing the beliefs and attitudes internalized from caregivers and one's culture, and the pole of ambitions, representing the assertive strivings that allow one to fulfill one's values, both must be transformed. With increasing age, the pole of values shifts from ideals involving action and achievement to ideals involving wisdom, mentoring, or advising. Accordingly, the pole of ambitions must be altered to incorporate these new ideals. Older adults who are unable to negotiate this transformation may become despairing or depressed. For example, one's self-esteem may be heavily invested in the ability to successfully *do* things, such as earn money or play tennis or care for others, to the point that one is unable to successfully negotiate the normative transition from doer to mentor or advisor.

Self psychology maintains that the cure or healing of psychopathology lies in the therapeutic relationship and the restitution of self/self object bonds. Two therapeutic goals are fundamental to self psychological approaches to treatment of older adults, irrespective of whether the therapy is conceived of as supportive (i.e., focused primarily on restoring a sense of equilibrium to a self that is significantly fragmented or in disarray) or insight-oriented (i.e., focused primarily on gaining a dynamic, historical understanding of the genesis of the patient's difficulties through a process of self-exploration). First, the therapist aims to establish a therapeutic bond that will provide the missing functions of the patient's fragmented self. The therapist assumes a consistently mirroring, supportive stance, providing infusions of self-worth to a patient otherwise depleted of self-esteem. For example, the therapist pays exquisite attention to the elder's unique background and history, frequently reflecting back to the patient the defining elements of his or her personal accomplishments, values, and identity. The patient is encouraged to bring in photos and other personal memorabilia that facilitate this process. The therapist allows the patient to develop a positive, idealized transference and offers demonstrations of admiration of the patient by making supportive telephone contacts or writing letters that reflect back to the patient the sense that he or she is valued and worthy of attention. To reinforce the self/self object bond, the therapist does not actively interpret the idealized transference or its roots in earlier relationships.

The second goal of therapy is to facilitate the transformation of values and ambitions from active, assertive ideals and strivings to those centered on the attainment of wisdom and the guidance of others. This often involves confrontation and interpretation of shame experienced by those elders who are no longer able to work or actively care for others. Some older adults view themselves as useless and burdensome to others in the face of their normative increase in dependency needs on the younger generations. These feelings and images must be actively explored in the context of the mirroring self/self object relationship with the therapist, a relationship that by its very nature contradicts the elder's distorted view of self as unworthy of attention or caring.

Life review therapy (Butler, 1963) is a psychodynamic approach consistent with the basic tenets of self psychology and the life cycle theory of development of Erik Erikson (1968). Erikson conceived of human development as a series of epigenetic stages, each characterized by dynamic tension between a positive and negative outcome (e.g., "basic trust versus mistrust," "autonomy versus shame"). The final developmental task, "ego integrity versus despair," involves the integration of life experiences and the resolution of old conflicts in order to face with equanimity the prospect of one's own impending demise. Butler noted that older adults engage in a natural process of reminiscence or "summing up," during which they take stock of their successes and failures, joys and disappointments. He suggested that psychotherapy capitalize on this natural process and developed life review therapy as a technique for helping elders construct a meaningful and sustaining personal story (Lewis & Butler, 1974). Consistent with the self object function that is central to self psychology, the stance of the life review therapist is one of a supportive, mirroring other who listens intently to the elder's life history and actively reflects back unique, defining elements to be integrated into the elder's own personal narrative.

Turning to the case of Mrs. S. as an illustration, the therapist used life review as a means of helping her resolve her grief about her sister's death (a precipitant of her depressive episode). The life review began when the therapist asked Mrs. S. if she would be willing to say more about her life, including her relationship with her sister. This discussion was framed as a means of "better understanding all that you have been through in life, leading up to your current problems." Mrs. S. complied with this request, revealing that she had been the second oldest of seven children growing up in a family with few financial resources. Her father was a salesman who died of a heart attack in his early 40s and her mother was hospitalized several times during Mrs. S.'s childhood and adolescence for what appeared to be a recurrent depressive illness. During these episodes, the children lived in various foster homes for periods of time lasting weeks or months. Mrs. S. and Harriet were actually the primary caretakers for their five younger siblings, as well as for their mother, who frequently took to her bed for days on end. Recounting this history, Mrs. S. began to grieve the loss of her sister, as well as the loss of her primary role as family caretaker. The therapist responded with empathic reflections of Mrs. S.'s profound pain and sorrow, while at the same time acknowledging how she and Harriet had sustained each other through remarkable hardship, relying on each other's resilience and strength through their entire lives. The therapist also reinforced the theme of Mrs. S.'s identity as a "caretaker who always tended to others," occasionally reflecting how difficult it must be now to be the one who needed help.

Interpersonal Psychology.   In addition to self psychology and life review approaches, another useful adaptation of classic psychoanalytic theory was formulated by Harry Stack Sullivan (1953). He underscored the pivotal importance of a patient's current social relationships in determining psychological health or distress. Building on this view, Klerman, Weissman, and Rounsaville (1984) developed interpersonal therapy (IPT) for unipolar ambulatory depression. This short-term psychodynamic treatment approach focused on four interpersonal risk factors that are especially relevant for older adults: grief, interpersonal role disputes, role transitions, and interpersonal deficits. IPT typically involves 12 to 16 weekly sessions focused on two sets of goals. First, the therapy aims to reduce depressive symptoms and improve self-esteem. Second, treatment is focused on the development of more effective strategies for dealing with current social and interpersonal problems. The therapist assumes a supportive, patient advocate stance while actively helping the patient focus on current areas of interpersonal difficulty and guiding the patient toward more adaptive resolution of these relationship problems. Like other psychodynamic approaches, IPT recognizes the importance of early developmental relationships and transference feelings toward the therapist, but uses this material only as it manifests in current relationships with significant others.

Effectiveness of Psychodynamic Approaches.   Evidence of the effectiveness of psychodynamic and self psychological treatment approaches to depression in older adults is limited largely to anecdotal case reports of longer-term treatments and a few empirical reports of the general effectiveness of life review and time-limited methods. Contrary to Freud's early admonitions against treating "older" patients (i.e., patients over 50 years) because of the supposed inflexibility of the mental processes with age, case-based reports have long since suggested that psychodynamic techniques can be used successfully with adults in the sixth through tenth decades of life (Muslin, 1992; Meyers, 1991). In fact, there is some evidence that older adults may be more compliant with therapy and less likely to drop out (Niederehe, 1994), perhaps because of a realization that there is a finite amount of time left to solve their problems.

Outcome studies of life review and related reminiscence approaches have been difficult to evaluate because of the wide variety of therapeutic techniques employed and the vast diagnostic heterogeneity of subjects sampled. There is some evidence that these approaches result in decreased levels of depressive symptoms in individuals with mild to moderate depression, but data are lacking regarding efficacy with severe depression (Bortz & O'Brien, 1997; Niederehe,

1994). Indeed, some clinical observers have reported negative effects of eliciting life review from individuals with severe, ruminative depression, obsessive tendencies, or life histories unlikely to yield a positive review. Brief, time-limited psychodynamic approaches have been more amenable to empirical study because they were developed with the goal of resolving clearly defined, circumscribed problems, such as depressive symptoms, self-esteem, or interpersonal functioning, rather than aiming to create lasting changes in insight or personality. One such study of brief psychodynamic therapy of older adults (Lazarus & Groves, 1987) replicated earlier findings of symptomatic relief and focal problem improvement without increased insight or self-understanding. Results indicated that the relationship with the therapist was used to reestablish a positive and stable sense of self in terms of normalcy and competence. Exploration of gender differences in this study revealed that women responded sooner, had a greater degree of improvement, and sustained improvements longer than men. Results of another study of 91 depressed patients age 60 years and older treated with brief psychodynamic, cognitive, or behavioral therapy revealed that patients in all treatment groups showed improvement relative to controls, with 52% of patients attaining full remission of major depression after treatment for 16–20 weeks (Thompson, Gallagher, & Breckenridge, 1987). The authors concluded that their findings supported the efficacy of psychotherapy as a treatment for depression in older adults.

IPT has received significant empirical attention, at least in part because it has a treatment manual specifically adapted for elderly patients. One randomized comparative treatment trial found IPT to be equally effective to nortriptyline (NTP) at 6 and 16 weeks in the treatment of older adults with depression, although IPT resulted in lower dropout rates than NTP (Schneider, Sloane, Staples, & Bender, 1986). Another study of 187 nonpsychotic elderly individuals with recurrent unipolar depression suggested that combined treatment with IPT and NPT was superior to either IPT or NPT alone in terms of preventing or delaying recurrence of depression (Reynolds, Frank, & Perel, et al., 1999). Moreover, the remission rates and time to remission in this study were comparable to those of a group of midlife patients with recurrent depression.

Cognitive and Behavioral Approaches
The comprehensive cognitive theory of Aaron Beck and colleagues (1976) maintained that depression was associated with a negatively distorted view of oneself, one's world, and one's future. Older adults may be especially prone to cognitive distortions, particularly regarding the true nature or prognosis of medical illnesses or their own perceived value to family members or friends. This tendency toward a negative appraisal of one's health or worth may be due in part to the ageist stereotypes of Western culture that old age is synonymous with frailty, dementia, and being a burden to others (Butler, Lewis, & Sunderland, 1998). Another related but distinct cognitive theory of depression is the social problem-solving model of Nezu and colleagues (Nezu, 1987; Nezu & Perri, 1989). This approach maintains that depression results from poor coping and problem-solving skills when one is under stress. Accordingly, problem-solving therapy

consists of five components, the first of which involves examination of beliefs and expectations about life's problems and one's own problem-solving skills. The remaining four components involve learning a set of skills: problem definition and formulation, generation of alternative solutions, decision making, and solution implementation and verification. Early reports have indicated that this model can be successfully applied to the treatment of late-life depression (Arean et al., 1993).

Behavioral theorists allow that distorted cognitions may play a role in depression, but posit that cognitions do not determine behavior in a causal sense. Instead, reinforcement contingencies are viewed as the primary determinants of behavior and behavior change. Lewinsohn's (1974) theory of depression emphasized the role of pleasant and unpleasant activities in determining positive or negative mood. Older adults may be especially vulnerable to experiencing fewer daily pleasant events because of age-associated stressors such as retirement, medical illness in self or others, and loss of significant others. Accordingly, behavioral assessment and treatment techniques have been developed specifically for depressed older adults (Teri, 1991) and older adults who have comorbid depression and dementia (Teri, 1994).

Drawing on both cognitive and behavioral theories and treatments, Gallagher and Thompson (1983) developed a cognitive-behavioral treatment model specifically for older adults with depression. Primary elements of the treatment included daily tracking of behavior (pleasant and unpleasant events), establishing the relationship between behavior and mood, identifying behavioral aspects of the older adult's life that are amenable to change, developing social and cognitive skills to increase the frequency of pleasant events and decrease the frequency of negative events, and developing a plan for change complete with methods of tracking one's progress. The cognitive skills in this approach include teaching the older adult to monitor negative self-statements and to correct the cognitive distortions on which they are based. These authors and others (Knight & Satre, 1999) encourage therapists to adapt their techniques to the needs of older adults by including a "socialization" process that clearly describes the collaborative, structured approach of cognitive-behavioral treatment. Accordingly, clients are told that they are expected to take an active role in setting treatment goals, monitoring their progress toward reaching goals, and changing negative patterns of behavior and thinking. This type of educational process at the outset of treatment may help older adults overcome their distrust of psychotherapy, a common attitude in this cohort of patients.

Cognitive-behavioral techniques were extremely useful in the beginning treatment sessions of Mrs. S. It was necessary to help her alter ruminative, negative self-statements and relax before she could benefit from other aspects of therapy. The therapist introduced these techniques by explaining the "strong connection between mind and body," helping Mrs. S. to understand that constantly thinking about her bowel only made her more anxious and depressed. As an example, the therapist asked Mrs. S. what kind of "self-talk" she engaged in during the morning, when she was most anxious. Mrs. S. was able to identify several anxiety-provoking self-statements, such as "Oh, I'm feeling sick this morning and it will only get worse" or "Oh, this bad bowel is going to kill me!" Moreover, Mrs. S. recognized that she felt noticeably more "sick" (i.e., anxious and depressed) when repeating these sentences. During the first few treatment sessions, Mrs. S. learned to identify her negative self-statements and to replace them with more neutral or positive self-statements (e.g., "Okay, I'm starting to feel sick, but this has never killed me before and it won't kill me now" and "I'm starting to feel anxious, but if I focus on my relaxation, this will get better"). During these initial sessions, the therapist also introduced progressive muscle relaxation as another means of interrupting negative cognitions and decreasing anxiety. This technique combined deep breathing with alternate tensing and relaxing of major muscle groups. By practicing relaxation twice daily and modifying her negative self-statements, she successfully decreased her morning anxiety and depression.

Empirical studies support the efficacy of cognitive and behavioral treatments of depression in older adults. Gallagher and Thompson (1983) compared cognitive, behavioral, and brief insight-oriented treatment approaches in a study of 38 adults age 55 years and older. They found all three treatments to be effective in reducing depressive symptoms, although the cognitive and behavioral treatment groups maintained more improvement at follow-up. As noted above, a subsequent study of 91 adults over the age of 60 found the same three therapies to be equally effective at the end of treatment and follow-up (Thompson et al., 1987). There is also evidence from this group that combining cognitive therapy with antidepressant medication was more effective than either treatment alone (Thompson et al., 1991).

SOCIAL THEORIES AND TREATMENTS

Although all of the psychological approaches to depression acknowledge the importance of social factors in the etiology and treatment of depression, they typically involve treatment of the individual patient in a setting distinct from the larger social system. Here we review approaches that conceptualize and treat the problems of the depressed older adult in the context of the family system or a group setting.

Family Systems Approaches

There are several well-developed theories of later-life family functioning and intervention (Hargrave & Anderson, 1992; Knight & McCallum, 1998; Qualls, 1995; Shields, King, & Wynne, 1995), yet there is little or no direct empirical evidence to support their applicability to the understanding and treatment of late-life depression. Most of these approaches conceive of the family as a system of interconnected "elements" such that change in any one individual's status or behavior will affect the behavior of other members in the system. For example, the strength-vulnerability model of Shields and Wynne (1997) views the mental health or illness of an individual as resulting from the interaction of individual and family life cycle processes. The family is conceived of as a system moving through time, encountering both predictable, normative transitions (e.g., retirement, grandparenthood) and unique, family-specific challenges (e.g., specific medical illnesses and losses).

Joseph Richman (1993) has written extensively on late-life suicide from a family systems perspective. He conceived of suicidal behavior as "a benevolent strategy of controlling change and coping with stress" within a family group characterized by lack of communication between generations and little tolerance for crisis or grief. According to this view, elders become depressed and suicidal as they become isolated from younger generations. In times of crisis or stress, when they require increased help or assistance, older adults may come to view themselves as burdensome and unwanted. Consistent with this view, King (in press) described a case of a supposedly "expendable elder" who was depressed and attempted suicide because of the mistaken impression that he was no longer wanted or needed by his extended family. Richman and Rosenbaum (1970) proposed that strained families of supposedly unwanted elders are actually the mediators of society's ageist attitudes, that is, that older adults are unwanted burdens at the level of culture and society. Although a comprehensive examination of societal attitudes toward the elderly is beyond the scope of this chapter, it is important to acknowledge the broader systems perspective that family attitudes toward older adults are shaped by society and culture, in the same way that older adults' self-perceptions are shaped by family attitudes.

Although empirical studies of families of older depressed adults are rare, the family literature on adult depression and suicide provides some indirect evidence for an association between impaired family functioning and increased levels of depression and/or suicidality. Families of severely depressed adults are characterized by high levels of criticism, impaired communication, and ineffective problem-solving, difficulties that in turn are associated with poor prognosis of the depression (Hinrichsen & Hernandez, 1993; Hooley & Teasdale, 1989; Keitner et al., 1995). One study revealed that high levels of expressed emotion (i.e., hostility, criticism, and emotional overinvolvement) from adult offspring of depressed older adults were associated with higher rates of relapse and lower rates of recovery from the depressive illness (Hinrichsen & Pollack, 1997). Similarly, a prospective study of suicide attempts in depressed older adults found that those who attempted suicide within one year after hospital admission had families characterized by more psychiatric symptoms, more strain in the relationship between the identified patient and family members, and more caregiving difficulties than older depressed patients who did not attempt suicide (Zweig & Hinrichsen, 1993).

Shields, King, and Wynne (1995; in press) and King, Shields, and Wynne (2000) proposed a comprehensive model for assessing and treating later-life families in a manner consistent with their level of relational development. Although outcome studies are lacking, the model has been applied to depressed older adults whose families are characterized by relational deficits in problem solving, communication, and attachment (King, in press). Critical features of this approach include a comprehensive family assessment of the following factors, summarized by the acronym LIFE: Life events or stressors experienced by the family and its individual members; Individual roles assumed by family members, especially those pertaining to caretaking, authority, and decision making; Family relational processes, including mutuality, problem solving, communication, and attachment (Wynne, 1984); and Ethnic or cultural factors that impact a family's interactional style.

Depending on the outcome of the family assessment, a level of intervention is chosen from several possible levels, each of which reflects work at successively deeper strata of family processes (Shields et al., 1995). Families with solid bonds of attachment, open and effective communication, and good problem-solving skills do not require intensive therapy but instead benefit from brief education and consultation regarding a late-life problem, such as serious medical or neurologic illness in an older family member. These families also may need support, grief work, and guidance in reorganizing the lines of authority and decision making in the family, especially if the late-onset illness has occurred in a previously capable family matriarch or patriarch (King, Bonacci, & Wynne, 1990). As noted above, families of severely depressed older adults may evidence high levels of hostility and criticism, indicative of communication problems and/or "deeper" problems in the basic bonds of attachment among family members. Attempts to help these families solve problems will be ineffective until the basic disturbance in communication or attachment is addressed. Often, weak or ambivalent bonds of attachment can be strengthened through a process of family life review, during which multiple generations of family members come together to weave a coherent intergenerational story (Hargrave & Anderson, 1992; Shields et al., 1995). This process allows younger adult family members to gain a different, more empathic perspective of the depressed older adult as they learn about the elder's early life circumstances and struggles. However, in some instances, the bonds among family members are too severely damaged, for example, in instances of physical or sexual abuse between generations, and the therapist must focus on preventing further family abuse by helping the concerned individuals adaptively limit their interactions and dependence on one another.

Family therapy was another important component of the treatment of Mrs. S. At the beginning of therapy, Mrs. S. consented to a session that would include her children, only two of whom agreed to attend. The therapist used this time to explain the "medical basis" of depression, an approach that lessened Mrs. S.'s resistance and helped her children gain a more sympathetic perspective on their mother's suffering. The therapist further explained that depression was "a family matter" that affected everyone and, by its very nature, caused frustrations and tensions in the family. Indeed, when her children began to vent frustrations or criticisms about their mother's behavior, the therapist diplomatically intervened to stop the negative interaction by commenting on how "frustrating depression can be," thus shifting the focus of blame off of Mrs. S. and onto her depressive illness. The therapist also asked the adult offspring whether they managed to take care of themselves while at the same time "working so hard to help" their mother. These initial interventions helped to educate the family about depression while at the same time structuring their patterns of communication so that there was less tension and conflict. Additionally, inclusion of family in the early stages of treatment helped to ensure that Mrs. S.'s children would be supportive of the initial treatment plan (which included antidepressant therapy, individual therapy, and periodic family sessions).

Later in the course of treatment, when Mrs. S.'s anxious, ruminative symptoms had improved so that she was better able to engage in interactive therapy, further family sessions were conducted to address the problematic bonds of attachment that were contributing to her depression. The therapist asked Mrs. S. if she wanted to invite her estranged son, Harry, to attend the session along with the two other children, Roger and Peggy. Mrs. S. was reluctant to "burden" Harry, but agreed to call after practicing her approach to the conversation with the therapist. Indeed, all three children attended the session, which began on a positive note with Roger and Peggy noting improvements in their mother's condition. Harry, however, was doubtful about his mother's gains and began to question aggressively whether she had truly improved. Rather than allowing a familiar negative interaction to ensue, the therapist turned the discussion to Mrs. S.'s early history by explaining that depression often has roots in one's early life struggles. With support and encouragement, Mrs. S. tearfully told her children for the first time the details of her mother's mental illness and the resulting foster placements. Through this process, it was clear that the children were able to gain a more empathic perspective on their mother. It was decided to conduct one or two more family sessions to facilitate their ability to grieve the many losses they had sustained together. In addition, more sessions were needed to help the family adjust to Mrs. S.'s role transition from an active caretaker to an elder who now needed some care herself. This component of therapy began with the therapist's reviewing the multigenerational family story that had been gathered so far (including Mrs. S.'s early history of loss and family chaos, her role as family caretaker, and the history of losses that they had all shared more recently). The therapist characterized the family as a group of "survivors," at which point Harry became more active and sadly recalled the details of his father's illness and death. It became clear that he had never adequately grieved his father, nor had he adjusted to his mother's aging and gradual role transition from an active caregiver to one who now needed his care. During the last family session, Mrs. S. was able to tell her children that she wanted more frequent visits, as well as help with shopping and medical appointments. All three children agreed that they wanted to help and began formulating plans to provide this support. The therapist reinforced these suggestions, noting that Mrs. S. needed help to "retire" from her role as active caretaker and to assume a new role as senior "advisor" on family matters.

Despite numerous accounts of successful family therapy with depressed older adults, there is great need for outcome studies that test the existing models of family treatment and seek to determine the most effective approaches for specific types and severity levels of depression. The limited research that does exist (Clarkin, Haas, & Glick, 1988) indicates that most serious mental health problems are treated more successfully when family members are involved. Although caution and clinical judgment must be exercised to determine the type and timing of family intervention for depression, there is substantial evidence that depression worsens or resolves less completely when conflictual or chaotic family environments are not addressed in the treatment.

Group Approaches

Unlike the other approaches reviewed thus far, group therapy is a treatment modality that draws on existing psychological theory. Theorists such as LeBon, McDougal, Freud, and Bion were among the first to write about the powerful influence of groups on the thoughts, feelings, and behavior of individuals. Joseph Pratt, a North American therapist in the early 1900s, is widely recognized as being the "father of group therapy" and one of the first to utilize groups for therapeutic benefit. The past 40 years have seen a proliferation of theoretical perspectives on group theory and technique. Although group therapy is frequently an intervention used with elderly patients, there is no overarching unitary theory of group process that offers etiologic explanations for mood disorders in older adults. Rather, group treatments build on the theoretical assumptions of psychodynamic, cognitive, and behavioral perspectives regarding the etiology of psychopathology. Group theory assists in understanding the dynamics and process of treatment groups so that appropriate intervention strategies can be utilized.

Regardless of the theoretical orientation, multiple factors and processes emerge in group therapy that may be especially useful for older adults experiencing the losses and social isolation often associated with the aging process. Group therapy offers opportunities for a sense of connectedness, support, hope, affect expression, socialization, insight, and skill acquisition (Yalom, 1995). Group treatment approaches aim not only to reduce psychiatric symptoms, but to counteract these common life stressors, teach the use of more effective coping strategies, facilitate problem-solving skills, and create a sense of worth, caring, and acceptance. For some, group therapy is sufficient for assistance in coping and relieving psychiatric symptoms. For others, group therapy is a useful conjoint form of treatment.

Group technique with the older population does not differ markedly from that of younger cohorts. Slight modification or adaptation of intervention strategies has been useful in making this modality more acceptable to older adults. For example, length of sessions may need to be decreased, sessions may need to be held more often, out-of-group socializing may be encouraged, and accommodation of physical limitations may be necessary (Lakin, 1988). Similar to other treatment approaches, clinicians may need to be more active and make efforts to decrease the perceived stigma associated with therapy held by this age cohort.

Research has documented the efficacy of group psychotherapy in the treatment of mood disorders in older adults (Beutler et al., 1987; Steuer et al., 1984; Tross & Blum, 1988). Empirical evidence indicates that group therapy for depressed older adults can be as effective as individual therapy in bringing about symptom relief (Scogin & McElreath, 1994). Although there are few studies comparing the relative effectiveness of different group therapy orientations or techniques, it appears that group therapy with older adults is effective regard-less of the particular form it takes (Leszcz, 1990).

CONCLUSION

Mood disorders in older adults are a significant public health problem. Major depression, the most prevalent mood disorder in elderly individuals, may be difficult to detect because of the frequency of comorbid psychological and medical conditions, as well as the common misconception that it is "normal" to become depressed with increasing age. Psychologists and other mental health professionals have sought to determine the biological, psychological, and social factors causing or contributing to late-life depression. Although it has not been conclusively determined that late-life depression is a clinical entity distinct from depression arising earlier in life, studies have revealed neuroanatomic and neurochemical changes that may be characteristic of depression in older adults. In addition, the aging process is associated with distinct psychological changes, including alterations in cognition and self-identity, and distinct family challenges.

Because it is widely acknowledged that depressed older adults suffer from a complex, interactive blend of illnesses and problems, treatment is based on comprehensive, multidimensional assessment and typically integrates multiple therapeutic approaches (Koenig, 1997; Marin, 1990; Sadavoy, 1994). This chapter reviewed various biological, psychological, and social systems approaches to treatment, many of which have been proven effective in treating mood disorders in older adults. The case of Mrs. S. was used to illustrate how multiple therapeutic modalities can be combined to treat late-life depression. From a biological point of view, Mrs. S. had a positive family history of depression and suffered severe melancholic symptoms likely to respond to antidepressant treatment. From a psychodynamic perspective, she carried an early vulnerability to depression stemming from loss of significant others and unstable family relationships in childhood. Her sister's death immediately prior to the onset of her depression deprived her of a lifelong ally, whom she was unable to grieve until she experienced the solid support of another self object in the form of the therapist. Additionally, the therapeutic relationship provided a secure context from which she could begin to address the necessary transition from active caretaker to a senior advisor or mentor of the younger members of her family. Through a process of family life review, her adult offspring were able to gain a more empathic understanding of her early and current struggles, thus becoming more able and willing to provide the support she needed to overcome her depressive illness.

STUDY QUESTIONS

1. List four common ways in which older adults' presentation of depression differ from their younger counterparts.

2. Summarize the major shortcomings of the large-scale epidemiological studies of mood disorders in the elderly population.
3. Describe the variation in prevalence rates that appear to exist in community-dwelling elderly populations versus institutionalized elders.
4. Summarize the findings regarding long-term prognosis for depressed elderly patients. In particular, what factors have been attributed to a recurrence or relapse of depressive symptoms?
5. Describe the differences that have been found when comparing rates of major depression versus clinically significant symptoms of depression.
6. What is the "diathesis stress model" of depression?

SUGGESTED READINGS

Arean, P.A., Perri, M.G., Nezu, A.M., Schein, R.L., Christopher, F., & Hiseog, T.X. (1993). Comparative effectiveness of social problem-solving therapy and reminiscence therapy for depression in older adults. *Journal of Consulting and Clinical Psychology, 61,* 1003–1010.

Caine, E.D., Lyness, J.M., & King, D.A. (1993). Reconsidering depression in the elderly. *American Journal of Geriatric Psychiatry, 1,* 4–20.

Chen, S.T., Altshuler, L.L., & Spar, J.E. (1998). Bipolar disorder in late life: A review. *Journal of Geriatric Psychiatry and Neurology, 11,* 29–35.

Hinrichsen, G.A., & Pollack, S. (1997). Expressed emotion and the course of late-life depression. *Journal of Abnormal Psychology, 106,* 336–340.

Knight, B.G., & McCallum, T.J. (1998). Psychotherapy with older adult families: The contextual, cohort-based maturity-specific challenge model. In I.H. Nordus & G.R. VandenBos (Eds.), *Clinical geropsychology.* (pp. 313–328). Washington, DC: American Psychological Association.

Leszcz, M. (1990). Towards an integrated model of group psychotherapy with the elderly. *International Journal of Group Psychotherapy, 40,* 379–399.

Lyness, J.M., Cox, C., Curry, J., Conwell, Y., King, D.A., & Caine, E.D. (1995). Older age and the underreporting of depressive symptoms. *Journal of the American Geriatrics Society, 43,* 216–221.

Reynolds, C.F., III, Frank, E., Perel, J.M., Imber, S.D., Cornes, C., Miller, M., Mazumdar, S., Houck, P., Dew, M.A., Stack, J.A., Pollock, B.G., & Kupfer, D.J. (1999). Nortriptyline and interpersonal psychotherapy as maintenance therapies for recurrent major depression: A randomized controlled trial in patients older than 59 years. *Journal of the American Medical Association, 28,* 39–45.

Shulman, K.I. (1996). Recent developments in the epidemiology, co-morbidity, and outcome of mania in old age. *Reviews in Clinical Gerontology, 6,* 249–254.

REFERENCES

Akiskal, H.S. (1996). Mood disorders: Introduction and overview. In H.S. Kaplan & B.J. Sadock (Eds.), *Comprehensive textbook of psychiatry* (pp. 1067–1079). Baltimore: Williams & Wilkins.

Alexopoulos, G.S. (1996). Mood disorders. In H.S. Kaplan & B.J. Sadock (Eds.), *Comprehensive textbook of psychiatry* (pp. 2566–2568). Baltimore: Williams & Wilkins.

American Psychiatric Association. (1994). *Diagnostic and statistical manual of mental disorders* (4th ed.). Washington, DC: Author.

Arean, P.A., Perri, M.G., Nezu, A.M., Schein, R.L., Christopher, F., & Hiseog, T.X. (1993). Comparative effectiveness of social problem-solving therapy and reminiscence therapy for depression in older adults. *Journal of Consulting and Clinical Psychology, 61*(6), 1003–1010.

Baker, F.M. (1996). An overview of depression in the elderly: A U.S. perspective. *Journal of the National Medical Association, 88*, 178–184.

Baxter, L.R., Schwartz, J.M., & Phelps, M.E. (1989). Reduction of prefrontal cortex glucose metabolism common to three types of depression. *Archives of General Psychiatry, 46*, 243–250.

Beck, A.T. (1976). *Cognitive therapy and the emotional disorders.* New York: International Universities Press.

Beutler, L.E., Scogin, F., Kirkish, P., Schretlen, D., Corbishley, A., Hamblin, D., Meredith, K., Potter, R., Bamford, C.R., & Levenson, A.I. (1987). Group cognitive therapy and alprazolam in the treatment of depression in older adults. *Journal of Consulting and Clinical Psychology, 55*, 550–556.

Blazer, D.G. (1994). Epidemiology of late-life depression. In L. Schneider, C. Reynolds, III, B. Lebowitz, & A. Friedhoff (Eds.), *Diagnosis and treatment of depression in late life: Results of the NIH consensus development conference* (pp. 9–19). Washington, DC: American Psychiatric Press.

Blazer, D.G. (1999). Depression. In W.R. Hazzard, J.P. Blass, W.H. Ettinger, Jr., D.B. Halter, & J.G. Ouslander (Eds.), *Principles of geriatric medicine and gerontology* (4th ed., pp. 1331–1339). New York: McGraw-Hill.

Bortz, J.J., & O'Brien, K.P. (1997). Psychotherapy with older adults: Theoretical issues, empirical findings, and clinical applications. In P.D. Nussbaum (Ed.), *Handbook of neuropsychology and aging: Critical issues in neuropsychology* (pp. 431–451). New York: Plenum Press.

Bowlby, J. (1977). The making and breaking of affectional bonds, I: Aetiology and psychopathology in the light of attachment theory. *British Journal of Psychiatry, 130*, 201–210.

Broadhead, J., & Jacoby, R. (1990). Mania in old age: A first prospective study. *International Journal of Geriatric Psychiatry, 5*, 215–222.

Butler, R.N. (1963). The life review: An interpretation of reminiscence in the aged. *Psychiatry, 26*, 65.

Butler, R.N., Lewis, M.I., & Sunderland, T. (1998). *Aging and mental health: Positive psychosocial and biomedical approaches* (5th ed.). Boston: Allyn & Bacon.

Caine, E.D., Lyness, J.M., & King, D.A. (1993). Reconsidering depression in the elderly. *American Journal of Geriatric Psychiatry, 1*, 4–20.

Caine, E.D., Lyness, J.M., King, D.A., & Conners, L. (1994). Clinical and etiological heterogeneity of mood disorders in elderly patients. In L.S. Schneider, C.F. Reynolds, III, B.D. Lebowitz, & A.J. Friedhoff (Eds.), *Treatment and diagnosis of depression in late life: Results of the NIH consensus development conference* (pp. 23–53). Washington, DC: American Psychiatric Press.

Chen, S.T., Altshuler, L.L., & Spar, J.E. (1998). Bipolar disorder in late life: A review. *Journal of Geriatric Psychiatry and Neurology, 11*, 29–35.

Clarkin, J.F., Haas, G.L., & Glick, I.D. (1988). *Affective disorders and the family.* New York: Guilford Press.

Coffey, C.E., Figiel, G.S., Djang, W.T., & Weiner, R.D. (1990). Subcortical hyperintensity on magnetic resonance imaging: A comparison of normal and depressed elderly subjects. *American Journal of Psychiatry, 147*, 187–189.

Conwell, Y. (1994). Suicide in elderly patients. In L.S. Schneider, C.F. Reynolds, III, B.D. Lebowitz, & A.J. Friedhoff (Eds.), *Diagnosis and treatment of depression in late life* (pp. 397–418). Washington, DC: American Psychiatric Press.

Delvenne, V., Delecluse, F., & Hubain, P. (1990). Regional cerebral blood flow in patients with affective disorders. *British Journal of Psychiatry, 157,* 359–365.

Engel, G.L. (1980). The clinical application of the biopsychosocial model. *American Journal of Psychiatry, 137,* 535–544.

Erikson, E.H. (1968). *Identity, youth, and crisis.* New York: Norton.

Freud, S. (1975). Mourning and melancholia. In J. Strachey (Ed.), *Standard edition of the complete psychological works of Sigmund Freud* (Vol. 4, p. 152). London: Hogarth Press.

Gallagher, D.E., & Thompson, L.W. (1983). Treatment of major depressive disorder in older adult outpatients with brief psychotherapies. *Psychotherapy: Theory, Research, and Practice, 19,* 482–490.

Gatz, M., Kasl-Godley, J.E., & Karel, M.J. (1997). Aging and mental disorders. In J.E. Birren & K.W. Schaie (Eds.), *Handbook of the psychology of aging* (4th ed., pp. 365–382). San Diego, CA: Academic Press.

Gerson, S.C., Plotkin, D.A., & Jarvik, L.F. (1988). Antidepressant drug studies, 1964–1986: Empirical evidence for aging patients. *Journal of Clinical Psychopharmacology, 8,* 311–322.

Goodwin, F.K., & Bunney, W.E. (1973). A psychobiological approach to affective illness. *Psychiatric Annals, 3,* 19.

Hargrave, T.D., & Anderson, W.T. (1992). *Finishing well: Aging and reparation in the intergenerational family.* New York: Brunner/Mazel.

Hinrichsen, G.A., & Hernandez, N.A. (1993). Factors associated with recovery from and relapse into major depressive disorder in the elderly. *American Journal of Psychiatry, 150,* 1820–1825.

Hinrichsen, G.A., & Pollack, S. (1997). Expressed emotion and the course of late-life depression. *Journal of Abnormal Psychology, 106,* 336–340.

Hooley, J.M., & Teasdale, J.D. (1989). Predictors of relapse in unipolar depressives: Expressed emotion, marital distress, and perceived criticism. *Journal of Abnormal Psychology, 98,* 229–235.

Jacoby, R.J., & Levy, R. (1980). Computed tomography in the elderly, 3: Affective disorder. *British Journal of Psychiatry, 136,* 270–275.

Kaslow, N.J., Reviere, S.L., Chance, S.E., Rogers, J.H., Hatcher, C.A., Wasserman, F., Smith, L., Jessee, S., James, M.G., & Seelig, B. (1998). An emperical study of the psychodynamics of suicide. *Journal of the American Psychoanalytic Association, 46,* 777–796.

Kaszniak, A.W., & Christenson DiTraglia, G. (1994). Differential diagnosis of dementia and depression. In M. Storandt & G.R. VandenBos (Eds.), *Neuropsychological assessment of dementia and depression in older adults: A clinician's guide* (pp. 81–118). Washington, DC: American Psychological Association.

Keitner, G.I., Ryan, C.E., Miller, I.W., Kohn, R., Bishop, D.S., & Epstein, N.B. (1995). Role of the family in recovery and major depression. *American Journal of Psychiatry, 152,* 1002–1008.

King, D.A. (in press). The care of the "expendable elder": Family therapy with an older depressed man. In S.H. McDaniel, D.D. Lusterman, & D. Seaburn (Eds.), *A casebook for integrating family therapy.* Washington, DC: American Psychological Association.

King, D.A., Bonacci, D.D., & Wynne, L.C. (1990). Families of cognitively impaired elders: Helping adult children confront the filial crisis. *Clinical Gerontologist, 10,* 3–15.

King, D.A., & Caine, E.D. (1996). Cognitive impairment and major depression: Beyond the pseudodemential syndrome. In I. Grant & K.M. Adams (Eds.), *Neuropsychological assessment of neuropsychiatric disorders* (pp. 200–217). New York: Oxford University Press.

King, D.A., Caine, E.D., Conwell, Y., & Cox, C. (1991). Predicting severity of depression in the elderly at six month follow-up: A neuropsychological study. *Journal of Neuropsychiatry and Clinical Neurosciences, 3*, 64–66.

King, D.A., Cox, C., Lyness, J.M., & Caine, E.D. (1995). Neuropsychological effects of depression and age in the elderly sample: A confirmatory study. *Neuropsychology, 9*, 399–408.

King, D.A., Shields, C.G., & Wynne, L.C. (2000). Interventions for families of older adults. In H.S. Kaplan & B.J. Sadock (Eds.), *Comprehensive textbook of psychiatry* (7th ed.). Philadelphia: Lippincott, Williams, & Wilkins.

Kivela, S., Luukinen, H., Koski, K., Viromo, P., & Pahkala, K. (1998). Early loss of mother or father predicts depression in old age. *International Journal of Geriatric Psychiatry, 13*, 527–530.

Klerman, G.L., Weissmann, M.M., & Rounsaville, B.J. (1984). *Interpersonal psychotherapy of depression*. New York: Basic Books.

Knight, B.G., & McCallum, T.J. (1998). Psychotherapy with older adult families: The contextual, cohort-based maturity-specific challenge model. In I.H. Nordus & G.R. VandenBos (Eds.), *Clinical geropsychology* (pp. 313–328). Washington, DC: American Psychological Association.

Knight, B.G., & Satre, D.D. (1999). Cognitive behavioral psychotherapy with older adults. *American Psychological Association, 188–200*.

Koenig, H.G. (1997). Mood disorders. In P.D. Nussbaum (Ed.), *Handbook of neuropsychology and aging: Critical issues in neuropsychology* (pp. 63–79). New York: Plenum Press.

Kohut, H. (1971). *Analysis of the self*. New York: International Universities Press.

Lakin, M. (1988). Group therapies with the elderly: Issues and prospects. In B.W. MacLennan, S. Saul, & M.B. Weiner (Eds.), *Group psychotherapies for the elderly*. Madison, CT: International Universities Press.

Lazarus, L.W., & Groves, L. (1987). Brief psychotherapy with the elderly: A study of process and outcome. In J. Sadavoy & M. Leszcz (Eds.), *Treating the elderly with psychotherapy: The scope for change in later life*. Madison, CT: International Universities Press.

Leszcz, M. (1990). Towards an integrated model of group psychotherapy with the elderly. *International Journal of Group Psychotherapy, 40*, 379–399.

Lewinsohn, P. (1974). A behavioral approach to depression. In R. Friedman & M. Katz (Eds.), *The psychology of depression: Contemporary theory and research* (pp. 157–176). New York: Wiley.

Lewis, M.I., & Butler, R.N. (1974). Life-review therapy: Putting memories to work in individual and group therapies. *Geriatrics, 29*, 165–173.

Lyness, J.M., Cox, C., Curry, J., Conwell, Y., King, D.A., & Caine, E.D. (1995). Older age and the underreporting of depressive symptoms. *Journal of the American Geriatrics Society, 43*, 216–221.

Marin, R.S. (1990). Geriatric populations. In M.E. Thase, B.A. Edelstein, & M. Hersen (Eds.), *Handbook of outpatient treatment of adults: Nonpsychotic mental disorders* (pp. 513–539). New York: Plenum Press.

Martinot, J.L., Hardy, P., & Feline, A. (1990). Left prefrontal glucose hypometabolism in the depressed state: A confirmation. *American Journal of Psychiatry, 147*, 1313–1317.

Massman, P.J., Delis, D.C., Butters, N., Dupont, R.M., & Gillin, C. (1992). The subcortical dysfunction hypothesis of memory deficits in depression: Neuropsychological validation in a subgroup of patients. *Journal of Clinical and Experimental Neuropsychology, 14*, 687–706.

Meyers, W.A. (1991). Psychoanalytic psychotherapy and psychoanalysis with older patients. In W.A. Meyers (Ed.), *New techniques in the psychotherapy of older patients.* Washington, DC: American Psychiatric Press.

Morris, P., & Rapoport, S.I. (1990). Neuroimaging and affective disorders in late-life: A review. *Canadian Journal of Psychiatry, 35,* 347–354.

Mulsant, B.H., & Sweeney, J.A. (1997). Electroconvulsive therapy. In P.D. Nussbaum (Ed.), *Handbook of neuropsychology and aging: Critical issues in neuropsychology* (pp. 508–514). New York: Plenum Press.

Muslin, H.L. (1992). *The psychotherapy of the elderly self.* New York: Brunner/Mazel.

Nezu, A.M. (1987). A problem solving formulation of depression: A literature review and proposal of a pluralistic model. *Clinical Psychology Review, 7,* 121–144.

Nezu, A.M., & Perri, M.G. (1989). Social problem-solving therapy for unipolar depression: An initial dismantling investigation. *Journal of Consulting and Clinical Psychology, 57,* 408–413.

Niederehe, G.T. (1994). Psychosocial therapies with depressed older adults. In L.S. Schneider, C.F. Reynolds, III, B.D. Lebowitz, & A.J. Friedhoff (Eds.), *Treatment and diagnosis of depression in late life: Results of the NIH consensus development conference* (pp. 293–315). Washington, DC: American Psychiatric Press.

Niederehe, G.T., & Schneider, L. (1998). Treatments for depression and anxiety in the aged. In P.E. Nathan & J.M. Gordon (Eds.), *A guide to treatments that work* (pp. 270–287). New York: Oxford University Press.

Nussbaum, P.D. (1994). Pseudodementia: A slow death. *Neuropsychology Review, 4,* 71–90.

Nussbaum, P.D. (1997). Late-life depression: A neuropsychological perspective. In P.D. Nussbaum (Ed.), *Handbook of neuropsychology and aging: Critical issues in neuropsychology* (pp. 260–270). New York: Plenum Press.

Nussbaum, P.D., Kazniak, A.W., & Allender, J. (1991). Depression and cognitive deterioration in the elderly: A follow-up study. *Journal of Clinical and Experimental Neuropsychology, 13,* 100–101.

Nussbaum, P.D., Kaszniak, A.W., Allender, J., & Rapcsak, S. (1995). Cognitive decline in elderly depressed: A follow-up study. *Clinical Neuropsychologist, 9,* 101–111.

Oakley Brown, M.A., Joyce, P.R., Wells, J.E., Bushnell, J.A., & Hornblow, A.R. (1995). Disruptions in childhood parental care as risk factors for major depression in adult women. *Australian and New Zealand Journal of Psychiatry, 29,* 437–444.

Pearlson, G.D., Rabins, P.V., & Kim, W.S. (1989). Structural brain CT changes and cognitive deficits in elderly depressives with and without reversible dementia ("pseudodementia"). *Psychological Medicine, 19,* 573–584.

Post, R.M. (1996). Mood disorders: Somatic treatment. In H.S. Kaplan & B.J. Sadock (Eds.), *Comprehensive textbook of psychiatry* (pp. 1152–1178). Baltimore: Williams & Wilkins.

Qualls, S.H. (1995). Clinical interventions with later-life families. In R. Blieszner & V.H. Bedford (Eds.), *Handbook of aging and the family.* Westport, CT: Greenwood Press.

Rabins, P.V., Pearlson, G.D., & Aylward, E. (1991). Cortical magnetic resonance imaging changes in elderly inpatients with major depression. *American Journal of Psychiatry, 148,* 617–620.

Reynolds, C.F., III, Frank, E., Dew, M.A., Houck, P.R., Miller, M., Mazumdar, S., Perel, J.M., & Kupfer, D.J. (1999). Treatment of 70+-year-olds with recurrent major depression. *American Journal of Geriatric Psychiatry, 7,* 64–69.

Reynolds, C.F., III, Frank, E., Perel, J.M., Imber, S.D., Cornes, C., Miller, M., Mazumdar, S., Houck, P., Dew, M.A., Stack, J.A., Pollock, B.G., & Kupfer, D.J. (1999).

Nortriptyline and interpersonal psychotherapy as maintenance therapies for recurrent major depression: A randomized controlled trial in patients older than 59 years. *Journal of the American Medical Association, 28,* 39–45.

Richman, J. (1993). *Preventing elderly suicide.* New York: Springer.

Richman, J., & Rosenbaum, M. (1970). A clinical study of the role of the hostility and death wishes by the family and society in suicidal attempts. *Israel Annals of Psychiatry and Related Disciplines, 8,* 213–231.

Roberts, R.E., Kaplan, G.A., Shema, S.J., & Strawbridge, W.J. (1997). Does growing old increase risk for depression? *American Journal of Psychiatry, 154,* 1384–1390.

Robinson, R.G., Morris, P.L., & Federoff, J.P. (1990). Depression and cerebrovascular disease. *Journal of Clinical Psychiatry, 51,* 26–33.

Robinson, R.G., & Starkstein, S.E. (1991). Heterogeneity in clinical presentation following stroke: Neuropathological correlates. *Neuropsychiatry, Neuropsychology, and Behavioral Neurology, 4,* 1–3.

Rubinow, D.R., Post, R.M., & Savard, R. (1984). Cortisol hypersecretion and cognitive impairment in depression. *Archives of General Psychiatry, 41,* 279–283.

Sackheim, H.A., Prohovnik, I., & Moeller, J.R. (1990). Regional cerebral blood flow in mood disorders, I: Comparison of major depressive and normal controls at rest. *Archives of General Psychiatry, 47,* 60–70.

Sadavoy, J. (1994). Integrated psychotherapy for the elderly. *Canadian Journal of Psychiatry, 39,* S19–S26.

Schildkraut, J.J. (1973). Norepinephrine metabolites as biochemical criteria for classifying depressive disorders and predicting responses to treatment: Preliminary findings. *American Journal of Psychiatry, 130,* 695.

Schneider, L.S., Sloane, R.B., Staples, F.R., & Bender, M. (1986). Pretreatment orthostatic hypotension as a predictor of response to nortriptyline in geriatric depression. *Journal of Clinical Psychopharmacology, 6,* 172–176.

Scogin, F., & McElreath, L. (1994). Efficacy of psychosocial treatments for geriatric depression: A quantitative review. *Journal of Consulting and Clinical Psychology, 62,* 69–74.

Shields, C.G., King, D.A., & Wynne, L.C. (1995). Interventions with later-life families. In R.H. Mikesell, D.D. Lusterman, & S.H. McDaniel (Eds.), *Integrating family therapy: Handbook of family psychology and systems theory.* Washington, DC: American Psychological Association.

Shields, C.G., & Wynne, L.C. (1997). The strength-vulnerability model of mental health and illness in the elderly. In T.D. Hargrave & S.M. Hanna (Eds.), *The aging family: New visions in theory, practice, and reality.* New York: Brunner/Mazel.

Shulman, K.I. (1996). Recent developments in the epidemiology, co-morbidity, and outcome of mania in old age. *Reviews in Clinical Gerontology, 6,* 249–254.

Snowdon, J. (1990). The prevalence of depression in old age (Editorial). *International Journal of Geriatric Psychiatry, 5,* 141–144.

Speedie, L.J., Rabins, P.V., & Pearlson, G.D. (1990). Confrontation naming deficit in dementia of depression. *Journal of Neuropsychiatry and Clinical Neurosciences, 2,* 59–63.

Starkstein, S.E., Bryer, J.B., Berthier, M.L., Cohen, B., Price, T.R., & Robinson, T.G. (1991). Depression after stroke: The importance of cerebral hemispheric asymmetries. *Journal of Neuropsychiatry and Clinical Neurosciences, 3,* 276–285.

Steuer, J.L., Mintz, J., Hammen, C.L., Hill, M.A., Jarvik, L.F., McCarley, T., Motoike, P., & Rosen, R. (1984). Cognitive-behavioral and psychodynamic group psychotherapy in treatment of geriatric depression. *Journal of Consulting and Clinical Psychology, 52,* 180–189.

Stroebe, M., van den Bout, J., & Schut, H. (1994). Myths and misconceptions about bereavement: The opening of a debate. *Omega Journal of Death and Dying, 29,* 187–203.

Sullivan, H.S. (1953). *The interpersonal theory of psychiatry.* New York: Norton.

Teri, L. (1991). Behavioral assessment and treatment of depression in older adults. In P. Wiscocki (Ed.), *Handbook of clinical behavior therapy with the elderly client* (pp. 225–243). New York: Plenum Press.

Teri, L. (1994). Behavioral treatment of depression in patients with dementia. *Alzheimer's Disease and Associated Disorders, 8*(3), 66–74.

Thompson, L.W., Gallagher, D., & Breckenridge, J.S. (1987). Comparative effectiveness of psychotherapies for depressed elders. *Journal of Consulting and Clinical Psychology, 55,* 385.

Thompson, L.W., Gantz, F., Florsheim, M., DelMaestro, S., Rodman, J., Gallagher-Thompson, D., & Bryan, H. (1991). Cognitive-behavioral therapy for affective disorder in the elderly. In W.A. Meyers (Ed.), *New techniques in the psychotherapy of older patients* (pp. 3–19). Washington, DC: American Psychiatric Press.

Tohen, M., Shulman, K.I., & Satlin, A. (1994). First-episode mania in late life. *American Journal of Psychiatry, 151,* 130–132.

Tross, S., & Blum, J.E. (1988). A review of group therapy with the older adult: Practice and research. In B.W. MacLennan, S. Saul, M.B. Weiner, J.E. Blum, M. Linden, & J. Skigen (Eds.), *Group psychotherapies for the elderly* (pp. 3–29). Madison, CT: International Universities Press.

Upadhyaya, A.K., Abou-Saleh, M.T., & Wilson, K. (1990). A study of depression in old age using single-photon emission computerized tomography. *British Journal of Psychiatry,* (Suppl. 9), 76–81.

Wynne, L.C. (1984). The epigenesis of relational systems: A model for understanding family development. *Family Process, 23,* 297–318.

Yalom, I. (1995). *The theory and practice of group psychotherapy* (4th ed.). New York: Basic Books.

Zubenko, G.S., Sullivan, P., & Nelson, J.P. (1990). Brain imaging abnormalities in mental disorders of late life. *Archives of Neurology, 47,* 1107–1111.

Zweig, R.A., & Hinrichsen, G.A. (1993). Factors associated with suicide attempts by depressed older adults: A prospective study. *American Journal of Psychiatry, 150,* 1687–1692.

CHAPTER 7

Sexual Dysfunctions in Later Life

CLAUDIA AVINA, WILLIAM T. O'DONOHUE, AND
JANE E. FISHER

CASE STUDY

Fred was a 77-year-old married man who was referred for psychological services after being discharged from the hospital, where he had undergone treatment for a severe infection. The infection had developed as a consequence of poor vascular function secondary to diabetes. While in the hospital, Fred's physician and nurses noted that his affect was severely depressed. He usually became tearful whenever he had visitors and when asked about his wife and children. He also was observed to make comments about his body being "good for nothing" and frequently complained that there was not much reason for him to "stick around," as he was "a burden" to his family and a "lousy" father and husband. At the recommendation of his physician and the insistence of his wife, he agreed to meet with a clinical psychologist to discuss the concerns he had about his health and the stress he was experiencing in managing his advanced diabetes.

During the first interview with the psychologist, it emerged that Fred was intensely distressed by what he characterized as "impotence." He reported that he had first experienced difficulty achieving an erection about a year earlier. Shortly afterward, he began to withdraw from his wife's gestures of affection. Over the course of the year, he eventually came to rebuff all of her approaches. During the course of the interview, he tearfully explained that he was concerned that he would not be able to perform sexually and he did not want her to find out that he was "impotent." He further reported that, although he no longer seemed able to achieve an erection, he still felt sexually desirous of his wife and had in fact experienced ejaculation and orgasm since developing the erectile difficulty. In response to his fears about his sexual performance, Fred had begun sleeping in a separate room and responded angrily anytime his wife expressed concern over his well-being or tried to engage him in a conversation regarding their relationship. He also began avoiding social contacts with friends and found that he was no longer experiencing pleasure from any of the hobbies he had enjoyed throughout adulthood.

With Fred's consent, his wife was invited to participate in subsequent sessions. She reported that she was at her "wit's end" and had tried everything she knew to cheer him and encourage him to reengage with their family, friends, and her. She reported that Fred had always been a private person, but she felt very hurt and increasingly angry by his rejection of her.

During the course of the assessment process, Fred was referred to a urologist for a thorough physical examination to rule out reversible organic conditions that might contribute to his erectile difficulties. He received a diagnosis of erectile dysfunction secondary to peripheral neuropathy.

In collaboration with Fred and his wife, a treatment plan was developed that included marital therapy targeted at improving their communication and increasing their knowledge and skill in noncoital methods of sexual pleasure. In addition, Fred participated in a brief course of individual cognitive-behavior therapy targeting his beliefs about his self-worth, his functioning as a husband and father, and his views about the future. The therapy also included a behavioral activation component that focused on increasing Fred's participation in pleasant activities, including his social contacts.

In this chapter, we review the literature concerning sexual dysfunction in the elderly. We discuss how the *Diagnostic and Statistical Manual of Mental Disorders (DSM-IV;* American Psychiatric Association [APA], 1994) diagnostic criteria for sexual dysfunctions are relevant to older adults, current epidemiological information, factors related to assessing sexual functioning in this population, and how certain societal features can play a role in undermining sexuality for elderly individuals. Then, we review the empirical status of possible assessment and treatment strategies for sexual problems in older populations.

Despite evidence of negative stereotypes about sexuality and aging (Mathias, Lubben, Atchinson, & Schweitzer, 1997; O'Donohue, 1987), research indicates that most of the elderly, given acceptable opportunities, are in fact sexually active and capable. Negative stereotypes may be accounted for in part by cohort effects, such as being raised in a sexually repressive environment without a technology of effective contraceptives and with limited or no sex education, and by the influences of a youth-oriented culture.

Barker (1968) explains that these myths may accurately reflect society's perceived role of the elderly. The asexual social role has the same influence as the sick or grandparent role. The social roles are reified by reinforcement for the behavior of older adults who exhibit asexual behavior and for individuals who behave in a manner consistent with these expectations. Institutionalized settings for the elderly (e.g., nursing homes) are structured in a manner that prevents sexual interactions by residents (Fisher & O'Donohue, 1991). They often lack privacy, and rarely does institutional management view sexual behavior as appropriate. It seems worthwhile to educate management of these institutions regarding the sexual interests and abilities of the elderly so that management would provide more outlets for appropriate sexual activity. This is an example of how the maintenance of false beliefs affects the sexual behavior of the elderly as well as actions taken by others to limit this kind of behavior.

Despite negative views about sexuality and aging, many elderly continue to have meaningful sexual relationships. When sexual activity for women is reduced, it is typically due to a lack of access to a partner, health problems of their male partners, or the death of their male partners.

DIAGNOSTIC CRITERIA

Sexual dysfunction manifests itself as a disruption in one or more of the first three of four phases of the sexual response cycle, which includes desire, excitement, orgasm, and resolution, or by pain associated with sexual intercourse. The 12 sexual dysfunctions recognized by the *DSM-IV* are hypoactive sexual desire disorder, sexual aversion disorder, female sexual arousal disorder, male erectile disorder, female orgasmic disorder, male orgasmic disorder, premature ejaculation, dyspareunia, vaginismus, sexual dysfunction due to a general medical condition, substance-induced sexual dysfunction, and sexual dysfunction not otherwise specified. Absence of or low desire, absence of or insufficient arousal (subjectively and physiologically), absence or delay of orgasm, genital pain, and involuntary vaginal spasms during intercourse characterize these disorders. The diagnostic criteria are the same across the life span; however, the specific criteria can be subjectively modified by the diagnostician. For example, the diagnosis of hypoactive sexual desire disorder requires the clinician to make a judgment of deficiency or absence, taking into account "factors that affect sexual functioning such as age, and the context of the person's life" (APA, 1994, p. 498). However, it provides no normative data regarding how this judgment is to be reliably made. Prevalence data indicate that approximately 24% of the U.S. population will experience a sexual dysfunction at some point in their lives.

EPIDEMIOLOGY

There are few epidemiological studies that document the prevalence of sexual functioning of healthy and unhealthy older adults, despite the value of this information for developing appropriate service delivery and allocation of resources (Fisher, Zeiss, & Carstensen, 1993; Laumann, Paik, & Rosen, 1999; Panser et al., 1995). To date, the general design of studies groups elder adults into one category that may include an age span of over 30 years (e.g., 65 and older) or exclude this population altogether (Laumann, Gagnon, Michael, & Michaels, 1994; Laumann et al., 1999).

Initial cross-sectional studies indicated that sexual activity generally declines across the life span (Kinsey, Pomeroy, & Martin, 1948; Kinsey, Pomeroy, Martin, & Gebhard, 1953). Panser et al. (1995) reported that sexual activity declined in men age 40–79 years in a survey of 2,115 subjects. In what is probably the best-designed epidemiological study, Laumann et al. (1994) investigated the data from the General Social Life Survey for 1988–1991 and for 1993 for older adults. They reported that as subjects aged, the percentage of no partnered sexual activity in the previous year increased. The percentages reported by women were 45% for those age 60–64; 75% for age 70–74, and 95% for age

80–84. The corresponding percentages for males were 16%, 40%, and 55%, respectively, for these same age ranges.

Several studies have also suggested that the prevalence of sexual dysfunctions increases with age, particularly erectile failure (Godschalk, Chen, Katz, & Mulligan, 1994; Rosen, Taylor, Leiblum, & Bachmann, 1993). Kinsey et al. (1948) reported the following rates of erectile difficulty: 18% at age 60, 27% at age 70, 55% at age 75, and 76% at age 80. Schiavi, Schreiner-Engel, Mandell, Schanzer, and Cohen (1990) investigated older men's difficulty in achieving vaginal insertion in 50% or more of coital attempts and reported the following rates: 23% at age 55–64 and 32% at age 65–74. Erectile problems appear to be less prevalent in younger age groups. Laumann et al. (1999) reports that 9% of males age 30–39 and 11% age 40–49 have trouble maintaining or achieving an erection. Sexual difficulties in women have been studied less frequently than in men, but findings have supported that sexual difficulties in women increase with age. In women age 80–102, vaginal dryness was one of the six most common problems reported by 30% of subjects (Bretschneider & McCoy, 1988). Brecher (1984) indicated a decrease in the proportion of women able to attain an adequate amount of vaginal lubrication from 48% of women in their 50s to 23% of women over 70 years.

Cross-sectional methodology, which compares subjects of different ages at a single point in time, confounds cohort and time of measurement effects and can provide information only about age difference, not aging effects. Results cannot be interpreted independent of cohort experiences. For example, results may indicate that the frequency of sexual activity may decline in elderly adults or that the frequency has always been lower in this particular older cohort. George and Weiler (1981) performed a longitudinal study with 278 men and women age 46–71. They suggest that the best predictor of the level of sexual behavior in the elderly is the level of sexual behavior when they were younger, unless a physical problem occurs. In this study, the trend was for sexual activity to maintain a steady level until a sudden decline occurred, generally due to changes in the male partner's health. More methodologically sophisticated studies are required to investigate the relationships among normal age-related changes, medical and cultural factors, and the onset of sexual dysfunction in the elderly.

The Laumann et al. study (1999) has recently received a lot of attention. It is a very well-designed study, as it captures a large, representative sample of the American population. The authors indicate that the sample represents 97% of the population between the ages of 18 and 59 years. One of the chief reasons it received so much attention is that the data reveal much higher rates of sexual problems in younger populations than many believed existed. For example, the study reports that 32% of women and 14% of men age 18–29 lack interest in sex, and 26% of women and 7% of men in this age group are unable to achieve orgasm. The percentages are similar for the 30–39-year-old age group. Although rates for older individuals were somewhat higher, Laumann et al. clearly dispelled the view that individuals in their 20s and 30s have generally unproblematic sexual functioning and that it is only with increased age that sexual problems occur at significant rates.

ETIOLOGY

Here we review several etiological pathways to sexual dysfunctions in the elderly. Masters and Johnson (1966) summarized the normal age-associated changes that occur in the sexual response cycle for older adults. Particularly for elderly males due to decreases in sensitivity, more direct penile stimulation is required to reach erection, and the erection may only be 70% to 80% of the size and rigidity achieved in younger years. Generally, the changes for older men and women include more intense stimulation needed to reach orgasm and a longer refractory period (i.e., the amount of time before arousal is sufficient for a further sexual encounter).

Studies have indicated that there exists a progressive reduction in nocturnal penile tumescence episodes (Karacan & Howell, 1988; Schiavi & Schreiner-Engel, 1988) and that these decreases are significantly correlated with decreased sexual desire, frequency of coital intercourse, and the prevalence of erectile problems in elderly males (Schiavi et al., 1990). Nocturnal penile tumescence refers to the fact that men who have no physical problems with the mechanisms responsible for erection will tend each night to have an erection. This phenomenon is sometimes used to make a differential diagnosis between organic and psychologically caused erectile dysfunction. Erectile dysfunction was a more predominant problem than ejaculation/orgasm problems for older males according to data from a specialized sexual dysfunction clinic (Hirst & Watson, 1996; Schiavi et al., 1990).

Menopause has been implicated as a strong predictor for the altered sexual performance of older females (Fisher, Swingen, & O'Donohue, 1997). Menopausal and postmenopausal women do not report a significant change in subjective sexual satisfaction (Bachmann, 1990), although menopause has been associated with decreases in the frequency of sexual activity and orgasm, sexual desire, and vaginal lubrication (Morokoff, 1993). Menopause can result in a decreased amount of sexual anxiety for females, as it frees them from worries concerning pregnancy. Menopause can result in reduced amount and rate of vaginal lubrication (Graber, 1993) and reduced vaginal elasticity (Gupta, 1990), making sexual intercourse painful unless estrogen replacement or an artificial lubricant is used (Fisher et al., 1993). McCoy, Cutler, and Davidson (1985) suggest that symptoms such as hot flushes and the reduction of estrogen may result in reduced sexual interest. In addition, a delay in reaction time of the clitoris (Wagner & Levin, 1978) and a decrease in vaginal blood flow (Tsai, Semmens, Semmens, Lam, & Lee, 1987) may result from normal age-associated changes.

An increase in the incidence of chronic illness and disease for older adults may also disrupt healthy sexual functioning. The *DSM-IV* (APA, 1994) mentions numerous medical conditions that may be implicated, such as neurological conditions like neuropathy and temporal lobe lesions, endocrine conditions (e.g., diabetes mellitus), vascular conditions, and genitourinary conditions (Fisher et al., 1997). Various neurological disorders, including Alzheimer's disease, Parkinson's disease, and multiple sclerosis, have been found to be associated with decreased sexual functioning (Zeiss, Davies, Wood, & Tinkleberg, 1990).

The side effects of disease treatment have been found to be the most frequent causes of erectile dysfunction in older males (Graber, 1993; Mulligan & Katz, 1989). These include treatment for diabetes mellitus (Fairburn et al., 1982) and stroke (Bray, DeFrank, & Wolf, 1981) that have been shown to affect orgasm and ejaculatory functioning. Also, hypertension and antihypertensives have been reported to be a common cause of erectile difficulties (Slag et al., 1983; Zeiss, Zeiss, & Dornbrand, 1989). Graber (1993) indicated that certain medical procedures, including prostatectomy, cystectomy, and rectal excision, are associated with erectile failures.

There is less research studying the etiology of sexual dysfunctions in women (Slag et al., 1983). Studies of women with diabetes have shown that Type I diabetes is not associated with sexual dysfunction but that Type II has negative effects on female sexual desire, orgasmic capacity, lubrication, sexual satisfaction, sexual activity, and relationship with sexual partner (Schreiner-Engel, Schiavi, Vietorisz, & Smith, 1987). Type I diabetes is a congenital condition in which one does not produce insulin, whereas Type II diabetes indicates the production of an insufficient amount of insulin. Schreiner-Engel (1988) hypothesizes that a woman's self-image may be affected by the introduction of a dietary and exercise regimen involved in the management of Type II diabetes, which thus has a higher probability of producing personal distress and marital tension.

Montamat, Cusack, and Vestal (1989) reported that older adults are the largest consumers of prescription and nonprescription medications. These authors also suggested that older adults are more likely than younger adults to engage in polypharmacy. An exhaustive description of how drug classes result in the physiological disruption of the sexual arousal cycle and sexual dysfunction is beyond the scope of this chapter (see Segraves, Madsen, Carter, & Davis, 1985, for a review). A few of the most important are noted below.

The majority of studies examining the role of drugs on older males' sexual dysfunction examine medications such as antihypertensives, diuretics, and antidepressants as causes for male erectile dysfunction (Segraves & Segraves, 1993). However, the results of a study by Rosen, Kostis, Jekelis, and Taska (1994) contradict previous studies. The study investigated 13 men age 39–70 years taking several hypertensive medications and experiencing sexual difficulties. The crossover design found a lack of consistent effect of antihypertensive medications on sexual response. These results are preliminary due to the small sample size and indicate that this area warrants further investigation.

Studies investigating the effect of medications on female sexual functioning have generally examined the effects of psychotropic drugs (Segraves & Segraves, 1993). Psychotropic medications such as trycyclic antidepressants and monoamine oxidase inhibitors have demonstrated the negative effect of inhibiting orgasm in women (Harrison et al., 1986; Segraves, 1988). Kaufman (1983) indicated that antihypertensives, anticholinergics, and antihistamines cause vaginal dryness. In contrast, Leiblum, Baume, and Croog (1994) reported that the anti-hypertensives atenolol, enalapril, and isradipine did not impact ratings of sexual interest in a sample of elderly hypertensive women.

ASSESSMENT

Due to the nature of sexual dysfunctions in any age group, it is vital for the assessment process to determine the relative contributions of medical versus psychological factors. A medical evaluation is useful for ruling out organic factors. The medical examination should not generally differ for older adults from that of other age groups. The medical evaluation should also include a sexual and psychiatric history (O'Donohue & Graber, 1996). Particularly for this cohort of elderly adults, sexual complaints more commonly present in a medical setting than they do at sexual dysfunction clinics or with mental health professionals (Hirst & Watson, 1996; Schover, 1988). Older adults initially seek services from medical professionals for their sexual difficulties and rarely approach a specialized clinic. This phenomenon may be cohort-related, as young and middle-aged cohorts who are socialized differently regarding mental health services may more frequently seek psychological solutions for sexual complaints (Fisher et al., 1997). Another plausible explanation is that due to the previously discussed beliefs that the aged should not consider sex to be important, they may be inhibited from articulating their problems in sexual functioning.

The psychological factors that may be causing or contributing to sexual dysfunction may be assessed by gathering information from the individual experiencing the sexual difficulties and collateral sources (e.g., current partner) through interviews, self-report instruments, and physiological measures. Specific formats and guidelines on sexual interviewing are available in L. LoPiccolo and Heimen (1978) and Pomeroy (1982). Morokoff (1988) recommends the use of the structured interview as the most important assessment technique in the area of sexual functioning. This is supported by studies demonstrating that more elderly men reported sexual problems in an interview than in a questionnaire (Solstad & Hertoft, 1993). However, currently, there are no structured interviews that assess sexual dysfunctions that are psychometrically valid (Avina & O'Donohue, 2000; Regev & O'Donohue, 2000).

The issue of comfort level in discussing and disclosing sexual concerns should be attended to in elderly populations as it is with younger persons. A sexual assessment interview should not differ across age groups. The interviewer should consider that attitudes toward disclosure regarding sexuality may vary widely across persons but not necessarily across ages. The interview is valuable in the assessment of client comfort because it affords the opportunity for observing verbal and nonverbal behavior. Consideration of a client's ease in discussing sexual issues is critical for interview questions and self-report inventories to assess the problem effectively and adequately.

Self-report inventories are available for the assessment of general sexual functioning (e.g., Derogatis Sexual Functioning Inventory; Derogatis & Melisaratos, 1979) and for specific areas of sexual functioning, including sexual arousal (e.g., Sexual Arousal Inventory for Women; Hoon, Hoon, & Wincze, 1976) and sexual desire (e.g., Sexual Desire Conflict Scale for Women; Kaplan & Harder, 1991). Conte (1983) provides a psychometric review of many of the existing instruments for assessing sexual function and dysfunction. Several of the current measures lack adequate psychometric properties, and others have not been tested psychometrically. Their use is problematic given that "no standardized paper-and-pencil questionnaires have been well accepted as measures of specific aspects of sexual functioning in women or men" (Morokoff, 1988, p. 444). The majority of existing instruments have poor psychometric validity (Avina & O'Donohue, 2000). Of the instruments that have some psychometric validity, rarely have any of these assessment inventories been normed with older populations (Fisher, Zeiss, & Carstensen, 2000). There are also specific factors relevant to older adults that should be considered, such as fatigue, sensory function (e.g., hearing or visual impairment), and the client's past experience with self-report inventories. Interpretation of data regarding sexual functioning can be confounded by the use of medication or the presence of illnesses. A source of current assessment instruments for sexual functioning is available in Davis, Yarber, Bauserman, Schreer, and Davis (1998).

TREATMENT

Few nonmedical interventions for sexual dysfunction in the elderly have been empirically investigated. Much of the literature regarding these interventions involves case studies or recommended modifications of treatments developed for younger populations experiencing sexual difficulties, such as cognitive-behavioral therapy (Crowther & Zeiss, 1999; Guarino & Knowlton, 1980; Kaas & Rousseau, 1983; Tsitouras & Alvarez, 1984). For example, Rowland and Haynes (1978) described a sexual enhancement program administered to 10 married elderly couples. The program was reported to increase sexual satisfaction, frequency of certain sexual activities, and improved attitudes toward marriage and life in general. The intervention was not directed toward treating problems in sexual functioning but rather aimed to provide information regarding this topic. Also, Crowther and Zeiss provide descriptions of cognitive-behavioral therapy (CBT) treatments and suggest special considerations when treating older adults, for example, sensitivity to health problems and changes in memory and information processing. These authors describe a case of a female client who presented with guilt concerning masturbation; she was treated with the CBT intervention, which specified clear goals for treatment, emphasized change rather than understanding, educated the client on techniques to be used, and taught her to use them independently.

A literature search revealed one treatment-outcome study related to nonmedical treatment of the elderly's sexual problems. Goldman and Carroll

(1990) conducted a study with 10 couples experiencing erectile dysfunction and 10 couples in a no-treatment control group. Participant inclusion criteria were: between 55 and 70 years of age, heterosexual, in an ongoing relationship for at least six months, had experienced secondary erectile dysfunction, and not exhibiting any major psychiatric disorder or severe marital distress. The measures included the Sexual Interaction Inventory (SII; J. LoPiccolo & Stegar, 1974), the Frequency of Sexual Behavior Form (Rowland & Haynes, 1978), and the Aging Sexual Knowledge and Attitude Scale (ASKAS; White, 1982). The instruments were administered at pre- and posttreatment. Treatment consisted of an educational workshop with the goals of (1) increasing knowledge about the sexual response cycle; (2) increasing knowledge about normal changes that occur in the sexual response cycle with aging; (3) increasing comfort level when talking about sexuality; (4) increasing satisfaction with participants' expression of sexuality in their relationship; and (5) increasing participants' acceptance of their sexual difficulties.

The treatment group demonstrated positive effects on knowledge and satisfaction after the workshop. There were no significant differences between groups at posttest, or between pre- and posttest for the experimental group on scores of the Frequency of Sexual Behavior Form. The authors reported a slight trend toward increased frequency for the experimental group and decreased frequency for the control group. There was a significant change in the experimental group's sexual satisfaction scores from the SII between pre- and posttest, but not for the control group. The significant difference between posttests indicated that the experimental group was more satisfied following treatment than was the control group. These results demonstrate that the educational workshop enhanced sexual satisfaction in older couples experiencing erectile dysfunction. Yet the conclusions that can be drawn from this study are limited, in that it cannot be concluded that this treatment differs from nonspecific treatment, due to the omission of a placebo control group. Also, the study did not evaluate the contribution of individual treatment components, which limits conclusions about the active ingredients.

O'Donohue, Dopke, and Swingen (1997) reviewed the empirical literature regarding psychotherapies for female sexual dysfunction. They reviewed 21 studies and concluded that none met minimal methodological criteria for validly drawing conclusions regarding causal efficacy of the treatments. O'Donohue, Dopke, and Regev (1999) reviewed psychotherapy outcome studies and reported that 80% of the reviewed studies did not meet methodological inclusion criteria. These reviews suggest that current psychotherapy technologies for the treatment of sexual dysfunctions are not well-established according to the criteria proposed by the Task Force on Promotion and Dissemination of Psychological Procedures (1995).

There is still much to be learned about the sexual behavior and problems of the elderly. Although sex is always an area in which there are many values and controversies concerning values, the sexual behavior of the elderly is a particularly value-laden topic. The values expressed by the authors of this chapter include recognizing the importance of sexual behavior for healthy, happy functioning in this group. Sex is an important way to seek pleasure and closeness with another human being. Sexual efficacy—including thinking one is sexually attractive and knowing that one can give another significant pleasure—can be an important component of a positive self-concept for individuals of all ages.

We know very little about how to assess sexual behavior (Avina & O'Donohue, 2000). More research needs to be done on developing valid measures of sexual functioning and dysfunction. We also know very little about the complicated nexus of what may cause sexual problems, although various theories have been developed (see Geer & O'Donohue, 1987; O'Donohue & Geer, 1993). Finally, much more research needs to be done regarding treatment outcome: what works to improve these problems. Federal funding sources need to be open to providing grants to support research in this area.

The mental health professional can serve as an advocate to help the elderly accept and achieve their sexual goals. Nursing homes can be redesigned to allow requisite privacy. Psychotherapists can explore the elderly's interest in pursuing these goals. The absence of desire should not be seen as the normative state in this population. A progressive trend in history demonstrates that certain groups (e.g., women, homosexuals) have increasingly been recognized as having sexual rights. We hope that older persons will make further progress in this regard.

CONCLUSION

Views about the sexual behavior of older adults reflect negative stereotypes as well as society's prescribed role for these individuals. These beliefs affect the elderly's sexual behavior and others' behavior to limit the elderly's sexual activity. Sexual disorders are characterized by absence of or low desire, absence of or insufficient arousal, absence or delay of orgasm, genital pain, and involuntary vaginal spasms. The frequency of sexual activity declines across the adult years and may be an influencing factor in the development of a sexual dysfunction. Also, chronic illness and disease that are prevalent in older adults may disrupt healthy sexual functioning. Elderly males commonly report erectile failure, and women commonly report vaginal dryness. However, recent epidemiological data also show that a significant percentage of younger adults experience sexual dysfunction.

A thorough assessment includes a medical examination in addition to a complete psychological evaluation. Although self-report inventories have been developed for assessing sexual dysfunctions, none have adequate psychometric properties or have been normed with older adults. The structured interview has been recommended as the most useful in eliciting verbal reports from elderly men.

There is a small amount of research documenting psychological treatments for sexual disorders in the elderly. Only one treatment-outcome study targeted this problem and population. The study demonstrated that an educational workshop produced positive changes in the sexual satisfaction scores of the experimental group. More research in the areas of etiology, assessment, and treatment are necessary to inform mental health professionals' decisions regarding sexual functioning in older adults.

STUDY QUESTIONS

1. Why is the existing research on the sexual functioning of older adults problematic?
2. What is considered the best predictor of the level of sexual behavior in later life?
3. Describe common changes in the sexual response cycle of men and women that may be related to sexual dysfunctions.
4. What important variables should be evaluated when assessing for sexual dysfunctions in an elderly population?

SUGGESTED READINGS

Davis, C.M., Yarber, W.L., Bauserman, R., Schreer, G., & Davis, S.L. (Eds.). (1998). *Handbook of sexuality-related measures.* Thousand Oaks, CA: Sage.

Fisher, J.E., & O'Donohue, W.T. (1991). Problems in (really) living: Behavioral approaches to the elderly's goals regarding dating, marriage, and sex. In P.A. Wisocki (Ed.), *Clinical behavior therapy for the elderly client.* New York: Van Nostrand-Reinhold.

Fisher, J.E., Swingen, D.N., & O'Donohue, W. (1999). Behavioral interventions for sexual dysfunction in the elderly. *Behavior Therapy, 28*(1), 65–82.

Geer, J.H., & O'Donohue, W.T. (Eds). (1987). *Theories of human sexuality.* New York: Plenum Press.

Leiblum, S.R., & Rosen, R.C. (Eds.). (1999). *Sexual desire disorders.* New York: Guildford Press.

O'Donohue, W.T. (1987). The sexual behavior and problems in the elderly. In L. Carstensen & B. Edelstein (Eds.), *Handbook of clinical gerontology* (pp. 66–75). New York: Pergamon Press.

O'Donohue, W.T., & Geer, J.H. (Eds.). (1993). *Handbook of the assessment and treatment of the sexual dysfunctions.* Boston: Allyn & Bacon.

Rosen, R.C., & Leiblum, S.R. (Eds.). (1999). *Case studies in sex therapy.* New York: Plenum Press.

Rosen, R.C., & Leiblum, S.R. (Eds). (1992). *Erectile disorders: Assessment and treatment.* New York: Plenum Press.

Rosen, S.R., Leiblum, R.C., & Rosen, R.C. (Eds). (1999). *Principles and practice of sex therapy: Update for the 1990s.* New York: Guildford Press.

REFERENCES

American Psychiatric Association. (1994). *Diagnostic and statistical manual of mental disorders* (4th ed.). Washington, DC: Author.

Avina, C., & O'Donohue, W. (2000). Book review of *Handbook of sexuality-related measures. Journal of Sex and Marital Therapy, 26*(1), 109–111.

Bachmann, G.A. (1990). Sexual issues of menopause. *Annals of the New York Academy of Sciences, 1*(592), 87–91.

Barker, R. (1968). *Ecological psychology*. Stanford, CA: Stanford University Press.

Bray, G.P., DeFrank, R.S., & Wolfe, T.L. (1981). Sexual functioning in stroke survivors. *Archives of Physical Medical Rehabilitation, 62*, 286–288.

Brecher, E.M. (1984). *Love, sex, and aging*. Boston: Little Brown.

Bretschneider, J.G., & McCoy, N.L. (1988). Sexual interest and behavior in healthy 80- to 102-year-olds. *Archives of Sexual Behavior, 17*, 109–129.

Conte, H.R. (1983). Development and use of self-report techniques for assessing sexual functioning: A review and critique. *Archives of Sexual Behavior, 12*, 555–576.

Crowther, M.R., & Zeiss, A.M. (1999). Cognitive-behavior therapy in older adults: A case involving sexual functioning. *Journal of Clinical Psychology, 55*, 961–975.

Davis, C.M., Yarber, W.L., Bauserman, R., Schreer, G., & Davis, S.L. (Eds.). (1988). *Handbook of sexuality-related measures*. Thousand Oaks, CA: Sage.

Derogatis, L.R., & Melisaratos, N. (1979). The DSFI: A multidimensional measure of sexual functioning. *Journal of Sex and Marital Therapy, 5*(3), 244–281.

Fairburn, C.G., Wu, F.C.W., McCulloch, D.K., Borsay, D.Q., Ewing, D.J., Clarke, B.F., & Bancroft, J.H.J. (1982). The clinical features of diabetic impotence: A preliminary study. *British Journal of Psychiatry, 140*, 447–452.

Fisher, J.E., & O'Donohue, W.T. (1991). Problems in (really) living: Behavioral approaches to the elderly's goals regarding dating, marriage, and sex. In P.A. Wisocki (Ed.), *Handbook of clinical behavior therapy with the elderly client* (pp. 203–223). New York: Plenum Press.

Fisher, J.E., Swingen, D.N., & O'Donohue, W. (1997). Behavioral interventions for sexual dysfunction in the elderly. *Behavior Therapy, 28*, 65–82.

Fisher, J.E., Zeiss, A.M., & Carstensen, L.L. (1993). Psychopathology in the aged. In P.B. Sutker & H.E. Adams (Eds.), *Comprehensive handbook of psychopathology* (2nd ed., pp. 815–842). New York: Plenum Press.

Fisher, J.E., Zeiss, A.M., & Carstensen, L.L. (2000). Psychopathology in the aged. In P.B. Sutker & H.E. Adams (Eds.), *Comprehensive handbook of psychopathology* (3rd ed.). New York: Plenum Press.

George, L.K., & Weiler, S.J. (1981). Sexuality in middle and late life: The effects of age, cohort, and gender. *Archives of General Psychiatry, 38*, 919–923.

Godschalk, M.F., Chen, J., Katz, P.G., & Mulligan, T. (1994). Prostaglandin E1 as treatment for erectile failure in elderly men. *Journal of the American Geriatrics Society, 42*, 1263–1265.

Goldman, A., & Carroll, J.L. (1990). Educational intervention as an adjunct to treatment of erectile dysfunction in older couples. *Journal of Sex and Marital Therapy, 16*, 127–141.

Graber, B. (1993). Medical aspects of sexual arousal disorders. In W. O'Donohue & J.H. Greer (Eds.), *Handbook of sexual dysfunctions: Assessment and treatment* (pp. 103–156). Needham Heights, MA: Allyn & Bacon.

Greer, J.H., & O'Donohue, W.T. (Eds.). (1987). *Theories of human sexuality*. New York: Plenum Press.

Guarino, S.C., & Knowlton, C.N. (1980). Planning and implementing a group health program on sexuality for the elderly. *Journal of Gerontological Nursing, 6*, 600–603.

Gupta, K. (1990). Sexual dysfunction in elderly women. *Clinics in Geriatric Medicine, 6*(1), 197–203.

Harrison, W.M., Rabkin, J.G., Ehrhardt, A.A., Stewart, J.W., McGrath, P.J., Ross, D., & Quitkin, F.M. (1986). Effects of antidepressant medication on sexual function: A controlled study. *Journal of Clinical Psychopharmacology, 6*, 144–149.

Hirst, J.F., & Watson, J.P. (1996). Referral aged 60+ to an inner-city psychosexual dysfunction clinic. *Sexual and Marital Therapy, 11*, 131–147.

Hoon, E.R., Hoon, P.W., & Wincze, J.P. (1976). The SAI: An inventory for the measurement of female sexual arousability. *Archives of Sexual Behavior, 5*, 291–300.

Kaas, M.J. (1978). Sexual expression of the elderly in nursing homes. *Gerontologist, 18*, 372–378.

Kaas, M J., & Rousseau, G.K. (1983). Geriatric sexual conformity: Assessment and intervention. *Clinical Gerontologist, 2*, 31–34.

Kaplan, L., & Harder, D.W. (1991). The Sexual Desire Conflict Scale for Women: Construction, internal consistency, and two initial validity tests. *Psychological Reports, 68*, 1275–1282.

Karacan, I., & Howell, J.W. (1988). Use of nocturnal penile tumescence in diagnosis of male erectile dysfunction. In E.A. Tanagho, T.F. Lue, & R.D. McClure (Eds.), *Contemporary management of impotence and infertility* (pp. 95–103). Baltimore: Williams & Wilkins.

Kaufman, S.A. (1983). The gynecologic evaluation of female excitement disorders. In H.S. Kaplan (Ed.), *The evaluation of sexual disorders* (pp. 122–127). New York: Brunner/Mazel.

Kinsey, A.C., Pomeroy, W.B., & Martin, C.E. (1948). *Sexual behavior in the human male.* Philadelphia: Saunders.

Kinsey, A.C., Pomeroy, W.B., Martin, C.E., & Gebhard, P.H. (1953). *Sexual behavior in the human female.* Philadelphia: Saunders.

Laumann, E.O., Gagnon, J.H., Michael, R.T., & Michaels, S. (1994). *The social organization of sexuality.* Chicago: University of Chicago Press.

Laumann, E.O., Paik, A., & Rosen, R.C. (1999). Sexual dysfunction in the United States: Prevalence and predictors. *Journal of the American Medical Association, 281*, 537–544.

Leiblum, S.R., Baume, R.M., & Croog, S.H. (1994). The sexual functioning of elderly hypertensive women. *Journal of Sex and Marital Therapy, 20*, 259–270.

LoPiccolo, J., & Steger, J.C. (1974). The Sexual Interaction Inventory: A new instrument for assessment of sexual dysfunction. *Archives of Sexual Behavior, 3*, 585–595.

LoPiccolo, L., & Heiman, J.R. (1978). Sexual Assessment and History Interview. In J. LoPiccolo & L. LoPiccolo (Eds), *Handbook of sex therapy.* New York: Plenum Press.

Masters, W.H., & Johnson, V.E. (1966). *Human sexual response.* Boston: Little Brown.

Mathias, R.E., Lubben, J.E., Atchinson, K.A., & Schweitzer, S.O. (1997). Sexual activity and satisfaction among very old adults: Results from a community-dwelling medicare population survey. *Gerontologist, 37*, 6–14.

McCoy, N.L., & Davidson, J.M. (1985). A longitudinal study of the effects of menopause on sexuality. *Maturitas, 7*, 203–210.

Montamat, S.C., Cusack, B.J., & Vestal, R.E. (1989). Management of drug therapy in the elderly. *New England Journal of Medicine, 321*, 303–308.

Morokoff, P.J. (1988). Sexual functioning. In E.A. Blechman & K.D. Brownell (Eds.), *Behavioral medicine and women: A comprehensive handbook* (pp. 440–534). New York: Guilford Press.

Morokoff, P.J. (1993). Female sexual arousal disorder. In W. O'Donohue & J.H. Greer (Eds.), *Handbook of sexual dysfunctions: Assessment and treatment* (pp. 157–199). Needham Heights, MA: Allyn & Bacon.

Mulligan, T., & Katz, P.G. (1989). Why aged men become impotent. *Archives of Internal Medicine, 149*, 1365–1366.

O'Donohue, W.T. (1987). The sexual behavior and problems in the elderly. In L.L. Carstensen & B.A. Edelstein (Eds.), *Handbook of clinical gerontology* (pp. 66–75). Elmsford, NY: Pergamon Press.

O'Donohue, W.T., Dopke, C.A., & Regev, L.G. (1999). Psychotherapy for male sexual dysfunction: A review. *Clinical Psychology Review, 19*, 591–630.

O'Donohue, W.T., Dopke, C.A., & Swingen, D.N. (1997). Psychotherapy for female sexual dysfunction: A review. *Clinical Psychology Review, 17*, 537–566.

O'Donohue, W.T., & Graber, B. (1996). Sexual dysfunction. In M. Hersen & V.B. Van Hasselt (Eds.), *Psychological treatment of older adults*. New York: Plenum Press.

O'Donohue, W.T., & Greer, J.H. (Eds.). (1993). *Handbook of the assessment and treatment of the sexual dysfunctions*. Boston: Allyn & Bacon.

Panser, L.A., Rhodes, T.R., Girman, C.J., Guess, H.A., Chute, C.G., Oesterling, J.E., Lieber, M.M., & Jacobsen, S.J. (1995). Sexual function of men ages 40 to 79 years: The Olmstead County Study of urinary symptoms and health status among men. *Journal of the American Geriatrics Society, 43*, 1107–1111.

Pomeroy, W.B. (1982). *Taking a sex history: Interviewing and recording*. New York: Free Press.

Regev, L., & O'Donohue, W. (2000). *Developing a structured interview for the sexual dysfunctions*. Manuscript in preparation.

Rosen, R.C., Kostis, J.B., Jekelis, A., & Taska, L.S. (1994). Sexual sequelae of antihypertensive drugs: Treatment effects on self-report and physiological measures in middle-aged male hypertensives. *Archives of Sexual Behavior, 23*(2), 135–152.

Rosen, R.C., Taylor, J.F., Leiblum, S.R., & Bachman, G.A. (1993). Prevalence of sexual dysfunction in women: Results of a survey study of 329 women in an outpatient gynecological clinic. *Journal of Sex and Marital Therapy, 19*, 171–188.

Rowland, K.F., & Haynes, S.N. (1978). A sexual enhancement program for elderly couples. *Journal of Sex and Marital Therapy, 4*, 91–113.

Schiavi, R.C., & Schreiner-Engel, P. (1988). Nocturnal penile tumescence in healthy aging men. *Journal of Gerontology: Medical Sciences, 43*, M146–M150.

Schiavi, R.C., Schreiner-Engel, P., Mandell, J., Schanzer, H., & Cohen, E. (1990). Healthy aging male sexual function. *American Journal of Psychiatry, 147*, 766–771.

Schover, L.R. (1988). Sexual problems. In L. Teri & P.M. Lewinsohn (Eds.), *Geropsychological assessment and treatment* (pp. 145–187). New York: Springer.

Schreiner-Engel, P. (1988). Diagnosing and treatment of sexual problems of diabetic women. *Clinical Diabetes, 6*, 126–134.

Schreiner-Engel, P., Schiavi, R.C., Vietorisz, D., & Smith, H. (1987). The differential impact of diabetes on female sexuality. *Journal of Psychosomatic Research, 31*, 23–33.

Segraves, R.T. (1988). Psychiatric drugs and inhibited female orgasm. *Journal of Sex Education and Marital Therapy, 14*, 202–207.

Segraves, R.T., Madsen, R., Carter, C.S., & Davis, J.M. (1985). Erectile dysfunction associated with pharmacological agents. In R.T. Segraves & H.W. Schoenberg (Eds.), *Diagnosis and treatment of erectile disorders* (pp. 23–63). New York: Plenum Press.

Segraves, R.T., & Segraves, K.B. (1993). Medical aspects of orgasm disorder. In W. O'Donohue & J.H. Greer (Eds.), *Handbook of sexual dysfunctions: Assessment and treatment* (pp. 225–252). Needham Heights, MA: Allyn & Bacon.

Slag, M.F., Morley, J.E., Elson, M.K., Trence, D.L., Nelson, C.J., Nelson, A.E., Kinlaw, W.B., Beyer, H.S., Nuttal, F.Q., & Shafer, R.B. (1983). Impotence in medical clinic outpatients. *Journal of the American Medical Association, 249*, 1736–1740.

Solstad, K., & Hertoft, P. (1993). Frequency of sexual problems and sexual dysfunction in middle aged Danish men. *Archives of Sexual Behavior, 22,* 51–58.

Task Force on Promotion and Disseminaton of Psychological Procedures. (1995). Training in and dissemination of empirically validated psychological treatments: Report and recommendations. *Clinical Psychologist, 48,* 3–23.

Tsai, C.C., Semmens, J.P., Semmens, E.C., Lam, C.F., & Lee, F.S. (1987). Vaginal physiology of postmenopausal women: pH value, transvaginal electropotential difference, and estimated blood flow. *Southern Medical Journal, 80,* 987–990.

Tsitouras, P.D., & Alvarez, R.R. (1984). Etiology and management of sexual dysfunction in elderly men. *Psychiatric Medicine, 2*(1), 43–55.

Wagner, G., & Levin, R.J. (1978). Vaginal fluid. In E.S.E. Hafez & T.N. Evans (Eds.), *The human vagina* (pp. 121–137). New York: Elsevier.

White, C.B. (1982). A scale for the measurement of attitudes and knowledge regarding sexuality in the aged. *Archives of Sexual Behavior, 11,* 491–502.

Zeiss, A.M., Davies, H.D., Wood, M., & Tinkleberg, J.R. (1990). The incidence and correlates of erectile problems in patients with Alzheimer's disease. *Archives of Sexual Behavior, 19,* 325–331.

Zeiss, A.M., Zeiss, R.A., & Dornbrand, L. (1989). *Treating sexual problems in older adults: Predictors of outcome.* Paper presented at the 23rd annual American Association for the Advancement of Behavior Therapy convention, Washington, DC.

CHAPTER 8

Schizophrenia and Related Disorders

SUZANNE MEEKS

Anne

Anne is a 60-year-old, Black, divorced, unemployed woman living on her own in a rented home. She was interviewed in her home as part of a research project. She has lived in the same home for approximately 12 years, and has recently taken on a boarder to help her with the rent. Her mother and sister live a few doors away, and she also has regular contact with four siblings, her sister-in-law, her three children, and five grandchildren. She is independent in all her instrumental and self-care activities of daily living. She describes her physical health as "good," although she reports having several chronic health problems, including arthritis, asthma, high blood pressure, diabetes, and heart trouble. She takes medication for the high blood pressure. During her interview, Anne voiced only minor complaints: worry about money, headaches, lack of energy, poor appetite, and a phobia of spiders. She had no other affective distress. She was quite pleasant and cooperative during the interview, and only with direct questioning did her psychosis become evident. She reported hearing auditory hallucinations for more than 30 years, including voices commenting on her actions, voices speaking to one another, and voices speaking to her, telling her they do not want her to go to heaven. She also reported both visual and somatic hallucinations, involving spirits appearing to her and crawling up and down her back. At times, she hears the devil telling her to do things. In addition to these voices, she is very suspicious that someone is out to harm her, poison her food, electrocute her, or steal her clothing. She shows very little emotion on her face when talking, and her speech is at times vague, rambling, and tangential in her responses to questions. Anne visits the community mental health center about every three months for medication counseling and is receiving daily oral and weekly depot injections of antipsychotic medication.

Anne completed 11 years of schooling, was married young, and gave birth to four children. Her psychiatric problems began shortly after the death of one of her children from lead poisoning, which, according to her family, occurred when she was 32. However, she reported first being hospitalized earlier, at about age 24. Apparently, she was separated and divorced some time during or after her first hospitalization. The earliest available hospital records are from age 40. From age 40 to the present, she has had 10 admissions to the local state hospital and one to a private psychiatric hospital. These records indicate that she had paranoid delusions and persecutory hallucinations in multiple modalities at each admission, very similar in content to those she currently displays. She was very agitated, hostile, and fearful, seeing dead relatives who told her they would eat her family, believing something was harmful in water, food, or medication. She attempted suicide at least once. At other times, she was seen carrying a weapon or wandering the neighborhood shouting and threatening others. Her admissions usually lasted two or three months, and she returned to her own home or that of her mother and did relatively well until she stopped taking her medication again. Since her last admission at age 47, she has been maintained with regular outpatient treatment. She has worked only briefly, as a waitress, and otherwise has been maintained on social security and supplemental security income.

Betty

Betty is a 74-year-old White woman who has been living in a personal care home for the past 25 years, although until recently, she lived more independently in one of the home's cottages. She has never been married. She was interviewed for a research study. She described her physical health as "excellent," with no chronic or acute diseases and no medication other than for psychiatric reasons. During the interview, she denied most symptoms, and the interviewer detected no overt signs of psychosis, although Betty did admit to a recent episode of believing her thoughts were broadcast aloud, following a stressful incident at the retirement community in which several cats she was fond of were removed. Her facial expressions were distinctly flat, showing little emotion, with long pauses between hearing a question and responding to it. She was quite odd to speak to; sometimes her thought processes seemed disorganized. She appeared to link her mental health experiences to either digestive processes or her menstrual cycle, and some of her somatic ideas were implausible. Her demeanor was childlike. She keeps mostly to herself, but does go to a few activities at the retirement center and is "sociable." She lists no significant others, friends, or family contacts. She is independent in self-care, but requires assistance with meal preparation, housework, and transportation. A guardian handles her finances.

Betty is originally from a wealthy family and was an excellent student in high school, with gifted musical talents. She attended an exclusive women's college in the northeast, but "failed" there because she was "unstable." She studied music in a northeastern city and played two seasons with orchestras, one before her initial breakdown and one afterwards. She was first treated for mental problems at age 25 and has been hospitalized a total of five times. She was in the hospital continuously between age 29 and 47, and was discharged from there to the retirement home where she now lives. She had several years of psychoanalysis in her youth and insulin shock and electric shock treatments while hospitalized. Since age 47, she has had one brief readmission, at age 65. Her symptoms are not well elaborated in hospital records, and she did not wish to talk about them. Apparently, she became disorganized in speech and thought, with hostility toward her father and persecutory delusions and hallucinations before her first admission. She also was quite withdrawn, flat, and inappropriate in her behavior. According to staff at the personal care home, her current functioning is the highest she has achieved since they have known her.

Carl

Carl is a 65-year-old, White, retired railroad worker who was brought to a psychiatric outpatient clinic by his sister. His sister reported that Carl had been "talking crazy," had barricaded himself in his apartment, was refusing to eat anything, and had not bathed in some time. Only with difficulty had she convinced him to come with her to get help. When interviewed, Carl was disheveled and had a strong body odor. His eyes darted from one corner of the room to another. He made no eye contact with the examiner, and his face showed very little emotion. When asked about his eating and bathing, he reported that someone had been poisoning his food and the water in his apartment was laced with acid. He had been drinking bottled water, but had not eaten anything for nearly three days. He had not bathed for about a week. Asked how he knew about the poison, he explained that he had heard a voice that told him to beware; the voice had been warning him for about a month. He was vague about who might be out to poison him, but made reference to the Mafia and to a "gang of thieves."

History was obtained from both Carl and his sister. Carl had graduated from high school and gone directly to work for the railroad. He had worked steadily until he had retired about two years ago. He had never married and has no children. His sister described him as "a loner," and he agreed that he had pretty much kept to himself all his life. He could name no good friends, though there were some guys at the local McDonald's with whom he talked over coffee. His sister was his closest confidante. She has lived in the same apartment building for about five years. She reported that he had always had some odd ways of thinking, that he had never trusted anyone much, but that he had always been a good worker and generous with his money, buying gifts for her children and their other nieces and nephews. She said he had become increasingly withdrawn over the past six months, had begun saying strange things about people being out to poison him, and then about two weeks ago, had started rearranging his furniture, pushing things up against the door whenever he was at home. Carl was started on an antipsychotic medication and seen weekly at the clinic for several months; he gradually returned to normal and, although he stayed on medication, phased out his clinic visits to quarterly.

DSM-IV CRITERIA FOR
SCHIZOPHRENIA AND RELATED DISORDERS

SYMPTOM DEFINITIONS

The three cases presented above, although quite different in their life histories and late-life presentation, all meet *DSM-IV* criteria for *schizophrenia*. Schizophrenia might be considered the quintessential "severe mental illness": it involves significant impairment in functioning, generally endures for a long period of time, and often, people suffering from the disorder appear "crazy" to others, hearing voices, believing outlandish things, and speaking and thinking oddly. Symptoms of schizophrenia fall into two general categories: *positive* and *negative* symptoms (American Psychiatric Association [APA], 1994). Positive symptoms include hallucinations, delusions, and disorganization of speech, language, and behavior (see Table 8.1). These symptoms are referred to as "positive" because they represent overt excesses in behavior or thinking: something is present in addition to normal behavior. Negative symptoms, by contrast, represent the absence of normally expected functioning. Examples of negative symptoms include affective flattening, withdrawal, avolition, and alogia (see Table 8.1). Although the positive symptoms are more visible to lay observers,

Table 8.1 Characteristics symptoms of schizophrenia.

System Names	Definition	Examples
Positive Symptoms		
Hallucinations	Experience of false perceptions, occurring in any sensory modality.	*Auditory:* Hearing voices speaking. *Visual:* Seeing visions. *Olfactory:* Smelling strange odors not identifiable to others. *Tactile/somatic:* Experience of being touched or having things crawling on one's skin.
Delusions	Convictions in beliefs that others can agree are not true; the beliefs are not shared with others in the person's cultural or religious group.	*Persecutory delusions (most common type):* Beliefs that others are tormenting or working to cause one harm. *Grandiose delusions:* Beliefs in extraordinary personal power or talent. *Delusions of reference:* Beliefs that ordinary events, such as TV commentary or hand gestures, convey some special meaning to the individual or are purposely directed at him or her.
Disorganized thought (formal thought disorder)	Inferred from speech: the person's speech is characterized by disorganization or incoherence; ideas do not follow each other, but shift about irrationally.	*Loosening of association:* The person shifts from one idea to another without logical connections. *Tangentiality:* Responses are marginally or completely unrelated to the original questions. *Word salad/incoherence:* speech is so disorganized as to make no sense.
Disorganized behavior	A constellation of possible behaviors including extreme, unpredictable agitation, grossly disheveled appearance, inability to engage in goal-directed behavior, or inappropriate silliness.	Aimless pacing and muttering in public places. Laughing aloud at inappropriate times or places. Standing on the street corner, dirty and ragged, swearing and preaching loudly.

Table 8.1 *(Continued)*

System Names	Definition	Examples
Catatonic behaviors	Decreased awareness of or responsiveness to the environment; in the extreme, complete lack of responsiveness.	*Catatonic stupor:* Complete unawareness. *Catatonic rigidity/posturing:* Takes rigid or bizarre postures or poses from which he or she cannot be moved, or can be moved as if made of wax ("waxy flexibility").
	Negative Symptoms	
Affective flattening	Restricted range of affective expression. Facial appearance is rigid or blank; facial expression and other gestures that are used to indicate emotional responsiveness are lacking or diminished.	Poor eye contact, "woodenness" of facial expression, lack of expressive gestures, does not smile at stupid jokes (*anhedonia*), decreased spontaneous movements.
Alogia	Speech productivity and content suggest a diminished content of thought.	Long pauses before answering; replies are very brief, may be only yes/no; replies are empty or vague; complete muteness.
Avolition	Inability to initiate goal-related behavior.	Personal hygiene is very poor in a person who has adequate physical ability to perform activities of daily living; long periods of time with no physical activity; cannot work on a simple job or participate in social groups.

both types of symptoms are critical to our understanding of schizophrenia and related disorders, and negative symptoms may be more disabling (e.g., Meeks et al., 1990; Meeks & Walker, 1990).

DSM-IV CRITERIA FOR SCHIZOPHRENIA

In the *DSM-IV*, there are three inclusion criteria (Criteria A, B, and C) for schizophrenia and three exclusionary criteria. Criterion A requires that two or more of the characteristic symptoms be present: delusions, hallucinations, disorganized speech, grossly disorganized behavior, and negative symptoms. If delusions are *bizarre*, or if hallucinations include hearing voices keeping a running commentary on the person's actions or thoughts or two or more voices in conversation with one another, only one of these symptoms is required. Although many people might find any delusion bizarre due to the fact that delusions involve fixed beliefs in things others generally find to be untrue, bizarre delusions are specifically defined as involving things that would be highly implausible or impossible in our everyday world. For example, believing that the Mafia is out to get you may be unrealistic, but it is possible. By contrast, believing that the Mafia has implanted wires in your brain to observe your thoughts from a microwave oven is both unrealistic and likely impossible, and therefore would qualify as bizarre.

Inclusion criteria B and C have to do with impairment and duration. The *DSM-IV* criteria specify that there must be significant impairment in functioning in at least one important area of living, such as social relationships, occupational or school functioning, or self-care. This impairment must be a clear change from the prior level of functioning. Note that in diagnosing older adults such as Anne and Betty, whose onset was many years prior, establishing a prior level of functioning may require some detective work. In Betty's case, there was clearly a marked and permanent decline from her adolescence and early adulthood; this is less clear in Anne's case, although it seems clear that she and her family noticed a change in her. Often, the necessity of hospitalization is used to infer a decline in functioning for the purpose of meeting Criterion B. Criterion C concerns duration: signs of the disorder must be present for at least six months, at least one month of which must involve active symptoms from Criterion A. During other months, the person may be displaying only negative symptoms, milder versions of positive symptoms, such as unusual beliefs or sensory experiences, or continued or prodromal disturbance in functioning. Individuals meeting Criteria A and B for schizophrenia along with the appropriate exclusionary criteria, but not C, would be diagnosed with schizophreniform disorder. For example, if Carl had been seen in the clinic immediately after his sister first heard him talk about delusional ideas, he could not have been diagnosed with schizophrenia but might instead have received a schizophreniform diagnosis.

The exclusionary criteria for schizophrenia involve differential diagnostic considerations concerning mood disorders, substance use and medical conditions, and pervasive developmental disorder. Some of these issues are discussed below in the section on differential diagnosis. In general, if the symptoms seen can be better accounted for by a mood disorder, medical condition, preexisting substance use disorder, or lifelong pervasive developmental disorder, then the diagnosis of schizophrenia is not given.

Once a diagnosis of schizophrenia is given, the *DSM-IV* requires that the longitudinal course of the disorder be classified. These course subtypes are new to *DSM-IV* and emerge from the research literature on longitudinal course in schizophrenia (e.g., Ciompi, 1980, 1987). It is first necessary to establish whether there have been single or multiple episodes. If there has been a single episode, one has to establish whether there has been a full or partial remission or the symptoms are continuous. If the disorder is episodic, one specifies whether there are residual symptoms between episodes. Finally, for any course type other than single episode in complete remission, one specifies whether there are prominent negative symptoms. These new course subtypes have an advantage from the perspective of gerontological work in that they force clinicians to view the disorder in its life span context, rather than at the limited cross-section of the clinical interview. In a new onset case such as Carl's, these specifications are relatively easy (Carl's course following treatment would most probably be *single episode, in full remission*). However, working with older adults who have long histories of disorder, it is sometimes difficult to make these specifications, because the historical data and reports of patients and families are often quite vague about functional levels between active treatment episodes. For example, would Anne be *continuous* or *episodic with interepisode residual symptoms?* Her history specifies she did "relatively well" between hospitalizations, but we know that she functions well currently with chronic delusions and hallucinations. Are these "prominent," as required by the *DSM-IV* designation of continuous course (APA, 1994, p. 286)? Much of Betty's course, on the other hand, might be characterized as *single episode, in partial remission,* although, lacking hospital records, we do not know during how much of her long hospitalization she was symptomatic. However, the history indicates that she did have an additional hospitalization some years after her discharge, suggesting there were in fact multiple episodes with significant residual symptoms in between. Clearly, her recent course suggests a long period of residual symptoms with no overt psychotic symptoms but with prominent negative symptoms.

In addition to the longitudinal course subtypes, *DSM-IV* has retained the older cross-sectional episode subtypes that were present in previous *DSM* versions. The most common subtype is paranoid, which involves a preoccupation with delusions or auditory hallucinations and the absence of flat or inappropriate affect and of disorganization in speech or behavior. The disorganized type involves the presence of flat or inappropriate affect, disorganized speech, and disorganized behavior. The catatonic subtype involves prominent catatonic symptoms (see Table 8.1), and undifferentiated is given when none of the other subtype criteria are clearly met. When a person presents with no prominent positive symptoms but is not in full remission, the subtype given is residual.

DIFFERENTIAL DIAGNOSIS IN LATE LIFE

Besides schizophrenia, there are six additional psychotic disorders specified in *DSM-IV,* and a seventh, "not otherwise specified" category: schizoaffective disorder, delusional disorder, brief psychotic disorder, shared psychotic disorder, psychotic disorder due to a medical condition, and substance-induced psychotic disorder. In the general population, these disorders are rare, probably occurring less frequently than schizophrenia, although extensive epidemiological data are lacking. In the limited space available here, rather than describing each of these diagnoses in detail, it seems more useful to describe the process of differential diagnosis one would follow for an older patient presenting with psychosis.

Because of the increased risk of physical disease in older adults, it is critical that a patient presenting with a new psychotic episode be evaluated medically as well as psychiatrically (Bartels & Mueser, 1999). Many symptoms of psychosis can be produced by medical illness, particularly in a person who is physically frail. Good differential diagnosis in late life requires a medical screening, medical history, psychiatric history, and information on the timing and nature of the illness onset. The likelihood that the psychotic episode is due to medical illness is high if the episode is the first ever, if it coincides with the onset of the medical illness or treatment for that illness, and if the person is frail. If the medical condition predates the psychosis and can provide a plausible explanation for it, the diagnosis given is psychosis due to a medical condition. However, even when a person has a long history of psychiatric illness, medical information can be valuable. A medical problem can lead to an exacerbation of psychosis. In Anne's case, for example, she has multiple chronic medical diseases that require ongoing medical management. Changes in any of these conditions, such as increased blood pressure or unstable blood sugar, might not come to the attention of her physicians but might lead to metabolic changes that exacerbate psychotic symptoms. A mental health clinician may miss the underlying cause of the exacerbation and treat the psychotic symptoms only. Note that such a situation may have a circular, escalating course. If the underlying medical symptoms are missed and the antipsychotic medication is increased, this might result in side effects that interact with the medical problems to increase their severity. Another type of circular pattern can also be a problem for older patients: symptoms of mental illness may lead to poor management of medical conditions and increased physical frailty, which in turn may lead to escalation of psychosis (Bartels & Mueser, 1999). When an older patient presents to a mental health clinic with psychosis, medical assessment should be routine.

Screening for cognitive impairment should also be routinely done for older adults. Dementia becomes increasingly common over the age of 65, and the damage to the brain due to dementia may lead to psychotic symptoms (see Chapter 9 for a discussion of dementia). At one time, it was assumed that all psychoses in later life could be attributed to central nervous system deterioration or arteriosclerosis (Mulsant et al., 1993). A landmark series of studies by British psychiatrists (see, e.g., Roth, 1955; Roth & Morrissey, 1952) significantly changed this conception, finding, instead, that late-life psychoses could be grouped into five categories: affective psychosis, late paraphrenia, acute confusion, and senile and arteriosclerotic psychoses. The latter three categories would overlap with delirium, psychoses due to medical illness, and dementias in *DSM-IV*. Under our current system, if the psychotic symptoms appear first and only in the presence of a diagnosis of dementia, the diagnosis is dementia and not one of the psychotic disorders listed above.

Once medical problems and dementia are ruled out, the differential diagnosis proceeds much as it would for younger adults. It is necessary to determine if there is a history of substance abuse, and whether that could explain the psychotic symptoms (substance-induced psychotic disorder). It is also important to evaluate for the presence and prominence of affective symptoms. Psychosis can occur in affective disorders, both bipolar and unipolar forms (see Chapter 6). When an episode of mood disorder is present along with the psychotic symptoms, the primary consideration concerns the duration of the mood episode relative to the psychosis. If the two overlap completely and there is no period when the psychosis is present without prominent mood symptoms for two weeks or more, the diagnosis of mood disorder with psychotic features is given. When there is only partial overlap, such that some time during the episode there are psychotic symptoms without prominent mood symptoms for two weeks, then the diagnosis is schizoaffective disorder, which has both bipolar and unipolar forms. Finally, if the mood symptoms meet criteria for major depressive episode but occur only with residual schizophrenia symptoms and the long-term course is primarily one of schizophrenia, the diagnosis given is schizophrenia with a secondary diagnosis of depressive disorder, not otherwise specified (see APA, 1994, p. 350).

Prior to the publication of the third edition of the *DSM* in 1980, patients with prominent psychotic symptoms often were diagnosed with schizophrenia, regardless of the presence of affective symptoms. This historical fact has significant implications for the evaluation of older patients with long psychiatric histories. Many of these patients may first have been diagnosed using *DSM-II* criteria (APA, 1968), and as such, may have diagnoses of schizophrenia in their medical records, when in fact current criteria would result in diagnoses of affective disorder. Clinicians may be strongly influenced by prior diagnoses in making current diagnostic and treatment decisions (Meeks, 1990) and consequently fail to assess or treat the affective symptoms (Francis, 1998; Meeks, Francis, Jackson, & Gibson, 1992). It is especially important to evaluate affective symptoms in older patients with psychosis and to consider alternative, affective diagnoses.

A final differential diagnosis, particularly when the first onset is in late life, is between schizophrenia and delusional disorder. When diagnostic criteria for schizophrenia or mood disorders are not met and there is a persistent delusion (lasting one month or more), the diagnosis is delusional disorder. In this disorder, there is not the impairment in functioning and behavior seen in schizophrenia, although responding to the delusion may cause some functional difficulties. The diagnosis of delusional disorder overlaps somewhat with the British concept of late paraphrenia, which has been conceptualized as involving paranoid delusions in a well-preserved premorbid personality, having a late (after age 45) onset (Roth, 1955). The issue of age of onset in late-life psychoses is discussed later in this chapter.

EPIDEMIOLOGICAL DATA

PREVALENCE AND INCIDENCE ESTIMATES

Estimates of prevalence of schizophrenia are variable, depending on study methods, diagnostic criteria used, and population sampled. The range of estimates in large studies is between 0.02% and 2%; the generally accepted estimate across populations is around 1% for both six-month and lifetime prevalence. Although there are some limited areas of high prevalence, prevalence estimates are relatively stable worldwide (APA, 1994). These estimates come from the most recent generation of epidemiological studies that used structured psychiatric interviews to improve diagnostic reliability across sites (e.g., Bland, Stebelsky, Orn, & Newman, 1988; Robins et al., 1984). Estimates for older adults are limited, but generally suggest that prevalence over the age of 65 is lower than for younger adults, with median estimates of 0.15% in one review (Bliwise, McCall, & Swan, 1987), and 0.32% in another (Babigian & Lehman, 1987). U.S. data from the Epidemiological Catchment Area study (ECA; Keith, Regier, & Rae, 1991) suggest the prevalence rate declines with age from around a peak of 1.5% at age 30–44 to 0.2% at age 65 and over. Decreased prevalence in older age groups may be partially attributed to the higher mortality risk for patients with psychotic disorders. For example, in addition to a higher risk for suicide, Babigian and Lehman (1987) found that psychoses were related to a twofold increase in the risk for respiratory and digestive disorders in their New York catchment area study. This differential mortality rate *decreased* with age, however, suggesting that older people with schizophrenia who survive to old age may be a hardier group than their younger peers.

Data from a large catchment area study in New York between 1965 and 1975 suggest a significant decline in annual incidence of schizophrenia and paranoid psychoses together, from around 1% in the youngest age category (under age 44) to 0.65% among those over age 65. This study did not separate schizophrenia from other types of paranoid psychoses, and therefore may overestimate the late-life incidence of schizophrenia. For example, in a study of an inpatient psychiatric population, the proportion of cases attributable to schizophrenia declined with age, whereas the proportion of other paranoid psychoses increased slightly (Siegel & Goodman, 1987). European research suggests that the vast majority of people with schizophrenia have an onset before age 40 (77%); 13% have onset between age 41 and 50, 7% between 51 and 60, and 3% have an onset after 60 (Harris & Jeste, 1988). Castle and Murray (1993) reported annual incidence rates for broadly defined schizophrenia and related disorders versus *DSM-III-R*–defined schizophrenia for a large catchment area in London. These figures show a clear decline with age in both the narrow and the broader categories.

Data on gender differences clearly demonstrate a change in gender distribution of schizophrenia in late life. Whereas in earlier age groups, schizophrenia is about evenly distributed between men and women (Kohn, Dohrenwend, & Mirotznik, 1998), there are more women than men with schizophrenia in older age groups (Bartels & Mueser, 1999; Davidson et al., 1995; Meeks & Murrell, 1997). This gender difference may reflect the general tendency for women to live longer than men. In addition, women have a mean age of onset of schizophrenia that is approximately five years later than that of men (Castle & Murray, 1993; Lewine, 1988). Possibly related to the later age of onset, women are also more likely to get married and be involved with their children and to have better social networks and social skills (Bartels & Mueser, 1999). These characteristics may afford a survival advantage to women over men.

Prevalence and incidence of other specific psychotic disorders in late life are difficult to estimate, because most studies have tended to group them together, often including affective and organic psychoses. Studies of paranoid *symptoms* suggest prevalence rates between 4% and 17% (Bliwise et al., 1987). Affective and organic (medical and dementia-related) psychoses accounted for the majority of these cases (e.g., Blessed & Wilson, 1982; Christie, 1982). One study suggests that the prevalence of delusional disorder was less than 1% in the youngest and oldest age groups, but somewhat higher (3.8%–7.5%) in the middle-aged and young-old groups (Heston, 1987). This would suggest a very low rate in the general population.

LONG-TERM COURSE OF SCHIZOPHRENIA AND RELATED DISORDERS

Because, for the majority of sufferers, schizophrenia has its onset in early adulthood, understanding schizophrenia in old age requires understanding something about the lifetime course of the disorder. Much of what we know about lifetime course comes from a number of long-term follow-up studies of schizophrenia and affective disorders published during the 1970s and 1980s. These studies have gone a long way toward changing our understanding of the outcomes of schizophrenia and other severe mental illnesses. Despite differing cultures, methodologies, and definitions of schizophrenia, the results of these studies have been remarkably consistent. Researchers have reached consensus particularly in two areas: the tendency for individuals diagnosed with schizophrenia to improve over time, and the heterogeneity of expected outcomes. These results are in direct contrast to original views of schizophrenia as a chronically debilitating illness with deteriorating course (Kraepelin, 1919/1971).

The focus of the long-term follow-up studies has been primarily on the "natural history," or natural course of the manifestations of schizophrenia. The results have generally been condensed and presented in terms of global and specific ratings of outcomes. The global outcomes can be summarized into three categories:

1. Approximately 20% to 25% of patients improve after a relatively short, usually fluctuating, and turbulent course. These are considered complete remissions (Harding et al., 1987; Huber, Gross, & Schuttler, 1975; Tsuang & Winokur, 1975; Vaillant, 1964). The percentage of remissions varies depending on the breadth of the definition of schizophrenia employed.
2. Approximately 10% remain chronically impaired and usually continue to reside in psychiatric hospitals; these are the "backward patients" (Bleuler, 1974).
3. Of the remaining 50% to 70%, a variety of courses have been observed, including revolving-door chronic and residual courses. It is among these patients that a gradual improvement in social contacts and a reduction of psychotic symptoms have been observed (Bleuler, 1974; Ciompi, 1980; Harding, Brooks, Ashikaga, Strauss, & Landerl, 1987).

Optimistic accounts of the general trend for improvement must be couched in the context of the equally general observation that outcomes for psychotic disorders are extremely heterogeneous. In fact, one of the most striking features of these attempts to describe the natural history of schizophrenia and related disorders is the failure to find one or two consistent patterns of outcome. For example, Ciompi (1980, 1987) identified eight separate courses, differing in types of onset, evolution, and end-state. When multiple dimensions of outcome are assessed for each subject, outcome domains are correlated but not identical in pattern (J.S. Strauss & Carpenter, 1972). Thus, to observe that there is general improvement in social relations would not necessarily imply an equivalent improvement in other domains. Until very recently, there was very little research attention paid to the various manifestations of schizophrenia in late life (Belitsky & McGlashan, 1993). The section below reviews recent literature describing clinical presentation and functioning in older people with schizophrenia.

CLINICAL PHENOMENOLOGY, PATIENT CHARACTERISTICS, AND FUNCTIONING IN LATE LIFE

J.S. Strauss and Carpenter (1972) have noted the independence of various outcome indicators for people with schizophrenia, including symptoms, social functioning, work functioning, and rehospitalization. The symptom-based diagnostic evaluation is insufficient to predict these indicators adequately because people meeting the diagnostic criteria of schizophrenia are heterogeneous (Andreasen & Carpenter, 1993). Adding to the heterogeneity of psychoses in late life are those individuals who do not meet strict criteria for schizophrenia, such as those with schizoaffective disorders or those who have atypical (late) onset. Strauss and his colleagues (see also J.S. Strauss, Kokes, Carpenter, & Ritzler, 1978) have argued that the course of schizophrenia should be considered in a developmental context. Implicit in vulnerability-stress models is the assumption that environmental factors interact with illness vulnerability to affect the course of illness. Aging itself may affect both vulnerability and the ability to cope with environmental stressors. Understanding schizophrenia in late life involves not only descriptive psychiatry, which has characterized much of the current literature, but also developmental models that look specifically at the impact of aging on living with schizophrenia and on the illness itself. As Strauss points out, such models must, at minimum, contain a combination of symptoms and their shifts over time, individual vulnerabilities and strengths, including but not limited to biological diathesis, and environmental characteristics.

One source of diversity among older people with schizophrenia is related to cohort differences in the availability of community treatment and neuroleptic medication. People who lived 20 or more of their adult years in psychiatric institutions are likely to be significantly more impaired in independent living skills than those who had the benefit of neuroleptics in early or mid-adulthood and were able to function at least part of the time in the community (Bartels & Mueser, 1999). Comparing the late-life outcomes of

Anne and Betty illustrates this point: their life histories suggest that Betty started life with significant advantages over Anne, but in old age, Anne is far more independent in her functioning.

Related to treatment cohort differences, there are a variety of additional changes that have taken place since the 1970s in mental health care in this country, resulting in greater homelessness, increased substance abuse, exposure to crime, and greater exposure to epidemics such as HIV infection. These events may also affect the service needs of the aging person with schizophrenia (Bartels & Mueser, 1999).

To date, most research on late-life psychosis has remained in the realm of descriptive psychiatry, and many studies have been carried out exclusively on inpatients. It is important to note in reviewing such studies that the majority of older adults with early-onset schizophrenia are not likely to be found in inpatient settings, but rather are living at least semi-independently in the community (Meeks et al., 1990). However, newer studies are beginning to give us a picture of the diverse characteristics of those who continue to suffer from psychosis in later life. Mulsant et al. (1993) studied consecutive admissions to a geriatric inpatient unit. Compared to patients with dementia and affective disorders, those with schizophrenia were more likely to have substance abuse and tardive dyskinesia (a medication side effect, discussed under "Treatment," below); also, their suicide attempt rate was higher than for dementia patients. Patients with late-onset schizophrenia were more symptomatic than early-onset patients, but recovered better with treatment. The authors noted the prevalence of positive symptoms, concluding that their evidence did not support the notion of late-life improvement in these symptoms, although they recognized that theirs was an inpatient sample, and they did not make comparisons to younger samples. In a study specifically addressing cross-sectional age differences in chronic schizophrenia, Davidson et al. (1995) noted a decline in positive symptoms with age. However, levels of positive symptoms still significantly exceeded clinically significant cutoffs. There were significant decrements in cognitive functioning in the older age groups, and an age difference in negative symptoms approached significance (see also Harvey et al., 1997). Overall severity of symptoms was not associated with age, which is not surprising, given that this was an inpatient sample. In our outpatient sample, the younger (middle-aged) cohort was significantly more symptomatic than the older sample across diagnoses, and the older participants showed better global functioning (Meeks & Murrell, 1997). These studies converge with the longitudinal data from long-term follow-up studies to suggest that there may be a shift in emphasis in late-life schizophrenia from positive symptoms to negative symptoms, but the majority of patients seen in treatment settings continue to exhibit significant psychological impairment (Meeks et al., 1990; Meeks & Murrell, 1997).

Depressive symptoms are common among people with schizophrenia and may be linked to poorer outcomes (Bartels & Drake, 1988). In our later-life sample (Meeks & Murrell, 1997), presence of superimposed affective syndromes that warranted Research Diagnostic Center (RDC) diagnoses of schizoaffective disorder was related to poorer functioning compared to people with affective disorders, but not poorer functioning than those with schizophrenia. Level of functioning depended on the primacy of affective *versus* schizophrenic symptoms. Within schizophrenia, depressive symptoms were not correlated with global functioning, overall impairment in the prior five years, level of psychosis, or functional impairment from symptoms, although they were marginally related to activities of daily living (ADL) functioning ($r = -.25$, $p = .054$). However, note that those with more depression had *better* ADL functioning.

Cohen, Talavera, and Hartung (1996) found a 44% prevalence of significant depressive symptoms among outpatients with schizophrenia. After comparing depressed to nondepressed patients, they concluded that depression in older people with schizophrenia is like depression in other older people. This conclusion is consonant with our findings (Jackson, 1997) that life events evoke affective distress among those with schizophrenia much as they do in nonpsychiatric older adults. These findings are significant in light of our additional finding that people with psychosis or mania are less likely to receive antidepressant medications (Meeks et al., 1992). Depressive symptoms and distress in people with schizophrenia should be dealt with as it would in nonpsychiatric older adults.

Another source of vulnerability in late-life mental illness appears to be cognitive impairment (Bartels & Mueser, 1999). Studies of late-life cognitive decline suggest that coexistent cognitive and functional deficits occur in about one-third of chronically hospitalized patients with schizophrenia (Harvey, Lombardi, et al., 1995; Harvey, Silverman, et al., 1999). This cognitive decline was not associated with dementing conditions, but rather appears to be integrally related to schizophrenia (see discussion of cognitive deficits in the next section). Cognitive impairment in samples of geriatric inpatients and nursing home patients predicts poorer adaptive functioning and overall outcomes (Harvey et al., 1998; Harvey, Parrella, et al., 1999). Cognitive deficits have been found to be related to negative symptoms but not to positive symptoms of schizophrenia (Harvey et al., 1996). These researchers found that cognitive impairments were relatively stable over time and did not predict changes in negative symptoms. Differences in cognitive impairment between younger and older people with schizophrenia are typically not large, suggesting that the persistent correlation between negative symptoms and cognitive impairment represents the characteristics of a negative-outcome subtype of the disorder (Davidson et al., 1995). Perhaps the greater importance of negative symptoms in later life may be due in part to the fact that the patients we see in this cohort are more likely to have this negative outcome subtype.

Because the availability of social supports is critical in determining who may remain independent in the community versus who ends up in institutions, older people with schizophrenia are particularly vulnerable. As compared to patients with other severe psychiatric disorders, those with schizophrenia are likely to be poorer, be more socially dependent, and have smaller social networks (Meeks & Murrell, 1997). Many of these people, especially the men, have never married (Meeks & Murrell, 1997) and therefore do not have spouses or children for support and have often relied on parents. In middle age, when their parents become ill and eventually die, they may lose their primary source of support. Sometimes, siblings are able to pick up the burden, but often, the burden must shift to outside the family. This distinguishes people with schizophrenia from older people with other chronic diseases requiring a great deal of social support, such as Alzheimer's disease (Bartels & Mueser, 1999). For most older people, family caregivers are the principal providers of support. Lacking critical social resources, older people with schizophrenia would seem to be an important group on which to focus our community support programs.

CONCEPTUAL ISSUES

CURRENT ETIOLOGICAL THINKING ABOUT SCHIZOPHRENIA

The earliest formulation of schizophrenia as a disease came from Kraepelin (1919/1971). Kraepelin adopted the label "dementia praecox" for the syndrome. Dementia praecox, roughly translated, means premature dementia, or premature loss of reason. The disease was defined by early onset of cognitive dysfunction, followed by a gradual decline in abilities across the life span, although he later acknowledged that there was not an inevitable deteriorating course. Both the notion of early onset and the notion of inevitable deteriorating course can now be challenged by modern research. However, current etiological models continue to emphasize the importance of cognitive deficits and hypothesized vulnerabilities related to early development.

The earliest conceptions of schizophrenia were of a biological, or "brain" disease, but only fairly recently has there been good evidence to support this idea. The modern era of understanding schizophrenia began in the 1950s, with the discovery of neuroleptic medication. Not only did this discovery revolutionize treatment of schizophrenia, it also changed etiological thinking and stimulated a wealth of research on physiological correlates of the disorder (Csernansky & Grace, 1998). During the two decades following the discovery of neuroleptic medications, research focused on neurotransmitter dysfunction, particularly the neurotransmitter dopamine, which is the neurochemical involved in the activity of the older antipsychotic medications. The thinking related to this research led to the popular idea of the "chemical imbalance" as a cause of schizophrenia. The dopamine hypothesis was that schizophrenia was related to an excess of dopamine, or hypersensitivity to its release at postsynaptic receptors (see Bowers, 1980, for a review). Although a naïvely simplistic view from today's standards, this was the beginning of the neuroscience era for the study of schizophrenia (Csernansky & Grace, 1998).

The dopamine hypothesis assumed that the chemical abnormality occurred in a structurally normal brain. As basic research began to map out the structure of the brain and the neuroanatomy of chemical communication within it, scientists began to appreciate the complexity inherent in any brain system. The availability of new imaging technology, beginning in the 1980s, began to demonstrate that there were a variety of abnormalities that could be identified in brains of people with schizophrenia. The newer models of pathophysiology of schizophrenia, therefore, are primarily models of neural circuitry abnormalities rather than neurochemical imbalance (Csernansky & Grace, 1998). Integrated into these models are concepts related to neurodevelopment. Specifically, many researchers now assume that the abnormalities seen in brain structure and circuitry may come about through problems with the development and programmed death of neurons during early childhood and adolescence (e.g., Andreasen, Paradiso, & O'Leary, 1998; Conrad & Scheibel, 1987; DeLisi, 1997).

There is no single accepted etiological model of schizophrenia, and the wealth of models and experimental research supporting them is beyond the scope of this chapter. It is broadly accepted that the onset of the clinical syndrome results from some combination of diathesis, or vulnerability, and environmental or biological stressors (e.g., Zubin & Spring, 1977). The diathesis is thought to be at least partially inherited (Kendler & Diehl, 1993) and, as mentioned above, related to neurodevelopmental processes. However, the clinical heterogeneity seen in schizophrenia, along with the many conflicting results in the experimental literature, suggest that schizophrenia as a clinical syndrome may be the result of more than one etiological process (Knoll et al., 1998). The study of schizophrenia in late life may be helpful to our developing etiological understanding of the disorder. Specifically, two bodies of research that have focused on older adults, work on late-onset schizophrenia and work on cognitive deficits in later life, provide some etiological insights.

RESEARCH ON LATE-ONSET SCHIZOPHRENIA

Although late-onset psychoses were studied as early as the 1940s in Europe, it was not until 1984 that the notion of late-onset schizophrenia appeared in the U.S. literature (Jeste et al., 1997). In that year, Rabins, Pauker, and Thomas (1984), published a paper describing patients with schizophrenia who had onset after the age of 44. This was in contradiction to the diagnostic criteria in use at the time (DSM-III), which defined schizophrenia as having an onset before age 45. This limit was eliminated in DSM-III-R and DSM-IV, based on research demonstrating that about 10% to 15% of patients meeting the other criteria for schizophrenia in fact have an onset after age 45 (Harris & Jeste, 1988). Research in the past decade suggests that late-onset patients diagnosed with schizophrenia are in fact a heterogeneous group, most likely incorporating some people with schizophrenia and others who have psychoses secondary to other types of brain dysfunction.

Jeste and his colleagues (Jeste et al., 1997) have suggested three possibilities for the origins of late-onset schizophrenia: (1) it is, like early-onset schizophrenia, a neurodegenerative disease; (2) it results from other types of brain injury, such as strokes or arteriosclerosis; or (3) it results from sensory deficits. Most of what we know about late-onset schizophrenia in this country comes from the work of this research group, comparing patients with late-onset schizophrenia to young and older early-onset schizophrenia patients and to other patients without psychiatric disorders.

From their data, Jeste and his colleagues concluded that late-onset schizophrenia is clearly neither a mood disorder nor dementia; late-onset and early-onset schizophrenia are presumed to have a common underlying (genetic) vulnerability to schizophrenia. Differences between late- and early-onset patients suggest that late-onset schizophrenia represents the predominantly paranoid type, more common among women, and involving fewer negative symptoms, less severe cognitive impairment, better premorbid functioning in adolescence and early adulthood, and better response to medications (Jeste et al., 1997). These characteristics are identical to those that describe better-outcome patients with early-onset schizophrenia. Perhaps, then, these individuals represent a group of people with shared vulnerability but who, because of protective factors or other advantages, have managed to make it to old age without triggering psychosis.

RESEARCH ON COGNITIVE DEFICITS IN LATE LIFE

Although diagnostic criteria for schizophrenia focus on clinically identifiable symptoms, 30 years of experimental literature has established that cognitive dysfunction is also an important feature of schizophrenia (Braff, 1993; M.E. Strauss, 1993). People with schizophrenia have trouble focusing their attention on relevant information and ignoring information that is distracting or irrelevant (see Braff, 1993, for a review). Much of the more recent neuroscience work has attempted to form connections between these dysfunctions and structural abnormalities, and these connections are also the focus of emerging etiological thinking (e.g., Andreasen et al., 1998). Because most of this work has been done with young patients, our understanding of both etiology and the effects of aging can be enhanced by the study of older patients with schizophrenia, and in fact, this work has begun to emerge.

An important question for this new body of research is whether poor cognitive functioning seen in older patients with schizophrenia is due to aging, dementia, schizophrenia, or some combination. Studies have shown that there is more cognitive impairment in older patients with schizophrenia than would be expected based on old age alone (e.g., Heaton et al., 1994). Autopsy studies suggest that dementia (AD) accounts for only a small portion of cognitive deficits, roughly corresponding to the incidence of AD in the general older population (Dwork et al., 1998; Jellinger & Gabriel, 1999). Normal aging patterns of cognitive decline also fail to explain cognitive deficits in late-life schizophrenia (McDowd, Filion, Harris, & Braff, 1993). Although there do seem to be some age-related changes in cognitive function and in associated structural abnormalities (Andreasen et al., 1990; Seno et al., 1997), these seem to be in addition to changes that are already seen in younger people with schizophrenia. The emerging evidence on cognitive deficits in older people with schizophrenia appears to support the neuro*developmental* model of schizophrenia: cognitive and structural changes that are apparent in young people with the disorder are also present and, in some cases, more pronounced in older patients. The increased deficits are more consistent with normal aging processes superimposed on a vulnerable nervous system than with the addition of a neuro*degenerative* process (Dwork et al., 1998; Harvey, White, et al., 1995; Lohr, Alder, Flynn, Harris, & McAdams, 1997; Olichney et al., 1998).

An important caveat in interpreting these studies is that they have been carried out mostly on chronic patients in inpatient settings; as pointed out earlier, these patients represent only a small proportion of people with schizophrenia. Even among inpatients there is considerable heterogeneity in cognitive functioning, and some researchers have argued that when subgroups are addressed, there continues to be evidence for a minority (mostly men) with a neurodegenerative psychosis (Knoll et al., 1998; O'Donnell et al., 1995). Taking a developmental view, and adopting developmental research methods, may ultimately lead us to integrate what now seem to be contradictory findings and hypotheses (e.g., DeLisi, 1997). Further work on psychosis across the life span will be helpful in increasing not only our understanding of the treatment implications of diverse clinical and neuropsychological presentation in late life, but also the implications for etiological models and diagnostic subgrouping.

TREATMENT

PHARMACOLOGICAL TREATMENT

The front line of treatment for psychoses is medication, specifically the class of antipsychotic medications known as *neuroleptics*. Table 8.2 lists the commonly used neuroleptic medications and their trade names. These medications have been available beginning in the 1950s, and an extensive body of research with young patients supports their effectiveness (see Kane & Marder, 1993, for a review). For the majority of patients coming to treatment with active positive symptoms such as delusions and thought disorder, treatment with neuroleptics reduces or eliminates those symptoms within a relatively short period of time. In addition, patients maintained on doses of these medications following the reduction or remission of their psychotic symptoms are less likely to have a relapse of active symptoms (Kane & Marder, 1993). This latter fact means that many people with schizophrenia and schizoaffective disorders are maintained on neuroleptics for long periods of time, and we might therefore expect older adults with early-onset schizophrenia to have been taking these medications for many years.

Very little of the effectiveness research has been carried out on older patients. In a review of the extant research, Jeste and his colleagues (Jeste, Lacro, Gilbert, Kline, & Kline, 1993) concluded that neuroleptics seem to be as useful with older patients as with the young. They seem to be effective with both late-onset and early-onset schizophrenia (Gregory & McKenna, 1994). Little is known about effectiveness in other classes of psychosis, but the prevailing

Table 8.2 Commonly used neuroleptic medications.

Trade Name	Generic Name
Thorazine	Chlorpromazine
Serentil	Mesoridazine
Mellaril	Thioridazine
Prolixin	Fluphenazine
Trilafon	Perphenazine
Stelazine	Trifluoperazine
	(Phenothiazines)
Haldol	Haloperidol
Taractan	Chlorprothixene
Navane	Thiothixene
	(Thioxanthenes)
Orap	Pimozide
Loxitane	Loxapine
	(Diphenylbutylpiperdines)
Moban	Molindrone

clinical wisdom suggests that psychotic symptoms, regardless of disorder, respond to neuroleptic treatment. Because of differences in how drugs are metabolized in elderly patients, dosages of medications may need to be reduced (Gregory & McKenna, 1994; Jeste et al., 1993), particularly if the individual has become physically frail. For the same reason, elderly patients may be especially sensitive to side effects of these medications.

There are three types of neuroleptic side effects that may be particularly problematic for older patients (Salzman & Nevis-Olesen, 1992). First, sedation may lead to increased confusion and agitation in older patients, and a negative cycle could result (Salzman & Nevis-Olesen, 1992). The second side effect of concern is orthostatic hypotension, which entails a sudden drop in blood pressure when changing position (e.g., getting up out of bed). Because of associated dizziness, this may lead to increased risk for falling and consequent bone fractures. The risk of both these side effects is highest with the low-potency drugs chlorpromazine, thioridazine, and chlorprothixene.

The third and largest group of problematic side effects are the *extrapyramidal side effects*, which occur most frequently with the high-potency neuroleptics, especially haloperidol and fluphenazine. Extrapyramidal side effects result from the action of neuroleptics on dopamine receptors in the brain. Older patients are at greater risk for these side effects because of decreased dopamine availability (Salzman & Nevis-Olesen, 1992). Three types have received particular attention: parkinsonism, akathisia, and tardive dyskinesia. Parkinsonism mimics the symptoms of Parkinson's disease: rigidity, tremor, and bradykinesia. Akathisia is a syndrome of extreme motor restlessness. Both parkinsonism and akathisia develop within the first few days of administration (or increased dosage). Parkinsonism can be treated with the addition of anticholinergic medication. However, those medications also have adverse side effects, including confusion

(Gregory & McKenna, 1994). The increased motor activity and accompanying patient distress associated with akathisia can be confused with agitation related to psychosis. This may lead to more problems if not immediately recognized, because the response to increased agitation may be raising the dosage of the offending medication. The usual solution for akathisia is dosage reduction or switching to another medication (Gregory & McKenna, 1994).

Perhaps the most serious of neuroleptic side effects is tardive dyskinesia (TD), which develops after a prolonged period of administration. TD entails involuntary, repetitive movements, most commonly involving the mouth or face, such as chewing, lateral jaw movements, or tongue rolling, but also occurring in other parts of the body. These movements are often highly visible and stigmatizing, and they also may not remit when medication is withdrawn. In human studies, age is the most consistent risk factor found for TD. TD occurs five to six times more frequently in older patients than in younger patients. There is also a reduced chance of remission following drug withdrawal (Jeste, Lohr, Eastham, Rockwell, & Caligiuri, 1998).

In addition to the older antipsychotics, a new group of "atypical" antipsychotic medications has been developed in the past decade. These medications, called atypical because their target of action is primarily serotonin rather than dopamine receptors, are shown in Table 8.3. One advantage of these newer medications is that they produce relatively fewer extrapyramidal side effects, and they therefore appear especially attractive for use with older adults (Sweet & Pollock, 1998). Not surprisingly, little is yet known about the effectiveness or safety of use of these medications with older adults. The same concerns regarding age-related changes in drug metabolism exist with these drugs, especially with regard to clozapine, which increases the risk for the potentially fatal condition agranulocytosis. Because of this risk, clozapine treatment requires more intensive monitoring with regular blood tests by a physician, and is therefore costly to administer. However, clozapine has been shown to be effective with patients who do not respond to neuroleptics, and therefore may have some value in treating older patients who have had chronic and unremitting courses of schizophrenia. The other atypical antipsychotic about which the most is known, risperidone, does not carry the same risk for agranulocytosis, and the limited evidence available suggests that it is well tolerated and effective with older patients (Sweet & Pollock, 1998). The remaining drugs have been available only for

Table 8.3   Atypical antipsychotic medications.

Trade Name	Generic Name
Risperdal	Risperidone
Clozaril	Clozapine
Zyprexa	Olanzapine
Seroquel	Quetiapine
Serlect	Sertindole
Zeldox	Ziprasidone

a short time, so their promise for treatment of late-life psychoses still awaits systematic examination.

PSYCHOSOCIAL TREATMENT

Although antipsychotic drugs are essential tools in the treatment of schizophrenia, problems with social adaptation and daily functioning are not specifically addressed by the medication, which means that most people with schizophrenia require some form of psychosocial treatment as well. There is extensive research on the types of psychosocial treatments that are available and effective with schizophrenia (see Bellack & Mueser, 1993; Mueser, Bond, Drake, & Resnick, 1998, for reviews). This research suggests that the best results emerge from comprehensive, community care models of treatment that provide assistance in a variety of life arenas, including daily living skills, medication management, vocational assistance, and counseling. Individual psychotherapy generally has not been shown to be effective, although some forms of cognitive interventions may have promise for treating persistent delusions and hallucinations. Social skills training has also been shown to be effective in improving social functioning, although the results do not generalize widely to other areas of living. Family interventions designed to improve communication styles among family members have also been shown to reduce relapse rates. None of these approaches has yet been evaluated for effectiveness with older adults. Given what we do know about psychosis in late life, it seems logical that some combination of community and family interventions would be appropriate for older patients. Stress-vulnerability models of schizophrenia suggest that outcomes should be improved by reducing environmental stress, or by enhancing skills to cope with that stress (Bartels & Mueser, 1999), so it would seem worth our while to try out some of the family and social skills-enhancing interventions that have been effective with younger patients. Community management needs to take place in the context of multidisciplinary collaboration because of the increased risk for health problems inherent in older patients. In developing treatment strategies, it is important to keep in mind the heterogeneity in late-life psychosis. People with lifelong schizophrenia are likely in need of very different approaches than people with newly developed psychoses. Clearly, there is a pressing need to evaluate appropriate treatment strategies for older adults with schizophrenia and related disorders.

CONCLUSION

Schizophrenia and related disorders in late life, as with younger persons, are a heterogeneous group of disorders that have in common certain symptom features (psychosis) but that are variable in terms of course, outcomes, and etiology. Heterogeneity is likely to increase with age, because of the interaction between varied life experiences and clinical course patterns. Understanding and treating these disorders in late life requires not only a solid understanding of diagnostic and clinical management issues relating to the disorders themselves, but also the willingness to take a life span perspective. New diagnostic features of *DSM-IV* encourage such a perspective by requiring us to provide course descriptors, but these descriptors are difficult to formulate without careful assessment. Differential diagnosis in late life is complicated by the increased probability of comorbid medical and cognitive difficulties. The use of a longitudinal assessment frame is essential; cross-sectional assessment is likely to be misleading. It is important to understand differences among people with the same diagnosis based on course projectories, treatment histories, aging processes, and social support systems. Use of a developmental, life span approach to schizophrenia should benefit not only clinical service, but also etiological research. Already, research on late-onset schizophrenia and on cognitive deficits in late-life schizophrenia has contributed to our understanding of this constellation of disorders. However, much remains to be known about these disorders in late life. Future research will benefit from a movement away from descriptive psychiatry based on select, inpatient samples to longitudinal designs employing broader samples. In addition, treatment studies will need to include both inpatient and outpatient older adults.

STUDY QUESTIONS

1. Imagine that you are a clinician seeing each of the cases presented in the beginning of the chapter for the first time. Answer the following questions about those cases:
   a. What are the specific diagnostic considerations, including course and subtype, for each case?
   b. In addition to reviewing symptoms and functioning, what other assessment approaches should be taken?
   c. How would you explain each of their disorders to concerned relatives? What would you say about the causes of the disorder, appropriate treatments, and expectations for functioning? In what way(s) are these cases typical or atypical of other patients with similar disorders?
2. Are older people at greater risk for psychotic disorders than younger people? What are the different types of psychotic disorders you might expect to see in a geriatric inpatient unit?
3. How can studying older people with schizophrenia enhance our knowledge about schizophrenia in general? What are the most pressing issues for future research on older adults with psychosis?

SUGGESTED READINGS

Miller, N.E., & Cohen, G.D. (Eds.). (1987). *Schizophrenia and aging: Schizophrenia, paranoia, and schizophreniform disorders in later life*. New York: Guilford Press.

Jeste, D.V., Lacro, J.P., Gilbert, P.L., Kline, J., & Kline, N. (1993). Treatment of late-life schizophrenia with neuroleptics. *Schizophrenia Bulletin, 19,* 817–830.

Jeste, D.V., Symonds, L.L., Harris, M.J., Paulsen, J.S., Palmer, B.W., & Heaton, R.K. (1997). Nondementia nonpraecox dementia praecox? Late onset schizophrenia. *American Journal of Geriatric Psychiatry, 5,* 302–317.

REFERENCES

American Psychiatric Association. (1968). *Diagnostic and statistical manual of mental disorders* (2nd ed.). Washington, DC: Author.

American Psychiatric Association. (1994). *Diagnostic and statistical manual of mental disorders* (4th ed.). Washington, DC: Author.

Andreasen, N.C., & Carpenter, W.T., Jr. (1993). Diagnosis and classification of schizophrenia. *Schizophrenia Bulletin, 19,* 199–214.

Andreasen, N.C., Paradiso, S., & O'Leary, D.S. (1998). "Cognitive dysmetria" as an integrative theory of schizophrenia: A dysfunction in cortical-subcortical-cerebellar circuitry? *Schizophrenia Bulletin, 24,* 203–218.

Andreasen, N.C., Swayze, V.W., Flaum, M., Yates, W.R., Arndt, S., & McChesney, C. (1990). Ventricular enlargement in schizophrenia evaluated with computed tomographic scanning. *Archives of General Psychiatry, 47,* 1008–1015.

Babigian, H.M., & Lehman, A.F. (1987). Functional psychoses in later life: Epidemiological patterns from the Monroe County Psychiatric Register. In N.E. Miller & G.D. Cohen (Eds.), *Schizophrenia and aging: Schizophrenia, paranoia, and schizophreniform disorders in later life* (pp. 9–22). New York: Guilford Press.

Bartels, S.J., & Drake, R.E. (1988). Depressive symptoms in schizophrenia: Comprehensive differential diagnosis. *Comprehensive Psychiatry, 29,* 467–483.

Bartels, S.J., & Mueser, K.T. (1999). Severe mental illness in older adults: Schizophrenia and other late-life psychoses. In M.A. Smyer & S.H. Qualls (Eds.), *Aging and mental health* (pp. 182–207). Malden, MA: Blackwell.

Belitsky, R., & McGlashan, T.H. (1993). The manifestations of schizophrenia in late life: A dearth of evidence. *Schizophrenia Bulletin, 19,* 683–685.

Bellack, A.S., & Mueser, K.T. (1993). Psychosocial treatment for schizophrenia. *Schizophrenia Bulletin, 19,* 317–335.

Bland, R.C., Stebelsky, G., Orn, H., & Newman, S.C. (1988). Psychiatric disorders and unemployment in Edmonton. *Acta Psychiatrica Scandinavica, 77* (Suppl.), 72–80.

Blessed, G., & Wilson, I.D. (1982). The contemporary natural history of mental disorder in old age. *British Journal of Psychiatry, 141,* 49–67.

Bleuler, M. (1974). The long-term course of schizophrenic psychoses. *Psychological Medicine, 4,* 244–254.

Bliwise, N.G., McCall, M.E., & Swan, S.J. (1987). The epidemiology of mental illness in late life. In E.E. Lurie, J.H. Swan, & Associates (Eds.), *Serving the mentally ill elderly: Problems and perspectives* (pp. 1–38). Lexington, MA: Lexington Books.

Bowers, M.B., Jr. (1980). Biochemical processes in schizophrenia: An update. *Schizophrenia Bulletin, 6,* 393–403.

Braff, D.L. (1993). Information processing and attention dysfunctions in schizophrenia. *Schizophrenia Bulletin, 19,* 233–259.

Castle, D.J., & Murray, R.B. (1993). The epidemiology of late-onset schizophrenia. *Schizophrenia Bulletin, 19,* 691–700.

Christie, A.B. (1982). Changing patterns in mental illness in the elderly. *British Journal of Psychiatry, 140,* 154–159.

Ciompi, L. (1980). The natural history of schizophrenia in the long term. *British Journal of Psychiatry, 136,* 413–420.

Ciompi, L. (1987). Review of follow-up studies on long-term evolution and aging in schizophrenia. In N.E. Miller & G.D. Cohen (Eds.), *Schizophrenia and aging* (pp. 206–213). New York: Guilford Press.

Cohen, C.I., Talavera, N., & Hartung, R. (1996). Depression among aging persons with schizophrenia who live in the community. *Psychiatric Services, 47,* 601–607.

Conrad, A.J., & Scheibel, A.B. (1987). Schizophrenia and the hippocampus: The embryological hypothesis extended. *Schizophrenia Bulletin, 13,* 577–587.

Csernansky, J.G., & Grace, A.A. (1998). New models of the pathophysiology of schizophrenia: Editors' introduction. *Schizophrenia Bulletin, 24,* 185–187.

Davidson, M., Harvey, P.D., Powchik, P., Parrella, M., White, L., Knobler, H.Y., Losonczy, M.F., Keefe, R.S.E., Katz, S., & Frecska, E. (1995). Severity of symptoms in chronically institutionalized geriatric schizophrenic patients. *American Journal of Psychiatry, 152,* 197–207.

DeLisi, L.E. (1997). Is schizophrenia a lifetime disorder of brain plasticity, growth, and aging? *Schizophrenia Research, 23,* 119–129.

Dwork, A.J., Susser, E.S., Keilp, J., Waniek, C., Liu, D., Kaufman, M., Zemishlany, Z., & Prohovnik, I. (1998). Senile degeneration and cognitive impairment in schizophrenia. *American Journal of Psychiatry, 155,* 1536–1543.

Francis, M.L. (1998). *Diagnosis, medication, and outcome: Their relationship in a community sample of older persons with bipolar disorder and schizoaffective disorder, bipolar type.* Unpublished doctoral dissertation, University of Louisville, Kentucky.

Gregory, C., & McKenna, P. (1994). Pharmacological management of schizophrenia in older patients. *Drugs and Aging, 5,* 254–262.

Harding, C.M., Brooks, G.W., Ashikaga, T., Strauss, J.S., & Landerl, P.D. (1987). Aging and social functioning in once-chronic schizophrenic patients 22–62 years after first admission: The Vermont Story. In N.E. Miller & G.D. Cohen (Eds.), *Schizophrenia and aging* (pp. 74–82). New York: Guilford Press.

Harris, M.J., & Jeste, D.V. (1988). Late-onset schizophrenia: An overview. *Schizophrenia Bulletin, 14,* 39–55.

Harvey, P.D., Howanitz, E., Parrella, M., White, L., Davidson, M., Mohs, R.C., Hoblyn, J., & Davis, K.L. (1998). Symptoms, cognitive functioning, and adaptive skills in geriatric patients with lifelong schizophrenia: A comparison across treatment sites. *American Journal of Psychiatry, 155,* 1080–1086.

Harvey, P.D., Lombardi, J., Kincaid, M.M., Parrella, M., White, L., Powchik, P., & Davidson, M. (1995). Cognitive functioning in chronically hospitalized schizophrenic patients: Age-related changes and age disorientation as a predictor of impairment. *Schizophrenia Research, 17,* 15–24.

Harvey, P.D., Lombardi, J., Leibman, M., Parrella, M., White, L., Powchik, P., Mohs, R.C., Davidson, M., & Davis, K.L. (1997). Age-related differences in formal thought disorder in chronically hospitalized schizophrenic patients: A cross-sectional study across nine decades. *American Journal of Psychiatry, 154,* 205–210.

Harvey, P.D., Lombardi, J., Leibman, M., White, L., Parrella, M., Powchik, P., & Davidson, M. (1996). Cognitive impairment and negative symptoms in geriatric chronic schizophrenic patients: A follow-up study. *Schizophrenia Research, 22,* 223–231.

Harvey, P.D., Parrella, M., White, L., Mohs, R.C., Davidson, M., & Davis, K.L. (1999). Convergence of cognitive and adaptive decline in late-life schizophrenia. *Schizophrenia Research, 35,* 77–84.

Harvey, P.D., Silverman, J.M., Mohs, R.C., Parrella, M., White, L., Powchik, P., Davidson, M., & Davis, K.L. (1999). Cognitive decline in late-life schizophrenia: A longitudinal study of geriatric chronically hospitalized patients. *Biological Psychiatry, 45,* 32–40.

Harvey, P.D., White, L., Parrella, M., Putnam, K.M., Kincaid, M.M., Powchik, P., Mohs, R.C., & Davidson, M. (1995). The longitudinal stability of cognitive impairment in schizophrenia: Mini-mental state scores at one- and two-year follow-ups in geriatric inpatients. *British Journal of Psychiatry, 166,* 630–633.

Heaton, R., Paulsen, J.S., McAdams, L.A., Kuck, J., Zisook, S., Braff, D.L., Harris, M.J., & Jeste, D.V. (1994). Neuropsychological deficits in schizophrenics: Relationship to age, chronicity, and dementia. *Archives of General Psychiatry, 51,* 469–476.

Heston, L.L. (1987). The paranoid syndrome after mid-life. In N.E. Miller & G.D. Cohen (Eds.), *Schizophrenia and aging: Schizophrenia, paranoia, and schizophreniform disorders in later life* (pp. 249–257). New York: Guilford Press.

Huber, G., Gross, G., & Schuttler, R. (1975). Psychiatric course of illness and prognosis. *Acta Psychiatrica Scandinavica, 52,* 49–57.

Jackson, E.S. (1997). *The relationship between life events and mental health functioning of severe mental illness.* Unpublished doctoral dissertation, University of Louisville, Kentucky.

Jellinger, K.A., & Gabriel, E. (1999). No increased incidence of Alzheimer's disease in elderly schizophrenics. *Acta Neuropathologica, 97,* 165–169.

Jeste, D.V., Lacro, J.P., Gilbert, P.L., Kline, J., & Kline, N. (1993). Treatment of late-life schizophrenia with neuroleptics. *Schizophrenia Bulletin, 19,* 817–830.

Jeste, D.V., Lohr, J.B., Eastham, J.H., Rockwell, E., & Caligiuri, M.P. (1998). Adverse neurobiological effects of long-term use of neuroleptics: Human and animal studies. *Journal of Psychiatric Research, 32,* 201–214.

Jeste, D.V., Symonds, L.L., Harris, M.J., Paulsen, J.S., Palmer, B.W., & Heaton, R.K. (1997). Nondementia nonpraecox dementia praecox? Late onset schizophrenia. *American Journal of Geriatric Psychiatry, 5,* 302–317.

Kane, J.M., & Marder, S.R. (1993). Psychopharmacologic treatment of schizophrenia. *Schizophrenia Bulletin, 19,* 287–302.

Keith, S.J., Regier, D.A., & Rae, D.S. (1991). Schizophrenic disorders. In L.N. Robins & D.A. Regier (Eds.), *Psychiatric disorders in America* (pp. 33–52). New York: Free Press.

Kendler, K.S., & Diehl, S.R. (1993). The genetics of schizophrenia: A current, genetic-epidemiologic perspective. *Schizophrenia Bulletin, 19,* 261–286.

Knoll, J.L., IV, Garver, D.L., Ramberg, J.E., Kingsbury, S.J., Croissant, D., & McDermott, B. (1998). Heterogeneity of the psychoses: Is there a neurodegenerative psychosis? *Schizophrenia Bulletin, 24,* 365–379.

Kohn, R., Dohrenwend, B.P., & Mirotznik, J. (1998). Epidemiological findings on selected psychiatric disorders in the general population. In B.P. Dohrenwend (Ed.), *Adversity, stress, and psychopathology* (pp. 235–284). New York: Oxford University Press.

Kraepelin, E. (1971). *Dementia praecox and paraphrenia* (R.M. Barclay, Trans.). Huntington, New York: Krieger. (Original work published 1919)

Lewine, R.J. (1988). Gender and schizophrenia. In H.A. Nasrallah (Ed.), *Handbook of schizophrenia* (Vol. 3, pp. 379–397). Amsterdam, The Netherlands: Elsevier.

Lohr, J.B., Alder, M., Flynn, K., Harris, M.J., & McAdams, L.A. (1997). Minor physical anomalies in older patients with late-onset schizophrenia, early-onset schizophrenia, depression, and Alzheimer's disease. *American Journal of Geriatric Psychiatry, 5,* 318–323.

McDowd, J.M., Filion, D.L., Harris, M.J., & Braff, D.L. (1993). Sensory gating and inhibitory function in late-life schizophrenia. *Schizophrenia Bulletin, 19,* 733–746.

Meeks, S. (1990). Age bias in the diagnostic decision-making behavior of clinicians. *Professional Psychology: Research and Practice, 21,* 279–284.

Meeks, S., Carstensen, L.L., Stafford, P.B., Brenner, L.L., Weathers, F., Welch, R., & Oltmanns, T.F. (1990). Mental health needs of the chronically mentally ill elderly. *Psychology and Aging, 5,* 163–171.

Meeks, S., Francis, M.L., Jackson, E.S., & Gibson, L.L. (1992, November). *Prevalence and treatment of affective symptoms among older severely mentally ill persons in the community.* Paper presented at the annual meeting of the Gerontological Society of America, Washington, DC.

Meeks, S., & Murrell, S.A. (1997). Mental illness in late life: Socioeconomic conditions, psychiatric symptoms, and adjustment of long-term sufferers. *Psychology and Aging, 12,* 296–308.

Meeks, S., & Walker, J.S. (1990). Blunted affect, blunted lives? Negative symptoms, ADL functioning, and mental health among older adults. *International Journal of Geriatric Psychiatry, 5,* 233–238.

Mueser, K.T., Bond, G.R., Drake, R.E., & Resnick, S.G. (1998). Models of community care for severe mental illness: A review of research on case management. *Schizophrenia Bulletin, 24,* 37–74.

Mulsant, B.H., Stergiou, A., Keshavan, M.S., Sweet, R.A., Rifai, A.H., Pasternak, R., & Zubenko, G.S. (1993). Schizophrenia in late life: Elderly patients admitted to an acute care psychiatric hospital. *Schizophrenia Bulletin, 19,* 709–721.

O'Donnell, B.F., Faux, S.F., McCarley, R.W., Kimble, M.O., Salisbury, D.F., Nestor, P.G., Bikinis, R., Jolesz, F.A., & Shenton, M.E. (1995). Increased rate of P300 latency prolongation with age in schizophrenia. *Archives of General Psychiatry, 52,* 544–549.

Olichney, J.M., Iragui, V.J., Kutas, M., Nowacki, R., Morris, S., & Jeste, D.V. (1998). Relationship between auditory P300 amplitude and age of onset of schizophrenia in older patients. *Psychiatry Research, 79,* 241–254.

Rabins, P., Pauker, S., & Thomas, J. (1984). Can schizophrenia begin after age 44? *Comprehensive Psychiatry, 25,* 290–293.

Robins, L.N., Helzer, J.E., Weissman, M.M., Orvaschel, H., Gruenberg, E., Burke, J.D., Jr., & Regier, D.A. (1984). Lifetime prevalence of specific psychiatric disorders in three sites. *Archives of General Psychiatry, 41,* 949–958.

Roth, M. (1955). The natural history of mental disorder in old age. *Journal of Mental Science, 101,* 281–301.

Roth, M., & Morrissey, J.D. (1952). Problems in the diagnosis and classification of mental disorders in old age, with a study of case material. *Journal of Mental Science, 98,* 66–80.

Salzman, C., & Nevis-Olesen, J. (1992). Psychopharmacologic treatment. In J.E. Birren, R.B. Sloane, & G.D. Cohen (Eds.), *Handbook of mental health and aging* (2nd ed., pp. 721–762). San Diego, CA: Academic Press.

Seno, H., Shibata, M., Fujimoto, A., Kuroda, H., Kanno, H., & Ishino, H. (1997). Computed tomographic study of aged schizophrenic patients. *Psychiatry and Clinical Neurosciences, 51,* 373–377.

Siegel, C.E., & Goodman, A.B. (1987). Mental illness among the elderly in a large state psychiatric facility: A comparison with other age groups. In N.E. Miller & G.D. Cohen (Eds.), *Schizophrenia and aging: Schizophrenia, paranoia, and schizophreniform disorders in later life* (pp. 23–34). New York: Guilford Press.

Strauss, J.S., & Carpenter, W.T., Jr. (1972). The prediction of outcome in schizophrenia. I. Characteristics of outcome. *Archives of General Psychiatry, 27*, 739–746.

Strauss, J.S., Kokes, R.F., Carpenter, W.T., Jr., & Ritzler, B.A. (1978). The course of schizophrenia as a developmental process. In L.C. Wynne (Ed.), *Nature of schizophrenia: New approaches to research and treatment* (pp. 617–630). New York: Wiley.

Strauss, M.E. (1993). Relations of symptoms to cognitive deficits in schizophrenia. *Schizophrenia Bulletin, 19*, 215–231.

Sweet, R.A., & Pollock, B.G. (1998). New atypical antipsychotics: Experience and utility in the elderly. *Drugs and Aging, 12*, 115–127.

Tsuang, M.T., & Winokur, G. (1975). The Iowa 500: Field work in a 35 year follow-up of depression, mania, and schizophrenia. *Canadian Psychiatric Association Journal, 20*, 359–365.

Vaillant, G.E. (1964). Prospective prediction of schizophrenic remission. *Archives of General Psychiatry, 36*, 724–739.

Zubin, J., & Spring, B. (1977). Vulnerability–a new view of schizophrenia. *Journal of Abnormal Psychiatry, 86*, 103–126.

CHAPTER 9

Dementia

JODY COREY-BLOOM

CASE STUDY

Mrs. J. is a 67-year-old woman who was brought to the clinic by her husband because of increasing forgetfulness. Mr. J. reports that his wife completed high school, two years of college, and a degree in interior design. She has worked as an interior decorator for over 30 years and has owned and managed her own company for most of that period. Confidentially, he reports that his wife has been having increased difficulty remembering appointments, clients' orders, and even conversations with coworkers over the past year or so. She has ceased making annual buying trips to Europe for her business because she cannot keep her itineraries and purchases straight. She has recently asked Mr. J. to help with the financial aspects of the business. He describes her reduced interest in clients' projects and withdrawal from many previous social activities. The patient used to be an avid golfer but stopped playing about six months earlier because of difficult keeping track of the score. Recently, Mrs. J. left food cooking on the stove, resulting in a small kitchen fire.

The patient has no significant current medical problems and takes no medications. The patient's older brother has recently been diagnosed with Alzheimer's disease and Mr. J. wonders if his wife might also have it.

There were no significant findings on physical examination. On mental status testing, the patient was not oriented to the exact date and demonstrated some mild naming problems. She had difficulty with serial 7s and calculations. Short-term verbal memory was impaired. Visuospatial abilities were intact. There was no right-left confusion. Vitamin B12 level and thyroid function tests were normal. Head CT was normal.

DSM-IV CRITERIA FOR DEMENTIA

The patient's history and mental status testing suggest a diagnosis of a primary progressive dementia. *DSM-IV* (American Psychiatric Association [APA], 1994) defines the term *dementia* as a syndrome (produced by many disorders) characterized by impairment from a previous higher level of intellectual functioning (see Table 9.1). The impairment involves memory and other cognitive domains (including language, orientation, constructional abilities, abstract thinking, problem solving, and praxis) and must be of sufficient severity to interfere with occupational or social performance or both; that is, there must be functional impairment. Changes in personality and affect are often noted, but a normal level of consciousness is preserved until very late stages of the disorder.

Patients with cognitive impairment without evidence of a functional decline do not strictly meet *DSM-IV* criteria for dementia. These patients are often classified in a variety of ways, such as "benign senescent forgetfulness," "age-associated memory impairment," and "at risk" for dementia. On follow-up, however, many of these individuals are found to have a progressive dementia (Morris et al., 1991).

EVALUATION OF DEMENTIA

For most clinicians, evaluating the older individual with memory complaints involves two levels of assessment. First, it is necessary to ascertain whether cognitive impairment exists and if that cognitive impairment meets criteria for dementia. If dementia is identified, the second step generally consists of those evaluations necessary to determine the etiology of the dementia and to grade its severity. A de novo diagnosis of dementia cannot be made when consciousness is impaired or if conditions exist that prevent adequate evaluation of mental status (e.g., impaired vision or hearing). Metabolic and other causes that usually present as delirium can manifest in a more chronic way and need to be distinguished.

Table 9.1 *DSM-IV* criteria for diagnosis of Alzheimer's dementia.

- Gradual onset and continuing decline of cognitive function from a previously higher level, resulting in impairment of social and occupational function.
- Impairment of recent memory and at least one of the following:
  —Language disturbances.
  —Word-finding difficulties.
  —Disturbances of praxis.
  —Disturbances of visual processing.
  —Visual agnosia.
  —Constructional disturbances.
  —Disturbances of executive function, including abstract reasoning, and concentration.
- Cognitive deficits are not due to other psychiatric disease, neurological diseases, or systemic disease.
- Cognitive deficits do not exclusively occur in the setting of delirium.

Source: American Psychiatric Association, 1994.

History

A skillfully taken history can reveal deficits in various areas of intellectual function and, when possible, should be substantiated by an informant, as in the case of Mrs. J. In taking a history, certain functional items, such as difficulty recalling recent events, preparing a balanced meal, playing games of skill (e.g., bridge, cards), filling out business forms (e.g., insurance), handling financial records (bills, checks, bank statements), and shopping alone, are helpful in confirming the presence of intellectual impairment (Pfeffer, Kurosaki, Harrah, Chance, & Filos, 1982) (see Table 9.2). It is also useful to inquire about a family history of Alzheimer's disease (AD) or other dementia.

The tempo of cognitive decline is extremely important in the evaluation of the demented patient. AD characteristically has an insidious onset. Acute or subacute onset of disability should raise the possibility of a dementia etiology other than AD. Rapid deterioration associated with fluctuating levels of alertness usually indicates delirium, which needs to be evaluated and treated before dementia can be considered.

Mental Status Testing

Cognitive testing is done according to the preference of the individual physician, but should include assessment of attention, orientation, recent and remote memory, language, praxis, visuospatial relations, calculations, and judgment. Brief mental status screening instruments that neurologists have

Table 9.2 Trigger symptoms that may indicate dementia.

- Does the person have increased difficulty with any of the activities listed below?*
  — *Learning and retaining new information.* Is more repetitive; has trouble remembering recent conversations, events, appointments; frequently misplaces objects.
  — *Handling complex tasks.* Has trouble following a complex train of thought or performing tasks that require many steps such as balancing a checkbook or cooking a meal.
  — *Reasoning ability.* Is unable to respond with a reasonable plan to problems at work or home, such as knowing what to do if the bathroom is flooded; shows uncharacteristic disregard for rules of social conduct.
  — *Spatial ability and orientation.* Has trouble driving, organizing objects around the house, finding his or her way around familiar places.
  — *Language.* Has increasing difficulty with finding the words to express what he or she wants to say and with following conversations.
  — *Behavior.* Appears more passive and less responsive; is more irritable than usual; is more suspicious than usual; misinterprets visual or auditory stimuli.
- In addition to a patient's failure to arrive at the right time for appointments, the clinician can look for a patient's difficulty discussing current events in an area of interest and changes in behavior or dress. It also may be helpful to follow up on areas of concern by asking the patient or family members relevant questions.

*Positive findings in any of these areas generally indicate the need for further assessment for the presence of dementia.
Source: Small et al., 1997.

found useful, and that may enhance clinical judgment, include the Mini-Mental State Examination (MMSE) (Folstein, Folstein, & McHugh, 1975; Giordani et al., 1990) (see Table 9.3). It should be emphasized, however, that age, education, ethnicity, and language of the respondent can influence responses to mental status test items, and the clinician must make allowances for each of these in assessing patients with cognitive difficulties (Bleecker, Bolla-Wilson, Kawas, & Agnew, 1988; Heeren, Lagaay, von Beek, Rooymans, & Hijmans, 1990; Mungas, Marshall, Weldon, Haan, & Reed, 1996; Murden, McRae, Kaner, & Bucknam, 1991; Uhlmann & Larson, 1991). Although cutoff points have been recommended for some of the standardized, well-known mental status tests, they are by no means definitive, and mildly demented patients may score in the "normal" range.

Test scores do not, of themselves, make a diagnosis of dementia, nor do they determine the etiology of the dementing illness. Although most of the standardized mental status tests are described primarily in relation to AD, scores on these screening tests may be abnormal when any form of dementia or cognitive impairment exists.

Table 9.3 Mini-mental state examination.

Area of Cognition	Potential Points	Specific Task
Orientation	10	Date, year, month, day of the week, season, current location (building), floor, town/city, county, state.
Immediate recall	3	Learn three unrelated words: "ball, flag, tree" (number of trials needed to learn all three: _____).
Attention and calculation	5	Counting backwards from 100 by 7 or spelling the word "world" backwards (the better performance is used to derive final score).
Recall	3	Recall three words: "ball, flag, tree."
Language	8	• Name "watch" and "pencil." • Repeat "No ifs, ands, or buts." • Follow three stage command: "Take paper in hand, fold paper in half, put paper on the floor." • Read and do what it says: "Close your eyes." • Write a spontaneous sentence.
Construction	1	• Copy a drawing of intersecting pentagons.
Deriving the Total Score	___	Add the number of correct responses. The maximum score is 30.

Source: Folstein et al., 1975.

Neurological Examination

The physical neurological examination does not help to assess the presence or absence of dementia. However, a thorough examination may reveal important clues to the etiology of the patient's dementia. Careful attention should be paid to the existence of focal abnormalities such as visual field cuts or hemiparesis, as these may suggest a focal brain lesion, such as from a stroke or tumor. In addition, evidence of parkinsonism (rigidity or bradykinesia), movement disorders, and abnormalities of gait may raise the possibility of other dementia etiologies.

Laboratory Testing

Clues to the differential diagnosis of dementia emanate from the history and examination as described, but diagnostic tests are also necessary to rule out metabolic and structural causes. The detailed workup depends on the suspected diagnosis, but generally includes a neuroimaging study—computed tomography (CT) or magnetic resonance imaging (MRI) of the brain—and the following blood tests: complete blood cell count, serum electrolytes (including calcium), glucose, renal function tests, liver function tests, thyroid function tests, serum vitamin B12 level, and syphilis serology (see Table 9.4). Other tests, though not recommended as routine studies, may be helpful in certain circumstances: sedimentation rate (ESR), HIV testing (where risk factors are present), chest X-ray (CXR), urinalysis, neuropsychological testing, cerebrospinal fluid (CSF) examination, electroencephalography (EEG), positron-emission tomography (PET), and single photon emission computed tomography (SPECT).

The utility of standard laboratory tests in the workup of dementia and the true incidence of potentially reversible etiologies have been questioned by many (Clarfield, 1988; Larson, Reifler, Sumi, Canfield, & Chinn, 1986). However, among patients who meet criteria for dementia, about 10% to 20% will be found to have a specific treatable or reversible etiology for their dementing syndrome. The most important examples are depression, prescription drugs, metabolic conditions such as thyroid disease and vitamin deficiencies, neurosyphilis, chronic infections, and structural brain lesions such as tumors, subdural hematomas, and hydrocephalus.

Table 9.4 Laboratory evaluation of patients with dementia.

Routine	*When Indicated*
CBC	ESR
Chemistry panel	HIV testing
Vitamin B_{12} level	CXR, urinalysis
Thyroid function tests	Neuropsychological testing
Syphilis serology	CSF examination
CT/MRI	EEG
	PET/SPECT

Source: Corey-Bloom et al., 1995.

DIFFERENTIAL DIAGNOSIS OF DEMENTIA

AD is the most frequent type of dementia in U.S. and European elderly, comprising about 50% to 80% of subjects presenting with dementing disorders in various clinicopathological series (Table 9.5). In contrast, vascular dementia may be more common in Scandinavia and certain non-European countries such as Japan, and the frequency with which AD and vascular dementia appear may depend to some degree on the age of the population.

Alzheimer's Disease

Although prevalence figures are not well established, currently two to four million individuals in the United States are estimated to be afflicted with AD, and that number will increase to at least seven million by the early 21st century (Brookmeyer, Gray, & Kawas, 1998; Evans et al., 1990; United States Congress & Office of Technology Assessment, 1987). AD is a major cause of disability and mortality, and the financial consequences are staggering (Katzman et al., 1994). The impact of AD on health care costs, including direct and indirect medical and social service costs, is estimated to be greater than $50 billion per year (Ernst & Hay, 1994; Huang, Cartwright, & Hu, 1988).

The diverse spectrum of symptoms of AD reflects dysfunction of widespread regions of the cerebral cortex. Symptoms begin insidiously, making it difficult to date precisely the onset of cognitive and functional decline. Progression is generally gradual and inexorable, with occasional pauses; however, reliable measurement of disease progression in AD is difficult because of variability between and within subjects.

Memory loss is the cardinal and commonly presenting complaint in AD. Initially, the patient has difficulty recalling new information such as names or details of conversation; remote memories are relatively preserved (Bondi, Salmon, & Butters, 1994). With progression, the memory loss worsens to include remote memory (see Table 9.6).

Table 9.5   Common causes of the dementia syndrome.

Alzheimer's disease.
Dementia associated with Lewy bodies.
Alzheimer's disease and vascular dementia (mixed dementia).
Vascular dementia.
Depression.
Metabolic disorders.
Drug intoxication.
Infections.
Structural lesions.
Dementia due to alcohol.
Hydrocephalus.
Parkinson's disease.
Pick's and other frontal dementias.

Table 9.6 Common clinical features of Alzheimer's disease by stage.

	Early	Intermediate	Late
Cognitive			
Memory	• Poor recall of new information. • Remote memories relatively preserved.	• Remote memories affected.	• Untestable.
Language	• Dysnomia. • Mild loss of fluency.	• Nonfluent, paraphasias. • Poor comprehension. • Impaired repetition.	• Near mutism.
Visuospatial	• Misplacing objects. • Difficulty driving.	• Getting lost. • Difficulty copying figures.	• Untestable.
Behavioral	• Delusions. • Depression. • Insomnia.	• Delusions. • Depression. • Agitation. • Insomnia.	• Agitation. • Wandering.
Neurological	• Abnormal face-hand test. • Agraphesthesia. • Frontal release signs.	• Abnormal face-hand test. • Agraphesthesia. • Frontal release signs.	• Muteness. • Incontinence. • Frontal release signs. • Rigidity. • Loss of gait. • ± Myoclonus.

Language is frequently normal early in AD, although reduced conversational output may be noted. As dementia progresses, many patients become more recognizably aphasic. Initially, this manifests as difficulty with naming and mild loss of fluency (Cummings, Benson, Hill, & Read, 1985). Later, language becomes obviously nonfluent until, terminally, the patient may be reduced to a state of near mutism (Murdoch & Chenery, 1987).

Visuospatial impairment in AD results in symptoms such as misplacing objects or getting lost, difficulty with recognizing and drawing complex figures, and deficient driving (Brouwers, Cox, Martin, Chase, & Fedio, 1984). Difficulty with calculation (affecting skills such as handling money) and apraxia and agnosia are further problems that develop in AD. Apraxia may impair activities such as operating appliances and dressing; as might be expected, more complex skills tend to break down first, while highly overlearned motor tasks (e.g., playing a musical instrument, using tools) may be retained until relatively late in the course (Rapcsak, Croswell, & Rubens, 1989). Agnosia develops in middle to late stages of AD, and includes features such as failing to recognize family members or spouse. Early in AD, judgment and abstraction are often impaired, suggesting involvement of the frontal lobes. Social comportment and interpersonal skills are often strikingly preserved in AD and may remain relatively intact long after memory and insight have been lost.

Behavioral and psychiatric symptoms occur frequently in AD. Over and above a general decline of activity and interest in virtually all AD patients, depressive symptoms occur in about 25%, although severe depression is uncommon (Becker, Boller, Lopez, Saxton, & McGonigle, 1994).

Delusions are common in AD, although they are rarely as systematized as in schizophrenia (Becker et al., 1994). They often have a paranoid flavor, with fears of personal harm, theft of personal property, and marital infidelity. "Phantom boarder" delusions, in which the patient believes that unwelcome individuals are living in his or her home, and misidentification syndromes also occur. Commonly, television characters are believed real or patients fail to recognize their own reflection in a mirror.

In addition to depression and psychotic symptoms, AD patients show a wide range of behavioral abnormalities, including agitation, wandering, sleep disturbances, and disinhibition (Becker et al., 1994). These often impose a significant burden on caregivers and may precipitate nursing home placement. In contrast to psychotic symptoms, behavioral disturbances are more clearly associated with the degree of dementia. Agitation includes physical aggression, verbal aggression, and nonaggressive behaviors. Physically nonaggressive behaviors, such as motor restlessness and pacing, are the most common forms of agitation in outpatients with AD. However, physical aggression is the most distressing behavior to caregivers, and occurs in about 20% of patients. Various factors appear to be important predictors of aggressive behavior, including premorbid history of aggression, a troubled premorbid relationship between caregiver and patient, and a greater number of social and medical problems. Wandering behavior affects 3% to 26% of AD outpatients. Insomnia and sleep disturbances are inconstant features of AD, and sexual disinhibition has been reported in fewer than 10% of patients. Thus, behavioral symptoms are a pervasive and poorly understood concomitant of cognitive deterioration in AD.

Excluding mental status testing, the neurologic examination is usually normal in AD, and the presence of significant or lateralizing abnormalities often suggests other diagnoses. Primitive reflexes (snout, glabellar, grasp), impaired graphesthesia, and an abnormal face-hand test are frequently encountered in AD (Becker et al., 1994). Variable features, including extrapyramidal signs (rigidity and bradykinesia), gait disturbances, and myoclonus, may occasionally be seen early in the course of AD and increase in prevalence with the severity of illness. The frequency of parkinsonian signs in patients with AD was as low as 12% to 14% in some series and as high as 28% to 92% in others, depending on the severity of dementia in patients who were studied (Bakchine, Lacomblez, Palisson, Laurent, & Derousne, 1989; Becker et al., 1994). In intermediate and advanced stages of dementia, patients often develop nonspecific impairment of gait and balance, leading to an increased risk of falls. Myoclonus develops late in the course of AD, and longitudinal studies report an increase in its frequency during follow-up. Its prevalence in AD has varied widely from 0 to 68%, although the usual reported rate is about 10% (Hauser, Morris, Heston, & Anderson, 1986).

As neuronal degeneration progresses in AD, all of the above symptoms worsen, and eventually patients become uncommunicative and unable to care for themselves, walk, or maintain continence. They require total care, including feeding, and are often institutionalized. In end-stage AD, death usually results from complications of being bedbound, such as aspiration pneumonia, urinary tract infections, sepsis, or pulmonary embolism (Molsa, Marttila, & Rinne, 1986).

The brain of a patient with AD shows marked atrophy, reflective of a widespread loss of neurons (Terry, Masliah, & Hansen, 1994). In addition, synapses, the connections between neurons, are diminished in number. The neuropathologic hallmarks of this disorder are neuritic plaques (NP) and neurofibrillary tangles (NFT). NP consist of a central core of fibrous protein known as amyloid, surrounded by degenerating nerve endings. NFT are found inside neurons and are composed of structures called paired helical filaments. Pathologic criteria for the diagnosis of AD at autopsy require the demonstration of a sufficient number of NP and NFT on microscopic examination. Because of the presence of amyloid in NP and to a variable degree in cerebral blood vessels in the AD brain, the role of this protein and its precursor peptide (beta amyloid precursor protein) has been widely investigated (Cummings, Vinters, Cole, & Khachaturian, 1998). The exact nature of their roles in the pathogenesis of AD remain unclear.

The two most widely used sets of criteria for the diagnosis of AD are those of *DSM-IV* and those developed by the National Institute of Neurological and Communicative Disorders and Stroke-Alzheimer's Disease and Related Disorders Association (NINCDS-ADRDA) joint task force (McKhann et al., 1984). According to *DSM-IV*, as noted above, primary degenerative dementia of the Alzheimer type requires an insidious onset, a generally progressive deteriorating course, and exclusion of all other specific causes of dementia. The more detailed NINCDS criteria reserve the designation of "definite" AD for cases with biopsy or autopsy confirmation. A diagnosis of "probable" AD is the maximum level of certainty possible without pathological confirmation and requires the insidious onset of decline in memory and at least one other area of cognition, a progressive course, preserved level of consciousness, and the exclusion of other conditions that could cause these symptoms. Patients with an atypical course, focal neurological findings, or coexistent disorders that by themselves may produce dementia are designated as "possible" AD. Using NINCDS-ADRDA or other criteria, with suitable laboratory and diagnostic studies, at least 80% to 90% accuracy in the clinical diagnosis of AD can be achieved (Gearing et al., 1995; Klatka, Schiffer, Powers, & Kazee, 1996).

In the future, biological markers to confirm AD during life may be available to permit early identification of the disease (Wahlund, 1996). In spite of many attempts to identify a biological marker to diagnose AD, this goal has remained elusive. Recent efforts have focused on CSF markers based on components of the neuropathologic lesions of AD (amyloid plaques and NFT) such as beta amyloid and tau protein. Although such markers would be highly desirable, at present, none have either been definitely proven or wholly excluded.

Dementia Associated with Lewy Bodies (DLB)

Dementia has also been described in association with cortical Lewy bodies, the neuropathological feature used to diagnose Parkinson's disease. Nosologically, this is a very complex area; however, despite variable nomenclature for this entity, these patients at autopsy are found to have an admixture of AD and parkinsonian pathology (including brainstem and also diffuse cortical Lewy bodies). Parkinsonian signs, including bradykinesia and rigidity, but usually lacking a resting tremor, are common on neurological examination (McKeith et al., 1996). Often, the parkinsonian signs appear early in the course and help to distinguish this entity from "pure AD." Many patients also have prominent psychiatric features (especially visual hallucinations) and a fluctuating level of consciousness, in addition to a history of antecedent falls. The cognitive deficits may be similar to those seen in AD; however, there is often greater visuospatial impairment and reduced verbal fluency. Several reports have suggested that these patients may progress more rapidly; unfortunately, the clinical and neuropsychological profiles of these patients have not been well characterized and accepted diagnostic criteria have only recently become available.

Vascular Dementia (VD)

About 5% to 10% of patients with dementia have evidence of clinically significant cerebrovascular disease. Symptoms appear when a certain volume of infarcted tissue is present or if small strokes are strategically placed.

Features suggestive of VD, such as sudden onset of dysfunction in one or more cognitive domains, with "patchy" distribution of deficits and a stepwise deteriorating course, are often sufficient to distinguish this entity from AD. Focal neurologic symptoms are frequently present on examination, including weakness of an extremity, exaggeration of deep tendon reflexes, an extensor plantar response, and gait abnormalities (del Ser, 1990). However, stepwise deterioration or focal findings need not be present; when present, focal findings do not rule out concomitant AD pathology. Affective changes and psychotic symptoms are also common complications of VD, with depression and delusions highly prevalent in these patients. As the disease advances, emotional incontinence and pseudobulbar palsy may be apparent. There is often a history of previous strokes, transient ischemic attacks (TIAs), and risk factors for stroke such as hypertension, coronary artery disease, or atrial fibrillation.

Diagnostic accuracy for VD has improved with the introduction of clinical criteria and neuroimaging techniques capable of demonstrating ischemic lesions, but remains much lower than that for AD (Chui et al., 1992; Erkinjuntti, 1994; Roman et al., 1993). The accuracy of the clinical diagnosis of VD in studies with postmortem follow-up varies from 25% to 85% (Gold et al., 1997). Further clinicopathologic studies will likely be necessary to confirm the usefulness of current criteria in the differential diagnosis between VD and AD. Nonetheless, documentation of infarctions is an important goal of imaging in dementia. The coexistence of AD and VD, called mixed dementia (MIX), is seen in roughly 10% of demented patients and further complicates the differentiation between AD and VD.

Other Dementias

Non-Alzheimer, nonvascular dementias comprise about 10% of some autopsy series. Although pathologically, and often clinically, distinct from AD, it can sometimes be difficult to recognize these unusual syndromes.

Frontotemporal Dementias.   When prominent alterations in emotion, affect, and behavior are the initial symptoms of dementia, Pick's disease and other frontal lobe dementias may be a more appropriate consideration (Neary et al., 1998). Typical early features include personality changes, withdrawal, lack of insight and disinhibited behavior (see Table 9.7). These subjects demonstrate significant disturbances in planning and "shifting set" but only modest difficulties in learning and recall.

Diagnostic criteria for the frontotemporal dementias have been described (Neary et al.); imaging studies, especially functional neuroimaging such as PET and SPECT, may be particularly helpful in these disorders (Miller et al., 1997). At autopsy, these subjects have focal cortical degenerative disease; however, other than Pick's disease, most are not terribly distinctive neuropathologically (Brun & Passant, 1996). In Pick's disease, intracytoplasmic argyrophilic inclusions known as Pick bodies are present. Other types of pathology, however, including swollen chromatolytic neurons, subcortical gliosis, or no distinctive histologic features, are significantly more common. Progressive aphasia is a related disorder characterized by a nonfluent language disturbance with relatively preserved comprehension and sparing of other cognitive abilities, including memory (Kertesz, Hudson, Mackenzie, & Munoz, 1994).

Dementias with Extrapyramidal Features.   Parkinsonian features are found in AD and DLB but may also be seen in other dementias such as PD, progressive supranuclear palsy (PSP), and corticobasal degeneration (Adler, 1999; Pillon, Dubois, Ploska, & Agid, 1991; Stoessl & Rivest, 1999) (see Table 9.8). Cognitive decline usually occurs late in the course of PD and may be seen in up to 50% of

Table 9.7   Clinical features of Alzheimer's disease and frontotemporal dementias.

Feature	Alzheimer's Disease	Frontotemporal Dementias
Age at onset	Most ≥ 65 years	Often 40–65 years
Presenting symptoms	Prominent memory loss; decline in category fluency	Inappropriate behavior and judgment; impaired planning (dysexecutive syndrome); relative paucity of anterograde amnesia
Language disturbance	Mild until more advanced stages	Early and prominent, with paraphasias and anomia
Social skills	Typically preserved until advanced stages	Often lost early

Table 9.8   Dementias with Parkinsonian features.

Alzheimer's disease
Dementia associated with Lewy bodies
Parkinson's disease
Progressive supranuclear palsy
Corticobasal degeneration
Striatonigral degeneration

cases prior to death, especially if patients are elderly and have severe motor impairment. Cognitive impairment typically is "subcortical," that is, characterized by mental slowing, markedly reduced attention and initiation, and improvement with cues, as in recognition memory testing (Savage, 1997). This pattern of cognitive deficits, seen also in PSP and corticobasal degeneration, differs significantly from that seen in "cortical" dementias such as AD and the frontotemporal dementias. The typical presentation of PSP involves loss of volitional vertical eye movements, rigidity, and gait instability with retropulsion (Litvan et al., 1997). Corticobasal degeneration is accompanied by a distinctive progressive apraxia (Pillon et al., 1995).

Other.   A rapidly progressive dementia with generalized myoclonus, especially to startle, and gait ataxia suggests Creutzfeldt-Jakob disease, a spongiform encephalopathy caused by genetically coded modifications of an endogenous protein called the prion protein (Korczyn, 1997; Mastrianni, 1998). A similarly rapid dementia is that seen with limbic encephalitis, a paraneoplastic syndrome most commonly described in association with primary lung carcinomas (Dropcho, 1998). The diagnosis of normal pressure hydrocephalus should be entertained for a subacute onset of dementia characterized by a pronounced frontal gait apraxia and urinary incontinence in the setting of greatly enlarged ventricles without a matching degree of cortical atrophy on neuroradiologic studies (Turner & McGeachie, 1988).

EPIDEMIOLOGY OF ALZHEIMER'S DISEASE

CLINICAL RISK FACTORS

Our understanding of the epidemiology of AD has advanced rapidly during the past decade with the emergence of various demographic, genetic, and exposure-related risk factors for its development. The most important clinical risk factors for the development of AD are shown in Table 9.9.

Age is clearly the major risk factor for AD, and many epidemiological studies have reported a striking increase in the prevalence of AD as a function of age (Jorm, Korten, & Henderson, 1987; Katzman & Kawas, 1994; Rocca et al., 1991). From age 65 to 85, the prevalence of AD doubles approximately every five years.

Table 9.9   Risk factors for Alzheimer's disease.

Age*
Genetic influences*
ApoE status*
Female gender
Lack of education
Head trauma
Myocardial infarction

* Most important.

In addition, genetic influences are important in AD, but their mechanism of action and whether they are operative in all cases of AD, remains unclear (Cummings et al., 1998; Katzman & Kawas, 1994). In some cases, AD is inherited ("familial AD") in an autosomal fashion with the gene linked to markers on three separate chromosomes (1, 14 and 21) (see Table 9.10). Familial AD families are those with multiply affected individuals in which the disease segregates in a manner consistent with fully penetrant autosomal dominant inheritance. These cases constitute fewer than 10% of all cases with AD; however, they reinforce the fact that genetic influences are important in AD, and it is likely that significant advances in our understanding of the molecular basis of AD will come from them.

Recently, the importance of an individual's apolipoprotein E (ApoE) status has received significant attention as an important genetic susceptibility risk factor for the development of AD. ApoE is a protein involved in cholesterol transport with three possible forms or alleles: e2 (rare), e3 (most frequent), and e4. Individuals who are homozygous and carry two ApoE e4 alleles have an increased probability (>90%) of developing AD by age 85 and do so about 10 years earlier than individuals carrying the e2 or e3 allelic variants. The exact mechanism by which this occurs and the utility of this for diagnostic purposes remain unsettled (Cummings et al., 1998).

Epidemiological studies have shown a higher prevalence of family history of AD in "sporadic" AD patients than in controls, suggesting that genetic factors are involved even in the sporadic form (Katzman & Kawas, 1994). A family history of AD in a first-degree relative (mother, father, brother, or sister) increases

Table 9.10   Alzheimer's disease: Genetic loci.

Chromosome	Gene	% of AD	Age at Onset
21	APP	<1	45–60
14	PS-1	1–5	30–60
1	PS-2	<1	50–65
19	ApoE	50–60	60+

APP = amyloid precursor protein; PS-1 = presenillin-1; PS-2 = presenillin-2; ApoE = apolipoprotein E.

the risk of developing dementia by approximately fourfold at any age. It is not clear if this holds for individuals over the age of 80.

Other demographic factors, including gender (women may be more susceptible to AD than men) and lack of education have emerged as putative risk factors for AD (Katzman & Kawas, 1994; Launer et al., 1999). Women, who constitute approximately two-thirds of the population over 75 years of age, may be at greater risk of developing AD, even when greater longevity is taken into account. In addition to differences in longevity, there are differences in education between men and women in many cohorts that have been examined, which might confound the findings because lack of education is a risk factor for dementia. An uneducated individual over age 75 has about twice the risk for dementia as one who has completed at least eight grades of school.

Head trauma, either a single episode leading to unconsciousness or hospitalization, or repeated head injuries, as in the case of boxers, appears to be a risk factor for AD (Katzman & Kawas, 1994; Mortimer et al., 1991). Head injury produces diffuse plaques in the brain similar to those detected in AD. Interesting preliminary data, which require verification, suggest that in the very elderly, myocardial ischemia may be a risk factor for dementia, particularly in women, again acting through the production of diffuse amyloid plaques.

Equally intriguing preliminary data suggest that exposure to estrogen replacement (Kawas et al., 1997; Waring et al., 1999) and possibly anti-inflammatory agents may reduce the risk of developing AD. Estrogen may have neurotrophic and neuroprotective effects on nerve cells. One recent study reported that a much smaller percentage of postmenopausal estrogen users developed AD compared to nonusers (Tang et al., 1996). Even controlling for education and ApoE genotype, the risk reduction for estrogen users was 60%. Risk reduction was greatest for those who had used estrogen for over one year. A large national prospective study, the Women's Health Initiative Memory Study, is currently underway to further look at the impact of estrogen on development of AD.

Inflammatory changes are common in the brains of patients with AD. This plus the finding of a lower frequency of AD in patients with arthritis has led to great interest in a possible ameliorating effect of anti-inflammatory agents in AD. A recent meta-analysis suggested the possibility of benefit of anti-inflammatory therapy in AD (McGeer, Schulzer, & McGeer, 1996). To date, there has been only one clinical trial of nonsteroidal anti-inflammatory agents (NSAIDs) in AD, the results of which must be considered very preliminary (J. Rogers et al., 1993). It is not currently possible to predict which drugs, or combination of drugs, might be useful in AD, because only limited data exist on the relative ability of various NSAIDs to reach the brain. Comprehensive trials are required to verify the purported protective effect of these agents.

CLINICAL PREDICTORS OF DISEASE PROGRESSION

It has been suggested that a number of factors affect the rate of decline in AD; however, this is a thorny issue because variables thought to have independent prognostic significance may simply be markers of the level of disease severity. For example, gender and level of education have been examined as predictors of decline in several studies but require further examination. Earlier age at onset of disease, however, may be a predictor of greater rate of cognitive and functional worsening (Teri, McCurry, Edland, Kukull, & Larson, 1995).

AD patients often develop parkinsonism, notably rigidity and bradykinesia, as dementia advances. Although it has been suggested that patients who develop parkinsonism have a faster rate of decline, many of the earlier studies likely included patients on neuroleptics and those with DLB. A more recent investigation reported no association between parkinsonism and cognitive decline in mildly to moderately demented AD patients free of neuroleptic medications (Lopez, Wisnieski, Becker, Boller, & DeKosky, 1997).

Whether neuropsychiatric symptoms superimposed on AD influence cognitive deterioration has also been examined by several authors. Although some reports have suggested that AD patients decline more rapidly when psychotic symptoms are present, opinion remains divided over the effect of neuropsychiatric symptoms on progression in AD (Chen, Stern, Sano, Mayeux, 1991; Chui, Lyness, Sobel, & Schneider, 1994; Stern et al., 1994). This obviously needs to be resolved by additional studies as these symptoms are potentially treatable.

Although the ApoE e4 allele is associated with both a high likelihood of developing AD and an earlier age of onset, there have been conflicting results with regard to the influence of ApoE genotype on the course of cognitive decline in AD. Several authors have found that the e4 allele is not associated with any change in rate of progression of dementia (Gomez-Isla et al., 1996), but this is not supported by others who report an accelerated rate of decline in e4 homozygotes with probable AD (Craft et al., 1998).

Whether estrogen or NSAIDs affect progression of AD also remains unclear. Analysis of longitudinal changes over one year revealed less decline among NSAID patients than among non-NSAID patients on measures of verbal fluency, spatial recognition, and orientation in a study of 210 patients with AD (Rich et al., 1995). Although several observational studies have suggested that estrogen replacement therapy may have a beneficial effect on cognitive performance in women with AD (Yaffe et al., 1998), many have substantial methodologic problems and, as is the case for NSAIDs, large placebo-controlled trials will be necessary to accurately address its role.

PREDICTORS OF NURSING HOME PLACEMENT

Most patients with AD reside in nursing homes or related institutions late in the course of the illness. The interval between the diagnosis of AD and the need for institutional placement has much practical and clinical importance, but is not easy to predict. Behavioral symptoms such as agitation, wandering, or aggression may preempt nursing home placement regardless of the level of cognitive impairment. Another variable that greatly influences the decision for institutional placement of a demented patient is social support.

Several studies have examined predictors of institutionalization in AD. As expected, the predictive factors are complex and, in addition to the time to institutionalization, vary greatly among studies. Several investigations have found that inability to speak coherently, loss of skills needed for bathing and grooming, urinary or fecal incontinence, and death or serious illness of a caregiver were major determinants of institutionalization (Hutton, Dippel, Loewenson, Mortimer, & Christians, 1985).

A prospective study of initially community-dwelling AD patients found that 12% with "mild AD" were in nursing homes after one year, and 35% after two years (Knopman, Kitto, Deinard, & Heiring, 1988). For "advanced AD," the figures were 39% at one year and 62% at two years. Incontinence, irritability, inability to walk, wandering, hyperactivity, and nocturnal behavioral problems were the leading reasons for placement cited by caregivers.

A recent study distinguished by an extremely large number of patients (n = 727) from 20 university medical centers found that the median time from enrollment to nursing home placement was 3.1 years, with significantly reduced times (2.1 years) for males who were unmarried (Heyman, Peterson, Fillenbaum, & Pieper, 1997). Disability, age at entry, and marital status predicted time to nursing home admission.

SURVIVAL

Length of survival with AD is highly variable, although an excess mortality has consistently been reported (Aevarsson, Svanborg, & Skoog, 1998; Jorm et al., 1987). Although mean survival after symptom onset may range from 2 to over 16 years, the observed survival rate among AD populations is generally significantly lower than the expected rate based on life expectancy tables (Walsh, Welch, & Larson, 1990). Depending on the study, survival at five years ranges from 10% to 40% in different AD populations. Of course, the most favorable survival rates are seen in mild cohorts followed up in outpatient settings, with lowest survival rates reported in relatively severely demented subjects from hospital series. The median duration of survival in one study from time of study entry was 5.9 years (Heyman, Peterson, Fillenbaum, & Pieper, 1996), which compares favorably to other reports of 5.3–5.8 years (Jost & Grossberg, 1995; Walsh et al., 1990).

The shortened survival of AD patients results from complications due to severe mental decline. Malnutrition, dehydration, pneumonia, and other infections occur frequently in the terminal stages, when patients are bed-bound, incontinent, and unable to communicate or feed themselves. Compared to other elderly individuals, AD patients are not especially predisposed to cancer or cerebrovascular or cardiovascular disease (Molsa et al., 1986).

Probably not surprisingly, the most consistent predictors of mortality in AD patients have been age, gender, and severity of dementia. Increasing age and male gender have been related to shorter survival in many studies (Aguero-Torres, Fratiglioni, Guo, Viitanen, & Winblad, 1998; Claus et al., 1998). As might be expected, patients with more severe dementia and greater functional disability at study entry have been reported to have shorter durations of survival (Claus et al., 1998; Heyman et al., 1996). Additional variables that may influence survival time in patients with AD have not been well established, including level of education, medical comorbidity, presence of an ApoE e4 allele, psychiatric or behavioral symptoms, and weight, among others.

TREATMENT OF DEMENTIA

Strategies for treating AD include treating the primary (cognitive) symptoms, treating the secondary (behavioral) symptoms, slowing the rate of dementia progression, delaying dementia onset, and preventing dementia occurrence.

TREATING THE PRIMARY SYMPTOMS OF AD

Although we currently have no therapy that can either cure or permanently arrest AD, the cholinesterase inhibitors represent an important first step toward delaying symptomatic decline and, in some, effecting temporary improvement of the core symptoms of memory impairment and functional loss.

Cholinergic agents are a rational approach to the palliative treatment of AD. Acetylcholine is an important neurotransmitter in the brain, and its decline is prominent in AD. Loss in cholinergic markers during the course of AD has been correlated with the degree of cognitive dysfunction. The most successful cholinergic strategy to date has comprised the class of compounds known as cholinesterase inhibitors. These agents reduce the metabolism of acetylcholine, thereby raising its levels at cholinergic synapses in the brain. Currently, the only FDA-approved cholinesterase inhibitors for AD are tacrine (Cognex) and donepezil (Aricept). However, several others are pending FDA approval or are in the final stages of clinical testing.

The first cholinesterase inhibitor to be approved for the treatment of AD by the FDA in September 1993 was tacrine. Although a clinically observable improvement was noted in 20% to 30% of treated patients participating in the multicenter, placebo-controlled trials, there was a high dropout rate in these studies (Knapp et al., 1994). In addition, a reversible elevation of liver enzymes was noted in about half of patients treated with tacrine.

More recently, donepezil has also been approved for the treatment of AD. In double-blind randomized trials, significant differences in favor of donepezil were seen on cognitive testing and global ratings by clinicians and caregivers (S. Rogers, Friedhoff, & Group, 1996). As expected, adverse effects were typically cholinergic, primarily gastrointestinal, and mild to moderate in intensity. The most frequently encountered adverse events were nausea, vomiting, diarrhea, dizziness, gastric upset, and constipation. Unlike tacrine, donepezil was not associated with any hepatotoxicity that would require clinical laboratory monitoring.

In general, cholinesterase inhibitors produce a measurable, albeit modest, improvement in cognition, as evidenced by treatment effects of 2.5 to 5 points on the Alzheimer's Disease Assessment Scale–Cognitive subscale (ADAS-Cog) over six months. In addition, a review of current cholinesterase inhibitor trials suggests treatment effects of about 0.3 on global scales such as the Clinician's Interview-Based Impression of Change (CIBIC). Recently, several studies of cholinesterase inhibitors have also begun to report improvements in the psychiatric and behavioral disturbances of AD (Levy, Cummings, & Kahn-Rose, 1999). Cholinergic treatment probably does not alter the progression of neurodegeneration in the brain; however, possible long-term benefits of cholinergic therapy include reduced rate of progression, delayed institutionalization, possible delayed mortality, and economic savings in the cost of patient care. It is likely that the next agents approved for the treatment of AD will also be cholinesterase inhibitors, with several new compounds becoming available in the next few years.

TREATING THE SECONDARY SYMPTOMS OF AD

Because the secondary behavioral disturbances of AD impair patients' function, increase their need for supervision, and often influence the decision to institutionalize them, their control is a priority in managing patients with this illness.

Psychotropic drugs, particularly neuroleptics, have been a mainstay in treating many of these symptoms, but carry a high risk of side effects. At present, treating secondary symptoms of AD is more an art than a science. For virtually every group of symptoms, older and newer classes of medications are available, with proven efficacy in nondemented patients and less clear results in AD patients. New agents, such as selective serotonin reuptake inhibitors and atypical neuroleptics, may herald the arrival of drugs that are both effective and better tolerated (Cummings & Knopman, 1999; Rabins, 1998). Until the appropriate trials are conducted in patients with AD, including comparative studies of different agents, it is recommended that clinicians choose a few medications from the suggestions in this review, know their pharmacokinetic and half-life profiles in depth, and follow the general principles that apply to using any medication in elderly patients.

The following is suggested as an overall approach to using psychotropic drugs for behavioral symptoms in AD and other dementia subjects:

- Define the most important behavior or symptom to target therapy clearly.
- Be aware of the natural history of the target symptom, as some symptoms such as agitation may be transient and stage-specific.
- Treat precipitating causes of behavioral symptoms (such as physical illness or medication side effects) whenever possible.
- Use environmental modification and nonpharmacological strategies whenever possible. For example, for mild degrees of pacing or wandering,

one can channel the patient's restlessness into physical activity by simplifying physical surroundings and providing an enclosed yard to walk in.

- Start drugs at very low doses and increase slowly, monitoring carefully for common and less frequent side effects.
- Recognize that medication toxicity is common in the elderly, who often take a large number of medications, thereby increasing the risk of interactions.
- Simplify dose schedules, use day-by-day pill dispensers, and enlist caregivers to supervise medications to ensure compliance.
- Consider tapering and withdrawing a drug that has produced symptomatic improvement, especially if the targeted symptom is one known to be stage-specific.

Depression

Symptoms of depression are more prominent early in AD, when patients have greater self-awareness and better communication skills. A new class of antidepressants, the selective serotonin reuptake inhibitors (SSRIs), such as fluoxetine, sertraline, paroxetine, and citalopram, may be especially useful in the treatment of geriatric depression because they are efficacious and well-tolerated (see Table 9.11) (Katz, 1998; Raskind, 1998). SSRIs are more expensive than cyclic antidepressants, and comparative studies of both classes of drugs in depressed AD patients would be helpful in guiding treatment choices. If depressive symptoms do not improve after three to four weeks, it is time to increase the medication. After an adequate dose has been attained, failure of symptoms to improve should prompt one to switch to another compound.

Psychosis, Agitation, and Insomnia

Neuroleptics have been a mainstay in managing this group of behavioral symptoms (see Table 9.12) (Rabins, 1998; Raskind, 1998); however, these agents

Table 9.11 Pharmacologic treatment of depression.

Drug	Recommended Dosage (mg/day)	Potential Side Effects
SSRI		
Fluoxetine (Prozac)	10–40	Nausea, insomnia, headache,
Sertraline (Zoloft)	25–100	restlessness, tremor.
Paroxetine (Paxil)	10–40	
Citalopram (Celexa)	10–40	
Tricyclics		
Nortriptyline (Pamelor)	10–100	Sedation, confusion, orthostasis,
Desipramine (Norpramin)	10–100	arrythmias, weight gain.
Other		
Venlafaxine (Effexor)	37.5–150	

Table 9.12 Pharmacologic treatment of psychosis and agitation.

Drug	Recommended Dosage (mg/day)	Potential Side Effects
Neuroleptics		
Haloperidol (Haldol)	0.5–3	Parkinsonism.
Thioridazine (Mellaril)	10–100	Sedation, anticholinergic effects.
Chlorpromazine (Thorazine)	10–10	Sedation, anticholinergic effects.
Atypical neuroleptics		
Risperidone (Risperdal)	1–3	Orthostatic hypotension, nausea.
Olanzapine (Zyprexa)	2.5–10	Weight gain, elevated liver tests.
Benzodiazepines		
Lorazepam (Ativan)	0.5–2	Lethargy, confusion, ataxia,
Oxazepam (Serax)	10–30	dependence.
Triazolam (Halcion)	0.0625–0.125	

may produce serious side effects, including parkinsonism, tardive dyskinesia, confusion, and falls. The initial neuroleptic dose in elderly subjects should be low, about one-quarter of that used in young adults, and the total daily dose should be gradually increased as needed, titrating against side effects such as cognitive deterioration, low blood pressure, and parkinsonism. The choice of drug can be tailored according to the clinical situation; for example, patients with marked nocturnal agitation or sundowning may benefit from the sedation produced by a low-potency agent given at night.

The risk of parkinsonism and tardive dyskinesia is a major problem confounding neuroleptic treatment. These findings may persist for weeks to months after cessation of neuroleptics and, even after neuroleptics are discontinued, may not remit in elderly patients. Because of the side effect profile of neuroleptics, some clinicians reserve these agents for patients whose behavioral symptoms do not respond to other classes of drugs. The newer atypical neuroleptics, such as risperidone and olanzapine, are effective in controlling psychosis and tend to produce parkinsonism only at high doses.

Benzodiazepines have been used in AD patients to promote sleep or control agitation. Short-acting agents, such as oxazepam and lorazepam, are preferred because they are less prone to produce daytime drowsiness and confusion than longer-acting agents. Benzodiazepines should be initiated at a low dose in patients with AD, roughly one-third to one-half the dose recommended for younger adults, and increased slowly as needed.

To enhance the onset of sleep, the benzodiazepine should be given 30 to 60 minutes before bedtime. As an adjunct to the management of insomnia in some demented patients, it is worthwhile to try nonpharmacological sleep hygiene measures, including sleep restriction and keeping patients awake during the day.

To treat sleep disorders in demented patients, nonpharmacological strategies supplemented by a short-acting benzodiazepine, neuroleptic, or sedating

Table 9.13 Pharmacologic treatment of insomnia.

Drug	Recommended Dosage (mg at bedtime—qhs)	Potential Adverse Effects
Tricyclics		
Nortriptyline (Pamelor)	10–75	Anticholinergic effects.
Benzodiazepines		
Lorazepam (Ativan)	0.5–1	Lethargy, confusion, dependence.
Oxazepam (Serax)	10–20	
Triazolam (Halcion)	0.0625–0.125	
Neuroleptics		
Haloperidol (Haldol)	0.5–1	Extrapyramidal symptoms (EPS).
Thioridazine (Mellaril)	10–50	Sedation, anticholinergic effects.
Chlorpromazine (Thorazine)	10–50	Sedation, anticholinergic effects.
Other		
Trazodone (Desyrel)	12.5–75	Orthostatic hypotension.

tricyclic antidepressant are recommended (see Table 9.13). In our experience, nortriptyline (10–75 mg) and trazodone (12.5–100 mg) are safe and effective choices for promoting sleep in AD. Uncontrolled studies also support the use of trazodone for agitation.

CONCLUSION

Our understanding of the neurobiology and epidemiology of dementia, and in particular AD, has advanced rapidly during the past decade. As a result, various demographic, genetic, and exposure-related risk factors have emerged for the development of AD, helping to change its status from an "untreatable" to a "treatable" condition. Although we currently have no agent that demonstrates a dramatic antidementia benefit, there is increasing promise that effective pharmacotherapy for dementia may soon become a reality. The need for such effective pharmacotherapy is underscored by the increasing prevalence of these dementing conditions and the staggering health costs attributed to them.

STUDY QUESTIONS

1. How does *DSM-IV* define dementia?
2. What are common causes of dementia in the elderly?
3. What are some of the clinical features of Alzheimer's disease?
4. Name some important risk factors for the development of Alzheimer's disease.
5. What laboratory tests are routinely ordered in a patient with suspected Alzheimer's disease to rule out other causes of dementia?

6. What pharmacologic treatment is currently available for the primary (cognitive) symptoms of AD? For the secondary (behavioral) symptoms?

SUGGESTED READINGS

Clarfield, A.M. (1988). The reversible dementias: Do they reverse? *Annals of Internal Medicine, 109,* 476–486.

Corey-Bloom, J., Thal, L.J., Galasko, D., Folstein, M., Drachman, D., Raskind, M., & Lanska, D.J. (1995). Diagnosis and evaluation of dementia. *Neurology, 45,* 211–218.

Cummings, J.L., & Benson, D.F. (1992). *Dementia: A clinical approach* (2nd ed.). Boston: Butterworth Heineman.

Cummings, J., Vinters, H., Cole, G., & Khachaturian, Z. (1998). Alzheimer's disease: Etiologies, pathophysiology, cognitive reserve, and treatment opportunities. *Neurology, 51*(Suppl. 1), S2–S17.

Friedland, R.P. (1993). Alzheimer's disease: Clinical features and differential diagnosis. *Neurology, 43*(Suppl. 4), S45–S51.

Geldmacher, D.S., & Whitehouse, P.J. (1996). Evaluation of dementia. *New England Journal of Medicine, 335,* 330–336.

Keefover, R.W. (1996). The clinical epidemiology of Alzheimer's disease. *Neurologic Clinics, 14,* 337–351.

Rabins, P. (1998). Alzheimer's disease management. *Journal of Clinical Psychiatry, 59*(Suppl. 13), 36–38.

Raskind, M. (1998). Psychopharmacology of noncognitive abnormal behaviors in Alzheimer's disease. *Journal of Clinical Psychiatry, 59*(Suppl. 9), 28–32.

Schneider, L.S., & Tariot, P.N. (1997). Update on treatment for Alzheimer's disease and other dementia. *Psychiatric Clinics of North America, 4,* 135–166.

Small, G.W., Rabins, P.V., Barry, P.P., Buckholtz, N.S., DeKosky, S.T., Ferris, S.H., Finkel, S.I., Gwyther, L.P., Khachaturian, Z.S., Lebowitz, B.D., McRae, T.D., Morris, J.C., Oakley, F., Schneider, L.S., Streim, J.E., Sunderland, T., Teri, L.A., & Tune, L.E. (1997). Diagnosis and treatment of Alzheimer disease and related disorders: Consensus statement of the American Association for Geriatric Psychiatry, the Alzheimer's Association, and the American Geriatrics Society. *Journal of the American Medical Association, 278,* 1363–1371.

van Duijn, C.M. (1996). Epidemiology of the dementias: Recent developments and new approaches. *Journal of Neurology, Neurosurgery and Psychiatry, 60,* 478–488.

REFERENCES

Adler, C. (1999). Differential diagnosis of Parkinson's disease. *Medical Clinics of North America, 83,* 349–367.

Aevarsson, O., Svanborg, A., & Skoog, I. (1998). Seven-year survival rate after age 85 years: Relation to Alzheimer disease and vascular dementia. *Archives of Neurology, 55,* 1226–1232.

Aguero-Torres, H., Fratiglioni, L., Guo, Z., Viitanen, M., & Winblad, B. (1998). Prognostic factors in very old demented adults: A seven-year follow-up from a population-based survey in Stockholm. *Journal of the American Geriatric Society, 46,* 444–452.

American Psychiatric Association. (1994). *Diagnostic and statistical manual of mental disorders* (4th ed.). Washington, DC: Author.

Bakchine, S., Lacomblez, L., Palisson, E., Laurent, M., & Derousne, C. (1989). Relationship between primitive reflexes, extrapyramidal signs, reflexive apraxia, and severity of cognitive impairment in dementia of the Alzheimer type. *Acta Neurologica Scandinavica, 79,* 38–46.

Becker, J., Boller, F., Lopez, O., Saxton, J., & McGonigle, K. (1994). The natural history of Alzheimer's disease: Description of study cohort and accuracy of diagnosis. *Archives of Neurology, 51,* 585–594.

Bleecker, M.L., Bolla-Wilson, K., Kawas, C., & Agnew, J. (1988). Age-specific norms for the Mini-Mental State Exam. *Neurology, 38,* 1564–1568.

Bondi, M., Salmon, D., & Butters, N. (1994). Neuropsychological features of memory disorders in Alzheimer disease. In R. Terry, R. Katzman, & K. Bick (Eds.), *Alzheimer disease* (pp. 41–64). Philadelphia: Raven Press.

Brookmeyer, R., Gray, S., & Kawas, C. (1998). Projections of Alzheimer's disease in the United States and the public health impact of delaying disease onset. *American Journal of Public Health, 88,* 1337–1342.

Brouwers, P., Cox, D., Martin, A., Chase, T., & Fedio, P. (1984). Differential perceptual-spatial impairment in Huntington's and Alzheimer's dementias. *Archives of Neurology, 41,* 1073–1076.

Brun, A., & Passant, U. (1996). Frontal lobe degeneration of non-Alzheimer type: Structural characteristics, diagnostic criteria and relation to other frontotemporal dementias. *Acta Neurologica Scandinavica, 168*(Suppl.), 28–30.

Chen, J.-Y., Stern, Y., Sano, M., & Mayeux, R. (1991). Cumulative risks of developing extrapyramidal signs, psychosis, or myoclonus in the course of Alzheimer's disease. *Archives of Neurology, 48,* 1141–1143.

Chui, H.C., Lyness, S., Sobel, E., & Schneider, L. (1994). Extrapyramidal signs and psychiatric symptoms predict faster cognitive decline in Alzheimer's disease. *Archives of Neurology, 51,* 676–681.

Chui, H.C., Victoroff, J.I., Margolin, D., Jagust, W., Shankle, R., & Katzman, R. (1992). Criteria for the diagnosis of ischemic vascular dementia proposed by the State of California Alzheimer's Disease Diagnostic and Treatment Centers. *Neurology, 42,* 473–480.

Clarfield, A.M. (1988). The reversible dementias: Do they reverse? *Annals of Internal Medicine, 109,* 476–486.

Claus, J., van Fool, W., Teunisse, S., Walstra, G., Kwa, V., Hijdra, A., Verbeeten, B.J., Koelman, J., Bour, L., & De Visser, B. (1998). Predicting survival in patients with early Alzheimer's disease. *Dementia and Geriatric Cognitive Disorders, 9,* 284–293.

Craft, S., Teri, L., Edland, S., Kukull, W., Schellenberg, G., McCormick, W., Bowen, J., & Larson, E. (1998). Accelerated decline in apolipoprotein E-epsilon4 homozygotes with Alzheimer's disease. *Neurology, 51,* 149–153.

Cummings, J., & Knopman, D. (1999). Advances in the treatment of behavioral disturbances in Alzheimer's disease. *Neurology, 53,* 899–901.

Cummings, J., Vinters, H., Cole, G., & Khachaturian, Z. (1998). Alzheimer's disease: Etiologies, pathophysiology, cognitive reserve, and treatment opportunities. *Neurology, 51*(Suppl. 1), S2–S17.

Cummings, J.L., Benson, D.F., Hill, M.A., & Read, S. (1985). Aphasia in dementia of the Alzheimer type. *Neurology, 35,* 394–397.

del Ser, T., Bermejo, F., Portera, A., Arredondo, J.M., Bouras, C., & Constantinidis, J. (1990). Vascular dementia: A clinicopathological study. *Journal of the Neurological Sciences, 96,* 1–17.

Dropcho, E. (1998). Neurologic paraneoplastic syndromes. *Journal of the Neurological Sciences, 153,* 264–278.

Erkinjuntti, T. (1994). Clinical criteria for vascular dementia: The NINDS-AIREN criteria. *Dementia, 5,* 189–192.

Ernst, R., & Hay, J. (1994). The U.S. economic and social costs of Alzheimer's disease revisited. *American Journal of Public Health, 84,* 1261–1264.

Evans, D.A., Scherr, P.A., Cook, N.R., Albert, M.S., Funkenstein, H.H., Smith, L.A., Hebert, L.E., Wetle, T.T., Branch, L.G., Chown, M.C., Hennekens, C.H., & Taylor, J.O. (1990). Estimated prevalence of Alzheimer's disease in the United States. *Milbank Quarterly, 68*(2), 267–287.

Folstein, M.F., Folstein, S.E., & McHugh, P.R. (1975). Mini-Mental State: A practical method for grading the cognitive state of patients for the clinician. *Journal of Psychiatric Research, 12,* 189–198.

Gearing, M., Mirra, S., Hedreen, J., Sumi, S., Hansen, L., & Heyman, A. (1995). The Consortium to Establish a Registry for Alzheimer's Disease (CERAD). Part X. Neuropathology confirmation of the clinical diagnosis of Alzheimer's disease. *Neurology, 45,* 461–466.

Giordani, B., Boivin, M.J., Hall, A.L., Foster, N.L., Lehtinen, S.J., Bluemlein, L.A., & Berent, S. (1990). The utility and generality of Mini-Mental State Examination scores in Alzheimer's disease. *Neurology, 40,* 1894–1896.

Gold, G., Giannakopoulos, P., Montes-Paixao, C., Jr., Herrmann, F., Mulligan, R., Michel, J., & Bouras, C. (1997). Sensitivity and specificity of newly proposed clinical criteria for possible vascular dementia. *Neurology, 49,* 690–694.

Gomez-Isla, T., West, H., Rebeck, G., Harr, S., Growdon, J., Locascio, J., Perls, T., Lipsitz, L., & Hyman, B. (1996). Clinical and pathological correlates of apolipoprotein E epsilon 4 in Alzheimer's disease. *Annals of Neurology, 39,* 62–70.

Hauser, W.A., Morris, M.L., Heston, L.L., & Anderson, V.E. (1986). Seizures and myoclonus in patients with Alzheimer's disease. *Neurology, 36,* 1226–1230.

Heeren, T.J., Lagaay, A.M., von Beek, W.C.A., Rooymans, H.G.M., & Hijmans, W. (1990). Reference values for the Mini-Mental State Examination (MMSE) in octo- and nonagenarians. *Journal of the American Geriatrics Society, 38,* 1093–1096.

Heyman, A., Peterson, B., Fillenbaum, G., & Pieper, C. (1996). The consortium to establish a registry for Alzheimer's disease (CERAD). Part XIV: Demographic and clinical predictors of survival in patients with Alzheimer disease. *Neurology, 46,* 656–660.

Heyman, A., Peterson, B., Fillenbaum, G., & Pieper, C. (1997). Predictors of time to institutionalization of patients with Alzheimer's disease: The CERAD experience, Part XVII. *Neurology, 48,* 1304–1309.

Huang, L.F., Cartwright, W.S., & Hu, T.W. (1988). The economic cost of senile dementia in the United States. *Public Health Report, 103,* 3–7.

Hutton, J.T., Dippel, R.L., Loewenson, R.B., Mortimer, J.A., & Christians, B.L. (1985). Predictors of nursing home placement of patients with Alzheimer's disease. *Texas Medicine, 81,* 40–43.

Jorm, A.F., Korten, A.E., & Henderson, A.S. (1987). The prevalence of dementia: A quantitative integration of the literature. *Acta Psychiatrica Scandinavica, 76,* 465–479.

Jost, B., & Grossberg, G. (1995). The natural history of Alzheimer's disease: A brain bank study. *Journal of the American Geriatrics Society, 43,* 1248–1255.

Katz, I. (1998). Diagnosis and treatment of depression in patients with Alzheimer's disease and other dementias. *Journal of Clinical Psychiatry, 59*(Suppl. 9), 38–44.

Katzman, R., Hill, L., Yu, E., Wang, Z., Booth, A., Salmon, D., Liu, W., Qu, G., & Zhang, M. (1994). The malignancy of dementia: Predictors of mortality in clinically diagnosed dementia in a population survey of Shanghai, China. *Archives of Neurology, 51,* 1220–1225.

Katzman, R., & Kawas, C. (1994). The epidemiology of dementia and Alzheimer disease. In R. Terry, R. Katzman, & K. Bick (Eds.), *Alzheimer disease* (pp. 105–122). New York: Raven Press.

Kawas, C., Resnick, S., Morrison, A., Brookmeyer, R., Corrada, M., Zonderman, A., Bacal, C., Lingle, D., & Metter, E. (1997). A prospective study of estrogen replacement therapy and the risk of developing Alzheimer's disease: The Baltimore Longitudinal Study of Aging. *Neurology, 48,* 1517–1521.

Kertesz, A., Hudson, L., Mackenzie, I., & Munoz, D. (1994). The pathology and nosology of primary progressive aphasia. *Neurology, 44,* 2065–2072.

Klatka, L., Schiffer, R., Powers, J., & Kazee, A. (1996). Incorrect diagnosis of Alzheimer's disease: A clinicopathologic study. *Archives of Neurology, 53,* 35–42.

Knapp, M., Knopman, D., Solomon, P., Pendlebury, W., Davis, C., & Gracon, S. (1994). A 30-week randomized controlled trial of high-dose tacrine in patients with Alzheimer's disease: The Tacrine Study Group. *Journal of the American Medical Association, 271,* 985–991.

Knopman, D.S., Kitto, J., Deinard, S., & Heiring, J. (1988). Longitudinal study of death and institutionalization in patients with primary degenerative dementia. *Journal of the American Geriatrics Society, 36,* 108–112.

Korczyn, A. (1997). Prion diseases. *Current Opinion in Neurology, 10,* 273–281.

Larson, E.B., Reifler, B.V., Sumi, S.M., Canfield, C.G., & Chinn, N.M. (1986). Diagnostic tests in the evaluation of dementia: A prospective study of 200 elderly outpatients. *Archives of Internal Medicine, 146,* 1917–1922.

Launer, L., Andersen, K., Dewey, M., Letenneur, L., Ott, A., Amaducci, L., Brayne, C., Copeland, J., Dartigues, J., Kragh-Sorensen, P., Lobo, A., Martinez-Lage, J., Stijnen, T., & Hofman, A. (1999). Rates and risk factors for dementia and Alzheimer's disease: Results from EURODEM pooled analyses. EURODEM Incidence Research Group and Work Groups: European Studies of Dementia. *Neurology, 52,* 78–84.

Levy, M., Cummings, J., & Kahn-Rose, R. (1999). Neuropsychiatric symptoms and cholinergic therapy for Alzheimer's disease. *Gerontology, 45*(Suppl. 1), 15–22.

Litvan, I., Campbell, G., Mangone, C., Verny, M., McKee, A., Chaudhuri, K., Jellinger, K., Pearce, R., & D'Olhaberriague, L. (1997). Which clinical features differentiate progressive supranuclear palsy (Steele-Richardson-Olszewski syndrome) from related disorders? A clinicopathological study. *Brain, 120,* 65–74.

Lopez, O., Wisnieski, S., Becker, J., Boller, F., & DeKosky, S. (1997). Extrapyramidal signs in patients with probable Alzheimer's disease. *Neurology, 54,* 969–975.

Mastrianni, J. (1998). The prion diseases: Creutzfeldt-Jakob, Gerstmann-Straussler-Scheinker, and related disorders. *Journal of Geriatric Psychiatry and Neurology, 11,* 78–97.

McGeer, P., Schulzer, M., & McGeer, E. (1996). Arthritis and anti-inflammatory agents as possible protective factors for Alzheimer's disease: A review of 17 epidemiologic studies. *Neurology, 47,* 425–432.

McKeith, I., Galasko, D., Kosaka, K., Perry, E., Dickson, D., Hansen, L., Salmon, D., Lowe, J., Mirra, S., Byrne, E., Lennox, G., Quinn, N., Edwardson, J., Ince, P., Bergeron, C., Burns, A., Miller, B., Lovestone, S., Collerton, D., Jansen, E., Ballard, C., de Vos, R., Wilcock, G., Jellinger, K., & Perry, R. (1996). Consensus guidelines for the clinical and pathologic diagnosis of dementia with Lewy bodies (DLB): Report of the consortium on DLB international workshop. *Neurology, 47,* 1113–1124.

McKhann, G., Drachmann, D., Folstein, M., Katzman, R., Price, D., & Stadlan, E.M. (1984). Clinical diagnosis of Alzheimer's disease. *Neurology, 34,* 939–944.

Miller, B., Ikonte, C., Ponton, M., Levy, M., Boone, K., Darby, A., Berman, N., Mena, I., & Cummings, J. (1997). A study of the Lund-Manchester research criteria for frontotemporal dementia: Clinical and single-photon emission CT correlations. *Neurology, 48,* 937–942.

Molsa, P.K., Marttila, R.J., & Rinne, U.K. (1986). Survival and cause of death in Alzheimer's disease and multi-infarct dementia. *Acta Neurologica Scandinavica, 74,* 103–107.

Morris, J.C., McKeel, D.W., Storandt, M., Rubin, E.H., Price, J.L., Grant, E.A., Ball, M.J., & Berg, L. (1991). Very mild Alzheimer's disease: Informant-based clinical, psychometric, and pathologic distinction from normal aging. *Neurology, 41,* 469–478.

Mortimer, J.A., van Duijn, C.M., Chandra, V., Fratiglioni, L., Graves, A.B., Heyman, A., Jorm, A.F., Kokmen, E., Kondo, K., & Rocca, W.A. (1991). Head trauma as a risk factor for Alzheimer's disease: A collaborative reanalysis of case-control studies. *International Journal of Epidemiology, 20*(Suppl. 2), S28–S35.

Mungas, D., Marshall, S., Weldon, M., Haan, M., & Reed, B. (1996). Age and education correction of Mini-Mental State Examination for English and Spanish-speaking elderly. *Neurology, 46,* 700–706.

Murden, R.A., McRae, T.D., Kaner, S., & Bucknam, M.E. (1991). Mini-Mental State Exam scores vary with education in blacks and whites. *Journal of the American Geriatrics Society, 39,* 149–155.

Murdoch, B.E., & Chenery, H.J. (1987). Language disorders in dementia of the Alzheimer type. *Brain Language, 31,* 122–137.

Neary, D., Snowden, J., Gustafson, L., Passant, U., Stuss, D., Black, S., Freedman, M., Kertesz, A., Robert, P., Albert, M., Boone, K., Miller, B., Cummings, J., & Benson, D. (1998). Frontotemporal lobar degeneration: A consensus on clinical diagnostic criteria. *Neurology, 51,* 1546–1554.

Pfeffer, R.I., Kurosaki, T.T., Harrah, C.H., Chance, J.M., & Filos, S. (1982). Measurement of functional activities in older adults in the community. *Journal of Gerontology, 37,* 323–329.

Pillon, B., Dubois, B., Ploska, A., & Agid, Y. (1991). Severity and specificity of cognitive impairment in Alzheimer's, Huntington's, and Parkinson's diseases and progressive supranuclear palsy. *Neurology, 41,* 634–643.

Pillon, B., Vidailhet, M., Deweer, B., Sirigu, A., Dubois, B., & Agid, Y. (1995). The neuropsychological pattern of corticobasal degeneration: Comparison with progressive supranuclear palsy and Alzheimer's disease. *Neurology, 45,* 1477–1483.

Rabins, P. (1998). Alzheimer's disease management. *Journal of Clinical Psychiatry, 59*(Suppl. 13), 36–38.

Rapcsak, S.Z., Croswell, S.C., & Rubens, A.B. (1989). Apraxia in Alzheimer's disease. *Neurology, 39,* 664–668.

Raskind, M. (1998). Psychopharmacology of noncognitive abnormal behaviors in Alzheimer's disease. *Journal of Clinical Psychiatry, 59*(Suppl. 9), 28–32.

Rich, J., Rasmusson, D., Folstein, M., Carson, K., Kawas, C., & Brandt, J. (1995). Nonsteroidal anti-inflammatory drugs in Alzheimer's disease. *Neurology, 45,* 51–55.

Rocca, W.A., Hofman, A., Brayne, C., Breteler, M., Clarke, M., Copeland, J., Dartigues, J., Engedal, K., Hagnell, O., & Heeren, T. (1991). Frequency and distribution of Alzheimer's disease in Europe: A collaborative study of 1960–1990 prevalence findings. The EURODEM-Prevalence Research Group. *Annals of Neurology, 30,* 381–390.

Rogers, J., Kirby, L., Hempelman, S., Berry, D., McGeer, P., Kaszniak, A., Zalinski, J., Cofield, M., Mansukhani, L., & Willson, P. (1993). Clinical trial of indomethacin in Alzheimer's disease. *Neurology, 43,* 1609–1611.

Rogers, S.L., Friedhoff, L.T., & the Donepezil Study Group. (1996). The efficacy and safety of Donepezil in patients with Alzheimer's disease: Results of a U.S. multi-centre, randomized, double-blind, placebo-controlled trial. *Dementia, 7,* 293–303.

Roman, G., Tatemichi, T., Erkinjuntti, T., Cummings, J.L., Masdeu, J.C., Garcia, J.H., Amaducci, L., Orgogozo, J.M., Brun, A., & Hofman, A. (1993). Vascular dementia: Diagnostic criteria for research studies. Report of the NINDS-AIREN International Workshop. *Neurology, 43,* 250–260.

Savage, C. (1997). Neuropsychology of subcortical dementias. *Psychiatric Clinics of North America, 20,* 11–31.

Stern, Y., Albert, M., Brandt, J., Jacobs, D.M., Tang, M.X., Marder, K., Bell, K., Sano, M., Devanand, D.P., & Bylsma, F. (1994). Utility of extrapyramidal signs and psychosis as predictors of cognitive and functional decline, nursing home admission and death in Alzheimer's disease. *Neurology, 44,* 2300–2307.

Stoessl, A., & Rivest, J. (1999). Differential diagnosis of parkinsonism. *Canadian Journal of Neurological Sciences, 26*(Suppl. 2), S1–S4.

Tang, M., Jacobs, D., Stern, Y., Marder, K., Schofield, P., Gurland, B., Andrews, H., & Mayeux, R. (1996). Effect of oestrogen during menopause on risk and age at onset of Alzheimer's disease. *Lancet, 348,* 429–432.

Teri, L., McCurry, S., Edland, S., Kukull, W., & Larson, E. (1995). Cognitive decline in Alzheimer's disease: A longitudinal investigation of risk factors for accelerated decline. *Journal of Gerontology, 50A,* M49–M55.

Terry, R., Masliah, E., & Hansen, L. (1994). Structural basis of the cognitive alterations in Alzheimer disease. In R. Terry, R. Katzman, & K. Bick (Eds.), *Alzheimer disease* (pp. 179–196). New York: Raven Press.

Turner, D., & McGeachie, R. (1988). Normal pressure hydrocephalus and dementia: Evaluation and treatment. *Clinics in Geriatric Medicine, 4,* 815–830.

Uhlmann, R.F., & Larson, E.B. (1991). Effects of education on the Mini-Mental State Examination as a screening test for dementia. *Journal of the American Geriatrics Society, 39,* 876–880.

United States Congress, & Office of Technology Assessment. (1987). *Losing a million minds: Confronting the tragedy of Alzheimer's disease and other dementias.* Washington, DC: Author.

Wahlund, L. (1996). Biological markers and diagnostic investigations in Alzheimer's disease. *Acta Neurologica Scandinavica 165*(Suppl.), 85–91.

Walsh, J.S., Welch, H.G., & Larson, E.B. (1990). Survival of outpatients with Alzheimer-type dementia. *Annals of Internal Medicine, 113,* 429–434.

Waring, S., Rocca, W., Petersen, R., O'Brien, P., Tangalos, E., & Kokmen, E. (1999). Postmenopausal estrogen replacement therapy and risk of AD: A population-based study. *Neurology, 52,* 965–970.

Yaffe, K., Sawaya, G., Lieberburg, I., & Grady, D. (1998). Estrogen therapy in postmenopausal women: Effects on cognitive function and dementia. *Journal of the American Medical Association, 279,* 688–695.

CHAPTER 10

Suicide

PAUL R. DUBERSTEIN AND YEATES CONWELL

CASE STUDY

Mr. A.'s body was discovered in the Genesee River on February 10, 1994, a week after he had unsuccessfully tried to kill himself by cutting his wrist and neck. (Details of this case were changed to protect the victim's identity.) He was a 76-year-old, never-married, White, 10th-grade educated, retired laborer who lived alone in a rooming house. Autopsy revealed severe calcific atherosclerosis of the coronary arteries (60%–80% narrowing), fatty changes of the liver, and evidence of emphysema. A toxicologic examination indicated that Mr. A. had been drinking alcohol shortly prior to death; there was no evidence that he had been taking antidepressant medications. A review of his medical chart revealed that Mr. A. had been diagnosed with prostatitis and degenerative joint disease, hypertension, cholelithiases, hiatal hernia, a history of esophageal ulcer and antral gastritis, diverticulosis, benign prostatic hypertrophy, benign positional vertigo, and arthritis. He last saw a physician less than a month prior to death. At that time, he presented to the emergency department complaining of difficulty voiding and suprapubic pains. Diagnoses were hematuria, prostatitis, and mild degenerative joint disease of the lumbar spine. He reported that he had had liaisons with prostitutes, was tested for HIV, and was scheduled to receive the results just a few days before his body was found in the river. It is not known whether he ever received these findings. In his seven-word suicide note, Mr. A. made no direct reference to the HIV testing, writing, "I can't stand the pain no more."

As part of a retrospective study of completed suicide that aims in part to determine the prevalence and nature of psychiatric disorders (American Psychiatric Association [APA], 1994) in a community sample of suicides, we conducted an interview with Mr. A.'s cousin, Ms. B. She indicated that Mr. A. was not clinically depressed when he ended his life. Ms. B. reported that her cousin did not have an appetite disturbance, difficulty concentrating, anhedonia, or feelings of worthlessness. Yet, Mr. A. did have a rather lengthy history of sleep problems, which worsened in the weeks prior to death. Ms. B. had requested that Mr. A. move in with her, but he refused, explaining that he "would walk the floors all night." Ms. B.

Work on this chapter was financially supported in part by United States Public Health Service grants K07-MH01135 and K24-MH01759.

observed that there had been changes in Mr. A.'s ability to function, despite the absence of an affective syndrome or prominent mood symptoms. Ms. B. described her cousin as "the sort of person who would always go out and go somewhere. He liked to walk." But in the weeks prior to death, functional impairments limited his walking. Taking the bus in the cold weather became more burdensome because it bothered his arthritis. Although his appetite was not disturbed, there were certain foods he would not eat in the weeks prior to death because they "would affect his stomach."

Mr. A. met criteria for a diagnosis of alcohol dependence. Although he stopped drinking alcohol and smoking cigarettes approximately six years prior to death, he began drinking again in September 1993. One month prior to death, his drinking worsened. Ms. B. stated, "He would drink and drink. All day and all night. He drank constantly." This relapse coincided with his belief that he had cancer. There was no objective indication on autopsy that he had that disease.

The victim had a number of anxiety-related symptoms. He did not like to travel and had not been out of town for nearly a decade. He never flew in an airplane and mentioned that he never would fly. He worried about everything, "little things that didn't make any sense." When not drinking alcohol he was a quiet person who did not like crowds and was also somewhat socially awkward and uncomfortable. When he drank, however, "he could talk all day and all night." Ms. B. recalled several episodes when the victim traveled to her home only to learn that she had visitors. Rather than enter her home and socialize as she requested, he refused. Later on, he would admit, "When you have someone over, I'm just not going to interfere."

On February 4, Mr. A. told his cousin that he had "lived long enough" and was going to kill himself by jumping into the river. Ms. B. never saw him again. Although she struggled with his desire to kill himself, she felt there was little she could do: "He was always on his own. Was not going to be pinned down somewhere. And I couldn't force him. . . . He never wanted anybody to be bothered with him. He always did things for himself. . . . He wouldn't ask you to do anything."

OVERVIEW OF CHAPTER

In the world of psychopathology research, the topic of suicide in older adults may sound like a remote outpost, but it lies at an intellectually vibrant intersection currently under construction: the crossroads of psychology, psychiatry, economics, public policy, epidemiology, public health, philosophy, primary care medicine, gerontology, sociology, and other disciplines too new to have names. Pioneering studies have shown that depression increases risk for completed suicide in older adults, leading to calls for interventions for that disorder. It is true that treating depression may lead to a decrease in the suicide rate. However, it must be acknowledged that treatment can be initiated only toward the *end* of a lengthy process that begins with health care professionals and their patients recognizing and labeling depressive symptoms and acknowledging that the symptoms are treatable. Older adults at risk for suicide pose special public health and clinical challenges because their psychiatric symptoms are not florid or obvious; by habit or genetic endowment, they, like Mr. A., tend not to seek help or attention; and their physical disease burden and functional limitations may lead their families and physicians to underappreciate their mental health needs. Thus, suicide prevention requires both better treatments *and* improved surveillance and diagnostic methods designed to increase the capacity of health care professionals and the public at large to identify and recognize depressive symptoms and other warning signs of suicide in themselves and others.

Indeed, the effectiveness of most prevention and intervention programs will hinge on adequate symptom recognition; this idea will be emphasized throughout the chapter. In surveying the literature on completed suicide, we explain why poor symptom recognition poses such a big obstacle to suicide prevention and discuss the methods proposed to deal with that problem. Following a brief discussion of some of the conceptual and methodological issues involved in research aimed at identifying risk factors for suicide, we review the disorders associated with suicide. Next, we summarize the epidemiological data. This is followed by a review of theories and interventions for suicidal behavior. We conclude by placing the concept of symptom recognition in a broader societal context. People may not recognize the warning signs of suicide in themselves or others unless they are also motivated to eliminate them. Educational initiatives and advertising campaigns are needed to dispel the myth that depression and suicidal ideation are a "normal" aspect of aging.

CONCEPTUAL AND METHODOLOGICAL ISSUES

WHY FOCUS ON COMPLETED SUICIDE?

Careful attention to terms and their meaning is essential to an understanding of the literatures on suicide and suicide prevention. Often, suicidal ideation, attempted suicide, and completed suicide are blended in discussions of suicidal behavior. Yet each has distinct implications for prevention. Variability in terms creates confusion, and leads to an inaccurate understanding of risk. Attempted suicide is an important topic of investigation because it is a source of preventable morbidity. Moreover, research on attempted suicide could, in theory, indicate possible directions for future studies of the pathogenesis and prevention of completed suicide. Still, the powerful urge to draw conclusions about completed suicide from research on attempted suicide must be resisted. The majority of suicide attempters seen in clinical settings will never die by their own hand, and only a minority of suicides have previously made a suicide attempt (Maris, 1992). In the most recent and comprehensive investigation of this issue, Isometsä and Lönnqvist (1998) reported that 56% of suicides in Finland ($n = 1,397$) had made no prior suicide attempt. Men were nearly 70% more likely than women to have their first attempt be their last. This gender difference is even greater when older men are compared with younger women. Given that he made a suicide attempt in the week prior to his suicide, Mr. A. was unusual; a substantial majority of older men who kill themselves made no prior suicide attempts.

Although many clinicians may have had experience with patients whose suicide attempts were nearly fatal had it not been for heroic efforts on the part of rescue or medical personnel, most attempted suicides are not "near misses." Moreover, the demographic risk factors for attempted and completed suicide differ; rates of attempted suicide are highest in young women (Kessler, Borges, & Walters, 1999), but it is older men who are at greatest risk for completed suicide (Centers for Disease Control and Prevention [CDC], 1999). The current director of the National Institute of Mental Health addressed this dilemma when he noted: "A study of unsuccessful suicide attempters would not illuminate the relationship between depression and completed suicide because it is well established that, despite overlap, the populations that attempt suicide and those that complete suicide are different" (Hyman & Arana, 1989, p. 171). This chapter focuses principally on completed suicide because it takes a significant but underacknowledged toll on individuals, their families, and society.

IDENTIFYING CLINICAL RISK FACTORS FOR COMPLETED SUICIDE

Two study designs can identify putative clinical risk factors for completed suicide: the prospective cohort design and the retrospective case-control. Prospective cohort studies identify and follow a cohort longitudinally. Cohorts have typically been constituted from populations of community dwellers, psychiatric patients, military conscripts, and college students. Variables that distinguish participants who eventually commit suicide from those who do not are labeled risk factors. A relatively new and important nomenclature seeks to differentiate causal, or modifiable, risk factors from correlates or fixed markers of risk (Kraemer et al., 1997). Still, for the sake of simplicity, we use the generic term "risk factor."

The prospective cohort design is one of the most powerful tools available to psychopathologists and developmentalists, mainly because it avoids hindsight bias (Henry, Moffitt, Caspi, Langley, & Silva, 1994). If employed over successive birth cohorts, prospective designs can attempt to tease apart birth cohort effects from maturational influences (e.g., Gallo, Rabins, & Anthony, 1999). They can also be used to determine whether different variables are associated with completed suicide at different intervals postintake (e.g., Fawcett et al., 1990). For example, a study of 954 depressed patients showed that alcohol abuse, anhedonia, anxiety, and global insomnia were all associated with suicide within 1 year of study entry, but not within 2 to 10 years. Data on hopelessness and suicidal ideation showed the opposite pattern. Both were associated with suicide in the longer term, but not within the first year of follow-up (Fawcett et al., 1990).

In contrast to retrospective designs, which rely heavily (if not exclusively) on data collected from informants, prospective strategies can use self-report data. They can therefore provide data on the completed suicide's *subjective experience*. Such information is vital to the design of psychotherapies. A subjective sense of hopelessness is a powerful indicator of future suicide risk. Prospective research established its clinical and prognostic significance (e.g.,

Beck, Steer, Kovacs, & Garrison, 1985; Fawcett et al., 1990). Retrospective research could not have done that.

Despite the advantages of the prospective design, the retrospective case-control is considered optimal for the study of suicide and other rare phenomena (Zahner, Hsieh, & Fleming, 1995). Its major strength is its capacity to yield large, representative samples. The hallmark of the case-control study of completed suicide is the informant interview, sometimes referred to as the "psychological autopsy" (Clark & Horton-Deutsch, 1992; Hawton et al., 1998). Researchers interview friends, caregivers, and relatives of suicides and controls. Risk factors are defined as those variables that distinguish the cases (suicides) from controls (e.g., community dwellers, accident victims). Because retrospective designs in theory could provide information about every suicide in a given community, their potential to contribute to prevention efforts is unique. Whereas prospective studies of clinical samples may be useful to clinicians who need information about risk factors among treatment seekers, the design of primary or universal prevention programs requires data on people who do not seek professional help.

Data gathered prospectively and retrospectively suggest that specific psychiatric disorders, personality traits, and physical disorders are associated with suicide. Few studies have focused exclusively on older adults, and no retrospective investigation has included contemporary control samples, comparable informant sources, or standardized instruments. Nor has any retrospective study controlled for the effects of various informant characteristics (e.g., relationship to deceased) that may skew the data provided. However, controlled retrospective studies of suicide in later life are now in progress in Great Britain, New Zealand, Sweden, and western New York State. These investigations will allow researchers to calculate odds ratios, risk ratios, or relative risks, and thus enable precise estimates of the potency of putative risk factors. In the meantime, research and practice in late-life suicide prevention must rely on a relatively incomplete knowledge base.

CLINICAL RISK FACTORS AND OBSCURED SYMPTOM RECOGNITION

Retrospective research conducted since the mid-1950s suggests that close to 90% of adults who complete suicide have a diagnosable psychiatric disorder (APA, 1994) at the time of death, most frequently major depression, alcohol abuse or dependence, or schizophrenia (Appleby, Cooper, Amos, & Faragher, 1999; Barraclough, Bunch, Nelson, & Sainsbury, 1974; Cavanagh, Owens, & Johnstone, 1999; Cheng, 1995; Conwell et al., 1996; Dorpat & Ripley, 1960; Foster, Gillespie, & McClelland, 1997; Henriksson et al., 1995; Rich, Young, & Fowler, 1986; Robins, Murphy, Wilkinson, Gassner, & Kayes, 1959; reviewed in Conwell & Brent, 1995). Prospective investigations conducted over roughly the same period have similarly highlighted the lethality of these disorders (reviewed in Harris & Barraclough, 1997). As a result, the topic of suicide—once the province primarily of religion and the law (Kushner, 1989)—has been recast to some extent as a public health problem. The language of psychopathology is now the lingua franca of suicidology; terms referring to psychiatric disorders and treatments are its shibboleths. Accompanying these developments is the too common belief that suicide represents "treatment failure": someone with a clearly defined, severe psychiatric disorder did not respond to psychotherapeutic or psychopharmacological treatments.

The solutions to this public health problem seem straightforward: develop and implement better treatments. The reality, however, is far more complex. Although solutions will ultimately entail better prevention strategies, a first priority must be improved symptom recognition and surveillance strategies to identify people at risk. For several reasons reviewed in this section, the concept of obscured symptom recognition is especially germane to older adults who commit suicide: their psychiatric symptoms are not florid or longstanding, and by habit or genetic endowment, they tend not to seek attention. Their comorbid medical disorders may lead their primary care physicians and other health care providers (e.g., emergency room physicians, in the case of Mr. A.) to concentrate on monitoring and treating their physical and functional problems and to underestimate their mental health needs. Indeed, it is possible that Mr. A.'s multiple physical problems and his apparent risk for AIDS may have increased his suicide risk, by leading his treaters to focus exclusively on his physical health.

Our emphasis in this chapter on symptom recognition is based on the finding that most (but not all) older people who commit suicide do so in the midst of psychological distress, if not frank psychiatric illness. Our approach is premised on the assumption that this distress or disorder confers risk for suicide and therefore is an appropriate target for intervention. Other perspectives must be acknowledged, however, if only to highlight the limitations of our approach. It can be argued that distress (or disorder) is a reasonable or expectable response to certain circumstances, such as terminal illness, and may not therefore be amenable to intervention. Questions may even be raised about the ethics of intervention in that context (Werth, 1999). As well, although suicidal ideation among seriously ill people is extremely rare in the absence of clinically significant mood disturbance (Brown, Henteleff, Barakat, & Rowe, 1986; Chochinov et al., 1995), it must be acknowledged that there is no consensus on the conceptualization and measurement of psychological distress or psychiatric disorder in the context of life-threatening illness.

PSYCHIATRIC DISORDERS

Retrospective research consistently shows a close association between suicide and psychiatric disorders in later life. Among victims 65 years of age and older, from 71% (Conwell et al., 1996) to over 90% (Henriksson et al., 1995) have diagnosable major psychiatric disorders (reviewed in Conwell, in press). In a study of 141 suicides in Monroe County, New York, older age at death was a significant predictor of the diagnosis of single episode, unipolar major affective disorder

(Conwell et al., 1996). Nonaffective psychoses (schizophrenia, schizoaffective illness, delusional disorder) and anxiety disorders appear to play a relatively small role in suicide among the elderly. However, symptoms of anxiety, like those experienced by Mr. A., are not uncommon. Although alcoholism and other substance use disorders are present in a relatively small proportion of completed suicides at older ages (Conwell et al., 1996), record-linkage research indicates that these disorders do place older people at significantly increased risk (Gardner, Bahn, & Mack, 1964). It is likely that Mr. A.'s heavy drinking in the month prior to his death contributed to his desire to kill himself. Interestingly, other data suggest that *remitted* alcohol and substance abuse disorders may also confer increased suicide risk (Conner et al., in press). People with histories of alcoholism and substance abuse may represent a population of special concern for late-life preventive intervention.

The most common psychiatric disorder of older suicide victims is a single episode of nonpsychotic, unipolar major depression of mild to moderate severity and without comorbid psychopathology (Conwell et al., 1996). This disorder may be more malignant in elders not because it is more severe, but because it is *less* severe and therefore more difficult to recognize. Indeed, older people are less likely to report depressed or sad mood than are younger people. This has been shown to be true in samples of psychiatric inpatients (Lyness, Cox, Curry, Conwell, King, & Caine, 1995; Wallace & Pfohl, 1995), general medical patients (Harper, Kotik-Harper, & Kirby, 1990), and community dwellers (Gallo, Anthony, & Muthen, 1994). Breaking the data down by gender is even more revealing. Older men, the demographic group at greatest risk for suicide, may be the least likely to report affective symptoms and crying spells (Allen-Burge, Storandt, Kinscerf, & Rubin, 1994). In addition, older inpatients (Duberstein et al., 1999) and community dwellers (Gallo et al., 1994) are less likely than younger people to report suicidal ideation. Taken together, these findings suggest that, by virtue of their age alone, elders may be less likely to present with two of the nine symptoms of major depressive disorder (APA, 1994), potentially making it more difficult for clinicians to recognize major depression in older patients. Worse, older suicide victims plan and implement their suicide attempts more carefully than their younger counterparts (Carney, Rich, Burke, & Fowler, 1994; Conwell et al., 1998) and are far less likely to express suicidal ideation within a week of their deaths (Conwell et al., 1998).

Consistent with the findings of a decrease in prevalence of major depressive disorder across the life course (Burvill, 1995), and the prominence of subsyndromal depressive symptoms in older primary care patients (Oxman, Barrett, Barrett, & Gerber, 1990), these age effects would drive depressive diagnoses toward the apparently less severe end of a diagnostic continuum, perhaps without decreasing risk for suicide or other causes of death. Mild to moderate symptoms in people with histories of adequate adjustment may be particularly difficult to detect, because health care providers, friends, relatives, and others in their social network are not cued into the possibility of imminent danger. But these symptoms may still confer risk, not just for suicide, but for other causes of death as well (Gallo, Rabins, Lyketsos, Tien, & Anthony, 1997;

Penninx et al., 1999). In one study, people who denied sadness or dysphoria, but who endorsed other symptoms of major depression, were at increased risk for psychiatric and physical morbidity and mortality at 13-year follow-up (Gallo et al., 1997).

PERSONALITY DISORDERS AND TRAITS

Approximately 30% to 40% of suicides are executed by individuals with personality disorders (Duberstein & Conwell, 1997). There is also substantial evidence for the notion that attention-getting traits of impulsiveness and dyscontrol contribute to suicide in people younger than 50 (Duberstein, Seidlitz, & Conwell, 1996). But people who are quiet about their suicide potential kill themselves, too. Some people are at increased risk because, as a rule, they do not seek help or attention—either from health care providers or members of their social network. Or, like Mr. A., they may quietly seek attention, but only up to a certain point, and then they withdraw. Mr. A. did not cut himself off completely from his cousin. He visited her occasionally and told her about some of his symptoms and concerns, but he declined her invitation to move in with her and thereby resisted her efforts to draw him nearer.

Reviews of the literature on personality and suicide reveal that avoidant personality disorder, schizoid personality disorder, self-consciousness, and social disengagement are all associated with completed suicide (e.g., Duberstein & Conwell, 1997). Our research suggests that people who obtain low scores on a questionnaire measuring a trait called *openness to experience* (OTE; Costa & McCrae, 1992) may also be at risk (Duberstein, Conwell, & Caine, 1994). People who are low in OTE tend to be relatively conventional in behavior and conservative in outlook. In contrast to those who are high in OTE, they have a relatively narrow range of interests, are less curious, and experience both positive and negative emotions less keenly (Costa & McCrae, 1992). They obtain relatively low scores on measures of personal growth and development (Schmutte & Ryff, 1997) and need for change (Costa & McCrae, 1988) and are less likely to report that they are considering changes in their work or family situations (Whitbourne, 1987).

Duberstein (1995) hypothesized that persons low in OTE may be at increased risk for suicide because their rigidly defined self-concept decreases their capacities to adapt to expectable age-associated changes in role, health, and function that accumulate over time. Recent findings have led to a refinement of this position: the theme of obscured symptom recognition is an essential element in the story of OTE and completed suicide. Given that people who are low in OTE may be relatively quiet about their suicide potential, their risk may not be recognized by members of their social network. Similarly, their health care providers may not be attuned to their risk potential.

Data collected in our Laboratory of Suicide Studies suggested this hypothesis. First, in a retrospective case-control study of 52 suicide victims, we reported that, in comparison to community-dwelling controls and suicide victims younger than 50 years of age, older suicides were characterized by low OTE (Duberstein et al., 1994), according to *informant-report.* Second, data collected on 81 depressed inpatients showed that those who obtained relatively low OTE scores on a *self-report* measure were less likely to report suicidal ideation (Duberstein et al., 2000). Finally, this latter finding was extended in a sample of 268 community-dwelling older adults (unpublished raw data).

How can the same trait be associated with a decreased likelihood of reporting suicidal ideation and an increased likelihood of completed suicide? Perhaps self-reported OTE and informant-reported OTE are not comparable constructs in older, depressed persons. That is unlikely, given the extensive literature supporting the relationship between self- and informant-report data (Costa & McCrae, 1992), even in depressed outpatients (Bagby et al., 1998). In our own sample of 57 depressed inpatients 50 years of age and older, the relationship between self- and informant OTE (intraclass correlation coefficient = .49) was moderately strong. Depressed people who are low in OTE have increased risk for completed suicide in part because they are less likely to report feeling suicidal and less likely to report feeling sad or dysphoric. This affective muting associated with low OTE may make suicide risk in many older adults more difficult to detect.

Physical Illness

Many assumptions are made about a causal link between physical illness and late-life suicide, but few data are available from rigorously controlled studies. The association seems important because physical conditions are so prevalent in older adults, and the heavily utilized primary care sector offers opportunities for intervention. In a review of 235 prospective studies with at least two years of follow-up and no more than 10% attrition, Harris and Barraclough (1994) calculated standardized mortality ratios for suicide in over 60 medical disorders and treatments. They concluded that HIV/AIDS, head and neck cancers, Huntington's disease, multiple sclerosis, peptic ulcer, renal disease, spinal cord injury, and systemic lupus erythematosus conferred increased suicide risk. The data on Parkinson's disease and several other disorders were suggestive but ultimately inconclusive. Given the limitations of the data, the mortality ratios could not be adjusted for the effects of comorbid affective disorders or personality traits that may have predated the onset of the physical disease.

In uncontrolled retrospective studies, Sainsbury (1955) estimated that physical illness contributed to suicide in 10% of younger victims but to more than 35% of elderly suicides. Dorpat and colleagues (Dorpat, Anderson, & Ripley, 1968) estimated that medical illness directly contributed to suicide in almost 70% of victims over 60 years of age. In a preliminary report using standardized measures and a matched control group, Conwell and colleagues (2000) demonstrated that greater physical illness burden and functional impairment significantly distinguished elderly primary care suicide victims from aged-matched primary care controls, even after controlling for mood disorders. Other analyses revealed that suicides were more likely to have a history of cancer or cardiovascular disease (Conwell et al., 1998).

Three interpretative frames may be applied to the data on suicide risk associated with specific medical conditions; each framework is premised on a different set of assumptions and has distinct implications for research. *Biological*
interpretations assume that there are pathophysiological pathways by which
a particular disorder affects brain function and thereby increases suicide
risk. Some tumors could have specific effects on the central nervous system
(McDaniel, Musselman, Porter, Reed, & Nemeroff, 1995), increasing risk for depression and subsequent suicide. Depression may increase risk for cardiovascular disease via dysregulated activity of the hypothalamic-pituitary-adrenal axis
or reduced heart rate variability (Musselman, Evans, & Nemeroff, 1998); the
pathophysiological changes accompanying cardiovascular disease may also increase risk for depression. Treatments for heart disease may decrease risk for
both depression and suicide, possibilities that could be examined empirically.

From a *social-constructionist* perspective, it is the symbolic meaning of the
disease, derived from societal norms as well as one's personal experiences, that
is potentially lethal. The diagnosis of cancer is often interpreted as a death
sentence, particularly among those who witnessed a relative succumb to the
illness (Conwell, Caine, & Olsen, 1990). Most of the diseases that seem to confer increased suicide risk (Harris & Barraclough, 1994) have no known cure,
and it may be the "perceived curability" of an illness, more so than its effects
on brain function, that confers risk. For many, a cure means control and certainty; no cure means being out of control and uncertainty. In the case of Mr.
A., it is possible that HIV testing represented a potential loss of control and
that his suicide was an attempt to regain control.

A third interpretation follows from the concept of symptom recognition.
Overburdened primary care physicians, striving to manage and treat patients
with several comorbid chronic illnesses, may underappreciate their patients'
mental health needs. A *public health* approach to the prevention of suicide in older
adults requires intensive research on how symptoms of mental disorders are reported, recognized, and treated in a variety of settings and contexts (primary
care, nursing home, other residential settings). Examples of such research include behavioral observation of communication patterns between patients and
members of their social network or physicians; identification of physician and
practice characteristics associated with the recognition of depressive symptoms;
and studies on the ability of family members to recognize facial and other nonverbal expressions of distress in older adults. As well, interventions designed to
increase the ability of primary care physicians to diagnose and treat depression
are also needed.

EPIDEMIOLOGICAL DATA

Each year, approximately 31,000 Americans take their own lives, leaving over
200,000 bereaved family members like Ms. B. wondering if they could have
done something to intervene. Contrary to what you might glean from your
nightly television news report, suicide is more common than homicide (Office

of the U.S. Surgeon General, 1999). It is the eighth leading cause of death in the United States, third among 15–24-year-olds (CDC, 1999). Firearms account for more than 60% of the suicides in the United States annually and close to 70% of the suicides among those 70 and older. Men are far more likely to use firearms than are women, and this gender difference appears to increase with age. In 1997, 2,857 men and only 237 women 70 years of age and older committed suicide by firearm in the United States (CDC, 1999).

AGE AND GENDER

Although the suicide rate is alarmingly high in adolescents and young adults it actually increases with age and is greatest in older adults (CDC, 1996). The rate among White males aged 85 and older is almost six times the nation's age-adjusted rate (CDC, 1999). In discussing suicide among older people, it is important to acknowledge the heterogeneity of this segment of the population; generalizations about suicide among older people should be made with caution. The risk factors for suicide in a 60-year-old and an 85-year-old probably differ considerably, but there are no firm data on this issue.

Men have higher rates than women, and Whites of both sexes have higher rates than Blacks (CDC, 1999). In the United States, rates for males increase with age, but rates for women peak in midlife and remain stable, or decline slightly, thereafter. In many other countries, however, later life is the time of highest risk for *both* men and women, according to statistics reported by the World Health Organization (Pearson & Conwell, 1995).

MARITAL STATUS

Suicide following the death of a partner may constitute a timeless theme in literature, folklore, and art, and was a focus of Robert Altman's 1999 film, *Cookie's Fortune*. It has been scientifically established since the nineteenth century that suicide rates for people who are single or widowed are higher than those for married people (Durkheim, 1897/1951). Trying to understand why suicide risk increases with marital loss, Duberstein, Conwell, and Cox (1998) compared widowed people whose suicides occurred more than four years after their spouse's death and those who took their lives after a shorter period of widowhood. The former had a higher rate of psychiatric treatment, prior suicide attempts, substance abuse/dependence, and early loss or separation (Duberstein et al., 1998). Four years was chosen as a cut-point because MacMahon and Pugh (1965) showed that suicide risk is elevated during the first four years of widowhood and decreases thereafter. Those who take their lives within four years are probably acting in the midst of complicated grief (Prigerson et al., 1995), but people who die by their own hand after a longer period may present with less florid symptoms and no previous psychiatric history, making their risk more difficult to detect.

SOCIOECONOMIC STATUS

There are well-established socioeconomic differences in all-cause mortality (Adler et al., 1994), but no firm data on the question of socioeconomic status and suicide. Media accounts may confuse rather than clarify this issue, reporting only the suicides of the rich and famous. Suicides of ordinary people receive no attention or are obscured in the standard obituary ("died suddenly"), presumably to respect the wishes of the family. It is possible that famous writers and other artists commit suicide at disproportionately high rates. It is also true that they constitute a tiny fraction of suicides; a plurality of older suicides are like Mr. A., who had a 10th-grade education and had worked as a laborer.

A case-control study of suicides and natural deaths of men between the ages of 25 and 64 in the United States showed that people with blue-collar occupations were more likely than white-collar employees to commit suicide (Kung, Liu, & Juon, 1998). Similar results emerged from a study of 175,000 deaths of men between the ages of 20 and 64 in England and Wales (Drever, Whitehead, & Roden, 1996), but a third investigation failed to support the notion that there is a relationship between socioeconomic status and health (Kagamimori et al., 1998). Our own data (Conwell et al., 2000) suggest that there may be a link between education, which is often conceived as a component of socioeconomic status, and suicide risk. Whereas a substantial majority of primary care patients 60 years of age and older had at least a high school education (165/196, 84%), only a minority of people who completed suicide had graduated from high school (19/42, 45%).

GEOPOLITICAL REGION

Data from countries throughout the world reveal that completed suicide is not randomly distributed across geopolitical region. We use the term "geopolitical" rather than geographic to emphasize that these differences may be ascribed not solely to bioclimatics, but to differences in laws, governance, economic arrangements, and other aspects of culture. In other words, these differences may be attributed to the cultural landscape as much as the natural landscape. Countries in Northern Europe (Sweden, Finland, Denmark, Norway, Iceland) have higher rates than countries in Southern Europe (Italy, Spain). Even in the United States, risk is not randomly distributed. The more densely populated states in the Middle Atlantic region (New York, New Jersey) and New England (Massachusetts, Rhode Island, Connecticut) have lower rates than the states in the more sparsely populated Mountain region (Nevada, Wyoming, Montana, Arizona). Acknowledging minor annual variations, the crude rates in the Mountain states are nearly twice that of the Middle Atlantic region. This difference is robust, but no compelling scientific hypotheses have been validated or even rigorously examined. Possible explanations include genetics, firearm availability, population density (which may be related to social support), religion, economics, and legislation.

TEMPORAL FLUCTUATIONS: PERIODICITY AND
HISTORICAL INFLUENCES

"Periodicity" is a term that has been used to refer to differences in rates as a function of time, defined as day-of-the-week, day-of-the-month, month-of-the-year, or season. In the early nineteenth century, Quetelet suggested that there is a spring peak in suicide rates, but Durkheim (1897/1951) concluded that rates were highest in the summer months—June, July, and August. Despite this difference, both agreed that rates in the northern hemisphere were higher during the warmer months than the colder months. Goodwin and Jamison (1990) ascribed the spring peak to differences in the rate of change in the brightness and duration of light.

In addition to bioclimatic hypotheses, social and socioeconomic explanations have been offered (Durkheim, 1897/1951). McCleary and colleagues (McCleary, Chew, Hellsten, & Flynn-Bransford, 1991) wondered whether certain demographic subgroups were more vulnerable to periodicity effects. Based on analyses of over 350,000 suicides from 1973 to 1985, they concluded that month-of-the-year effects are found exclusively in males, particularly in teenagers and in individuals 60 years of age and older. Rates among older men were elevated from late spring through the summer; teenagers had higher rates in the autumn and winter. Day-of-the-week effects are seen almost exclusively in individuals between the ages of 41 and 55, with a peak on Mondays. Bioclimatic hypotheses cannot accommodate this finding. It may be attributable in part to the social, economic, and symbolic significance of Mondays for middle-aged Americans.

Among the general population, suicide rates have remained relatively stable throughout the second half of this century, but rates among older people declined by up to 50% between 1930 and 1980 (McIntosh, Santos, Hubbard, & Overholser, 1994). That variation may reflect technological developments, such as the greater availability of more effective antidepressant treatments (Conwell, 1994). Alternatively, the decrease in rates may be ascribed to birth cohort effects. A birth cohort is a group born within a specific time frame. Due to shared "exposures"—for example, to life-defining events (e.g., economic depressions, wars, or political upheaval) or child-rearing practices— some birth cohorts may have an increased or decreased vulnerability to suicide. Individuals born before 1865 had higher rates of suicide at all points in the life course than did those born in later cohorts. At all ages, the large post–World War II "baby boom" cohort has had substantially higher suicide rates than preceding generations. However, the size of the baby boom generation may benefit that cohort in later life through greater political influence and accumulated resources (McIntosh, 1992). Moreover, historical shifts toward greater emotional expressiveness in the United States and other Western nations as well as decreased stigma attached to suicide may also mitigate risk. Perhaps reflecting these changes, the U.S. Congress passed resolutions in 1997 and 1998 declaring suicide prevention a national problem (Congressional Record, 1997, 1998). Senator Harry Reid (D-NV) introduced the Senate resolution and courageously went "on record" as a suicide survivor, indicating that his father, a retired hardrock miner with an 8th-grade education, died by his own hand in 1972.

RELEVANT THEORIES
AND INTERVENTIONS

Theories are meant to be clinically and empirically heuristic. In other words, they ought to be practical and useful. It is inaccurate to think of theories in the social sciences as solely right or wrong or proven or unproven. Rather, theories should be judged by how generative they are in terms of advancing debate, discussion, clinical practice, and science. In suicidology, two broad classes of relevant theories can be distinguished: theories of etiology and theories of prevention. The former attempt to explain suicide in terms of underlying "causes," or, more modestly, risk factors and correlates. Theories of prevention are aimed primarily at developing and testing measures designed to decrease the risk of suicide.

THEORIES OF ETIOLOGY

Three well-established theoretical perspectives dominate scientific theorizing about the etiology of suicide, each roughly corresponding to a different level of analysis: psychological, sociological, and biological. Within each level, there are numerous theories (or microtheories), all of which share basic assumptions. This section focuses on the most prominent theories and is not designed to be an exhaustive theoretical overview. For a more detailed discussion, see McIntosh et al. (1994).

Psychological
Although Sigmund Freud never wrote a paper exclusively focused on suicide and did not intend to characterize all suicides, he was vexed by the act and the problems it posed for his theory. One of his papers, *Mourning and Melancholia*, has profoundly influenced generations of clinicians and theorists interested in the topics of depression, suicide, and self-destruction. In that paper, Freud (1917/1957) argued that the combination of loss and hostility can be lethal. This formulation of suicide recognizes the interactive roles of an enduring disposition (hostility), a stressful circumstance (loss), and acute responses to that stressor (depression, regression).

Most psychological theories of suicide take this general form, differing only slightly in content and emphasis (Baumeister, 1990; Beck et al., 1985; Shneidman, 1986). Shneidman emphasizes lifelong coping problems (disposition), pain, perturbation and psychache (acute response), and press (stressful circumstances). Beck and colleagues emphasize cognitive rigidity (disposition) and hopelessness (acute response). There is substantial empirical support for the notion that hopelessness increases suicide risk, but little investigation of the role of stressful events in triggering suicidal hopelessness in vulnerable individuals.

There are no psychological treatments designed specifically to decrease the risk of completed suicide. It is generally assumed that treatments for depression will decrease suicide risk, but this has not been sustained. Of all available psychotherapies, Linehan's (1993) Dialectical Behavior Therapy most closely resembles a treatment specifically for self-destructive behavior. There is compelling evidence for its ability to decrease the risk of parasuicide (suicide attempts), but it is not known whether it decreases risk of completed suicide. Psychoanalytically oriented therapy offered in the context of a partial hospital program may also decrease risk of parasuicide (Bateman & Fonagy, 1999). No study of treatments for suicidal behavior has been completed on a sample of patients 50 years of age and older, but several relevant multisite investigations are currently in progress.

Sociological

In his classic text, Durkheim (1897/1951) outlined three major types of suicide. *Anomic suicide* results when persons cannot manage cultural changes that reorganize behavioral norms and prescriptions. (Anomie, literally translated, means lack of rules.) Anomic suicide may be particularly relevant for older adults. Whereas the roles of young adulthood (worker, spouse, parent, employee) have evolved over a comparatively long period of time and are relatively well structured, there is less consensus on the "tasks" and roles of later adulthood. Consequently, there is less structure, less cultural constraint, and more ambiguity (Kuypers & Bengston, 1973). The resulting paucity of structure may force the older person to increased dependency on external (societal) labels, many of which imply that the elder is deficient, incompetent, unproductive, and an economic liability. Not all elders are equally vulnerable to the effects of negative labels. Those who may be especially vulnerable have an external locus of control, for whom the source of all good and evil is external to the self.

Egoistic suicide springs from "excessive individualism" (Durkheim, 1897/1951, p. 209). Weak family ties and lack of involvement in society and its institutions increase suicide risk. For Durkheim, there is nothing particularly magical or mysterious about marriage, religion, or other societal institutions that confer protective effects. Rather, these institutions compel people to abide by certain rules and norms. Suicide is explicitly prohibited in many institutional contexts and is implicitly proscribed as well. If you're married and have children, you're not supposed to kill yourself because your spouse and children depend on you. Some have speculated that this proscription may be taken more seriously by women than by men. This constraint was not relevant to Mr. A., who never married and did not have children. *Altruistic suicide* results when individuals who are completely absorbed in societal institutions (family, work) kill themselves for the common good. A contemporary example of this may be the older adult who kills himself rather than receive extensive medical treatment and put his family into debt.

Durkheim's lasting contribution is probably not his typology, but rather the broader notion that suicide risk is associated with societal norms and rules. It is the structure of his argument that is compelling, not its particular emphases on anomie, altruism, and egoism. Whereas psychological theories point to psychological interventions targeting at-risk individuals (and occasionally their families), sociological theories suggest that modifications in public policy may affect the suicide rate in a given population. For example, to the extent that society provides older adults with well-structured roles and functions, the place of elders in society will be less ambiguous, and they will be less vulnerable to the adverse effects of labeling. Similarly, programs designed to disabuse the public of ageist stereotypes may also have an effect on the rate of suicide in older adults.

Biological

Abundant evidence supports an association between suicidal behavior and altered function of the central nervous system (CNS) monoamine neurotransmitter serotonin (5-hydroxytryptamine; 5-HT, see Mann, Oquendo, Underwood, & Arango, 1999, for a review). Among the earliest findings were diminished levels of 5-HT and its metabolite, 5-hydroxyindoleacetic acid (5-HIAA), in the brains of suicide victims compared with controls. Methodological limitations of working in postmortem tissue with unstable neurochemical compounds subsequently led investigators to study 5-HT receptors. $5-HT_2$ receptors are located on the postsynaptic membrane. With few exceptions, studies have repeatedly found increased binding of radiolabeled $5-HT_2$ receptor ligands in the frontal cortex of suicides compared with controls. 5-HT reuptake sites are marked by receptors on the presynaptic membrane. Although results have been mixed, several reports have noted significantly decreased binding at these sites in suicides compared with controls.

Most contemporary psychological and sociological theories of suicide risk are based on the premise that the psychological or social attributes are nonspecifically associated with morbidity or cause of death. The combination of loss and hostility not only increases risk for suicide, but it probably increases risk of death from other causes as well. In contrast, some recent biological theorizing has taken a different approach to the problem of specificity. For example, Gross-Isseroff and colleagues (Gross-Isseroff, Biegon, Voet, & Weizman, 1998) have argued that suicidal behavior has specific neurochemical characteristics. Unfortunately, relatively little is known about changes in most neurochemical systems with normal aging. Nor has age been adequately considered as a relevant variable in postmortem tissue studies of suicide victims and controls. The limited available data suggest, however, that the dopaminergic, GABAergic, and opiate systems, as well as the hypothalamic-pituitary-adrenal (HPA) axes, should be considered potentially significant to suicide in the elderly (see Conwell, Raby, & Caine, 1995, for a review). It may be premature to focus on any one neurochemical system.

Biological theorizing and research on suicide etiology appear to hold much promise for intervention and prevention, because they may pave the way for the development of new medications. Acknowledging that medical comorbidity complicates treatment because of medication interactions and side effects, it is commonly assumed that 70% to 80% of patients with single-episode unipolar major depression will respond to available somatic therapies, including medications and electroconvulsive therapy (ECT), or psychological therapies. There are incontrovertible data on the safety and effectiveness of antidepressant medications for older adults with a form of depression that is recurrent, moderate to severe, and characterized by relatively brief interepisode intervals (e.g., Reynolds et al., 1999). Still, Niederehe and Schneider (1998) maintained that no firm conclusions can be drawn about the benefits of either medication or ECT for older people with "milder and subclinical forms of depression" (p. 279)—subtypes of depression that are common among elders who take their lives. The authors of a recent meta-analysis similarly admonished against the use of heterocyclic drugs and selective serotonin reuptake inhibitors (SSRIs) for patients with milder depression (McCusker, Cole, Keller, Bellavance, & Berard, 1998).

Questions have been raised about the safety and effectiveness of pharmacological treatments (Fisher & Greenberg, 1997; Valenstein, 1998), the methodology and interpretation of data from controlled clinical trials of pharmacotherapies (Ader, 1997), and the extent to which researchers' preconceived notions about the superiority of a particular treatment approach may lead to biased interpretations of findings (Luborsky et al., 1999). Ideally, rigorous research on the effectiveness of particular treatments for older adults with milder forms of depression will be responsive to these and other questions. Even under optimal conditions, these studies will not be able to address one stubborn fact: the majority of older people who complete suicide never receive any mental health treatment, and many of those who do, receive inadequate care (Waern, Beskow, Runeson, & Skoog, 1996). Developing mechanisms to get these at-risk elders into some form of effective treatment is as pressing a public health need as tailoring specific treatments to specific groups of patients.

THEORIES OF PREVENTION

In addition to aggressive interventions when an older person is recognized to be suicidal, measures must be developed that are aimed at preventing completed suicide. Two theoretical approaches to suicide prevention have been identified: population-based strategies and high-risk models (Lewis, Hawton, & Jones, 1997).

Population-Based Strategies

Population-based strategies advocate universal prevention through interventions or initiatives that have a potential impact on large segments of a society. Some of these public health initiatives, such as gun control legislation, are politically controversial; others, such as the detoxification of domestic gas and restrictions on access to drugs with a low index of lethality, seem relatively irreproachable

(Gunnell & Frankel, 1994). Many, such as advertising campaigns designed to increase public awareness of mental health issues and disabuse the public of stereotypes about aging, may improve overall quality of life. However, they may be too weak to decrease suicide risk absent improvements in treatment. A distinguished group of British researchers concluded that restricting access to lethal means and crafting economic policies that reduce unemployment may decrease the suicide rate; treating people at high-risk is a less promising strategy (Lewis et al., 1997).

High-Risk Strategies

High-risk strategies are appealing in part because they are less controversial than population-based approaches. By definition, they affect a smaller segment of society. Among the elderly, two high-risk approaches to suicide prevention have been proposed: interventions in primary care settings designed to improve recognition and treatment of depressed and suicidal older patients, and community outreach to socially isolated elders. Although both strategies are promising, it must be acknowledged that there is no single cause for any suicide, and no two suicides can be understood to result from exactly the same constellation of factors. As no single factor is universally causal, no single intervention will prevent all suicide deaths. Still, attempts to prevent suicide in older people by improved recognition and treatment of its most potent risk factor, depression, will result in a host of other "ancillary" benefits, such as decreased depression-related morbidity and all-cause mortality (Conwell, in press).

Interventions in Primary Care.   There are systemic barriers to mental health care access, but the majority of older people at greatest risk for suicide probably have access to health care services in which preventative intervention should be feasible (Conwell, in press). Studies conducted in Great Britain and the United States have demonstrated that 43% to 76% of older people who took their lives saw a primary care provider within 30 days of death (Barraclough, 1971; Carney et al., 1994; Conwell, 1994). Mr. A. visited the emergency department of a local hospital within a month of his suicide. Primary care offices and other "frontline" settings may be suitable contexts for the development of initiatives designed to decrease the toll of completed suicide.

Depression is the most common psychiatric disorder associated with suicide in late life and the most prevalent mental disorder seen among older patients in primary care settings. Yet primary care physicians have difficulty recognizing treatable depression in their patients (Coyne, Schwenk, & Fechner-Bates, 1995; Crawford, Prince, Menezes, & Mann, 1998; Tiemens, Ormel, & Simon, 1996). Characteristics of the patient may obscure symptom recognition, and factors relating to the physician and setting exacerbate that problem. Physicians spend less time on average with older adults than with their younger patients (Keeler, Solomon, Beck, Mendenhal, & Kane, 1982); time spent in mental health diagnosis and intervention is reimbursed at a proportionately lower rate, providing further disincentive. Physicians may assume that depression is a "natural" consequence of aging and related stressors (Callahan, Nienaber, Hendrie, & Tierney,

1992), or they may avoid diagnosing a mood disorder out of concern for stigma-tizing and alienating their patients (Rost, Smith, Matthews, & Guise, 1994).

One influential but uncontrolled study tested the hypothesis that improved recognition and treatment of depressive disorders reduces rates of suicide. On the Swedish island of Götland, an educational intervention to improve the abil-ity of physicians to recognize and treat depression was associated with reduced sick leave for depressive disorders, decreased inpatient care days for depression, increased number of antidepressant prescriptions, and lower suicide rates com-pared both to contemporary rates in other parts of Sweden as well as rates on Götland before the educational program took place (Rutz, von Knorring, & Walinder, 1992). Further analyses suggested that the effect was time-limited and largely confined to women (Rutz, von Knorring, Pihlgren, Rihmer, & Walinder, 1995). Other questions have been raised about the methodology of the Götland study, and research conducted in the United States showed that educating pri-mary care physicians about treating depression does not lead to lasting improve-ments (Lin et al., 1997).

Active collaborations between mental health professionals and primary care practitioners may be a more realistic and effective approach to decreasing the morbidity and mortality associated with late-life mental disorders. Schulberg and colleagues (1996) tested whether care provided by mental health profession-als to depressed patients in primary care practices was superior to treatment as usual. Young adult and middle-aged depressives treated with either an antide-pressant, nortriptyline (NT), or interpersonal psychotherapy (IPT) had signifi-cantly better outcomes at eight-month follow-up than patients who received treatment as usual. There were no differences between the NT and IPT groups in depression severity or recovery rates (Schulberg et al., 1996). Further analyses showed that patients randomized to NT improved more rapidly than patients randomized to IPT, but this effect was observed only among patients who were more depressed. Treatment type was not related to clinical course among more severely depressed patients (Schulberg, Pilkonis, & Houck, 1998).

In a randomized controlled trial in a general adult population, Katon and colleagues (1996) tested a collaborative care model in which both mental health professionals and primary care physicians provided treatment for depression. Subjects with serious suicidal ideation were excluded, as were patients whose depressions were not recognized by their primary care physicians. The inter-vention involved patient and physician education, cognitive behavioral therapy delivered by psychologists, antidepressant therapy prescribed by physicians, and regular ongoing consultation between the two disciplines. Patients with major depression showed significant improvement in adherence to medica-tions, satisfaction with care, and reduction of depressive symptoms at four and seven months after the initiation of treatment. However, results for patients with minor depression were ambiguous, with most analyses showing no sig-nificant differences between intervention patients and usual care patients (Katon et al., 1996). Similarly, collaborative care produced a modest increase in the cost-effectiveness of care for patients with major depression, but not for pa-tients with minor depression (Von Korff et al., 1998). At 19-month follow-up, there was a substantial rate of relapse (Lin et al., 1998) and no difference in mental health outcomes between the enhanced intervention and comparison groups for patients with major depression (Lin et al., 1999).

These findings raise questions about the long-term effectiveness of collaborative treatments, but they also cast doubt on the effectiveness of these treatments for people with milder forms of depression—even in the short term. The collaborative care model produced short-term improvements in patients with major, but not minor, depression. This was true for all outcomes examined, ranging from percent reduction in symptom severity (Katon et al., 1996) to cost-effectiveness (Von Korff et al., 1998). It seems counterintuitive, but perhaps people with milder depressions are more difficult to treat than those with more severe symptoms. Or perhaps it is simply more difficult to demonstrate statistically that people with milder depressions respond to treatment. Further research is needed on this topic, especially given that milder depressions are associated with significant morbidity as well as mortality. Knowledge is needed on the risk factors (e.g., personality traits, medical disorders) and treatments for mild major depression, minor depression, and subsyndromal depression.

No studies have been conducted to test the effectiveness of collaborative models for detection and treatment of depression among older people in primary care. Nor is it known whether collaborative treatment models reduce the risk of completed suicide in older adults. For now, aggressive attempts to recognize and treat depression in older adults should be expected to lower suicide rates. Treatment for depressed older adults at risk for suicide may best be initiated in the context of primary care delivery. Ideally, primary care physicians will determine that a patient has significant affective symptoms and then initiate treatment either in their offices or in close collaboration with mental health care providers.

Community Outreach.   Initiatives in primary care settings promise to provide access for prevention to the majority of older people at risk for suicide. However, outreach is required to recognize and treat depressions among those without resources to pay for care, or who are homebound and physically unable to access care. One such low-cost model has been tested in Padua, Italy (De Leo, Carollo, & Dello Buono, 1995), a country unlike our own in size, religion, ethnicity, and other parameters relevant to suicide risk. Social service and health care workers identified older people at risk for suicide. Research personnel gave each elder a portable alarm system assuring emergency response capability and engaged them in regular supportive telephone contacts. There was no control group. After four years of service, the authors found only one death by suicide among the elderly clients, a significantly lower rate than would have been expected in the elderly population of that region. Although older adults may be reluctant to use crisis or "hot" lines, telephone support systems should be tested in controlled studies in the United States.

The effectiveness of telephone services as a suicide prevention measure hinges in part on the availability of methods for case finding and the capability to mount acute, multidisciplinary in-home assessments. The Spokane Mental

Health Center, Elder Services Division has developed such a program, combining a method for reaching at-risk elders living in the community, known as the Gatekeeper model (Florio et al., 1996), and a comprehensive clinical case management system. The Gatekeeper model relies on nontraditional community referral sources to identify older individuals at risk for self-harm. Meter readers, utility workers, bank personnel, apartment and mobile home managers, postal carriers, and others likely to observe older people in their homes and the community during the course of their routine business serve as gatekeepers. With a small amount of education and training, they refer elders whom they judge to be at risk to the Clinical Case Management Program. That program is equipped to respond with clinical referrals; in-home medical, psychiatric, family, and nutritional assessments; medication management and respite services; and crisis intervention.

In combination, the Gatekeeper case-finding strategy and the clinical management model were designed to eliminate problems of access, fragmentation, and lack of coordination of aging and mental health services for this high-risk population of older adults (Florio, Jensen, Hendryx, Raschko, & Mathieson, 1998). An important element of the program's apparent success is its collaborative funding and support by the region's consortium of aging services providers and the mental health system. Approximately one-third of the service's referrals were by gatekeepers, who tended to identify socially isolated individuals, particularly those diagnosed with a substance use disorder, bipolar disorder, or schizophrenia. Lacking a control sample, the impact of the Gatekeeper model on suicide risk and other outcomes remains speculative. Moreover, enthusiasm for the Gatekeeper model must be weighed against the sobering findings from a rigorously conducted British study (Clarke, Clarke, & Jagger, 1992). The investigators sought to decrease social isolation among older (75+ years of age) community dwellers who lived alone. Elders ($n = 523$) were randomly assigned to a control group or an experimental intervention aimed at providing support in five domains: social, financial, medical, housing, and nursing. Remarkably, 50% of those in the experimental group declined repeated offers of help. More data are needed to address the question of whether the socially isolated elderly are willing to participate in outreach efforts, and under what circumstances. Still, preliminary evidence from the Gatekeeper program may be cause for optimism. Whereas the suicide rate of persons aged 60 years and over rose significantly in the state of Washington during the years in which the Gatekeeper program has operated, rates for that age group in Spokane County decreased (R. Rashko, personal communication).

CONCLUSION

Older adults at risk for suicide pose specific public health challenges because their risk may not be recognized by health care professionals and members of their social network. This possibility suggests the need for a new way of thinking about and implementing suicide prevention programs. High-risk approaches, based either in primary care or community settings, hold much promise. In emphasizing the concept of obscured symptom recognition and ascribing it to psychiatric symptoms (mild, not florid), personality (affectively muted, stoic), and medical conditions (chronic and complicated, diverting physician's attention away from mental health issues) that characterize older suicides, we have deliberately narrowed our focus. However, this emphasis ignores other issues, one of which must be broached at least briefly to connect this chapter with a broader question in gerontology and psychopathology: What are some of the societal barriers to the recognition and treatment of depressive symptoms in elders at risk for suicide?

The decision to seek mental health treatment is complex. Symptoms must first be identified, recognized, and labeled. Any attempt to understand this process is incomplete without examining the role of motivation. It is clear that people will not be motivated to seek treatment unless they believe they are impaired or symptomatic; these beliefs are multidetermined, reflecting both objective signs of disease or dysfunction and also subjective impressions. People also differ in the extent to which they are motivated to recognize, label, and report symptoms and functional impairments. People may not label their abnormally low mood "sadness" unless they are also motivated to get back to normal. This will depend in turn on the individual's definition of normal or expectable. It is possible that the attitudes of older people toward mental illness, aging, and suicide discourage early recognition and treatment of symptoms. To paraphrase Edwin Shneidman (1986), many may think of suicide as an autonomous, action-oriented solution to a problem. The prospect of growing old in a body that steals one's independence, in a society that questions one's ability to solve problems and provides few opportunities for achievement past the retirement party increases the appeal of suicide. These attitudes, woven so deeply into the fabric of our culture (Bellah, Madsen, Sullivan, Swidler, & Tipton, 1991), represent attitudinal and motivational barriers to suicide prevention.

Removing these attitudinal barriers will require mass advertising and the infiltration of some of our most cloistered subcultures, those of higher education. Legislation may also be useful. Coupled with educating health care providers about the signs, symptoms, and risk factors for depression and suicide, a campaign should be mounted to educate the public about these issues as well. Print and electronic advertisements and other educational materials could inform the public of the benefits of available treatments and dispel the myths that depression and suicidal ideation are a "normal" aspect of aging. The campaign should be coupled with the development of community-based risk-identification programs that are linked to systems capable of providing a full range of interventions and services.

There is unprecedented enthusiasm in the United States and other nations for suicide prevention, as exemplified by the remarkable growth of grassroots organizations such as the Suicide Prevention Advocacy Network, passage of Senate Resolution 84 and House Resolution 212 declaring suicide prevention to be a national public health priority (Congressional Record, 1997, 1998), and the availability of funds for suicide research (CDC, 1999; National Institutes of Health, 1997). But more than vision and energy will be required to remove ageist attitudes and other insidious barriers to suicide prevention.

STUDY QUESTIONS

ESSAY/SHORT ANSWER QUESTIONS

1. Discuss the advantages and disadvantages of the high-risk and public health approaches to suicide prevention.
2. The research designs that have been used to learn about the risk factors for completed suicide are the prospective cohort design and the retrospective case-control. Discuss the strengths and weaknesses of each.
3. Primary care physicians often fail to diagnose depressive disorders in their older patients. This problem can be ascribed in part to the way patients present themselves, but it may also reflect the attitudes and behaviors of physicians. Explain.
4. The relationship between physical illness and suicide can be understood from three different theoretical perspectives: biological, social constructionist, and public health. Describe each.
5. Discuss the bioclimatic and socioeconomic hypotheses that have been offered to explain the periodicity of the suicide rate. Explain.

FOR CLASS DISCUSSION

1. The chapter notes that suicide rates vary across geopolitical region. What do you think accounts for these differences?
2. It is now commonly believed that primary care physicians can play a critical role in the prevention of suicide in older adults. Do you think that primary care physicians can play a significant role in preventing suicides in teenagers and young adults? Why?
3. The authors recommend an advertising campaign designed to increase public awareness of the signs, symptoms, and lethality of depressive disorders in older adults. Do you think such an approach would be helpful? Why? Could it be harmful?
4. In an op-ed piece published in the *Wall Street Journal* on August 3, 1999, a lawyer with the International Anti-Euthanasia Task Force wrote, "When it comes to suicide, America is Dr. Jekyll and Mr. Hyde. Oregon voters legalized physician-assisted suicide, but when newspapers run headlines about the state's soaring suicide rate among adolescents, nobody connects the dots." Do you think there is a relationship between the legalization of assisted suicide and the risk of suicide among adolescents and young adults? Do you think that young adults whose grandparents requested and

received assisted suicide would themselves be more likely to request an assisted suicide in their old age? Do media reports of suicide machines, physician-assisted suicides, forecasts for prolonged dependency at the end of life, and predictions for increased suicide rates among the elderly increase suicide risk in older adults? If so, is the risk increased only among those with specific personality traits or vulnerabilities? Or is the risk increased randomly throughout the population?

5. Does the falling rate of elderly suicide through most of the 20th century reflect "cohort" changes in certain personality traits, such as stoic individualism? If changing societal conditions (e.g., size of birth cohort) contribute to fluctuations in the suicide rate, are some persons more "vulnerable" and others more "protected" by these changes?

6. The gender difference in suicide rates has perplexed scholars for decades. Acknowledging that it is probably multidetermined, what do you think accounts for this difference? Is it possible to design a study to test your hypothesis?

7. The media and mass-market books may have a tendency to romanticize suicide, and view it as a fitting end to a life full of drama and intrigue. In an interview with Bob Dylan reported in the *Village Voice* on March 25, 1965, the following exchange took place:

Q: Bob, what about the situation of American poets? Kenneth Rexroth has estimated that since 1900 about 30 American poets have committed suicide.

A: 30 poets! What about American housewives, mailmen, street cleaners, miners? Jesus Christ, what's so special about 30 people that are called poets? I've known some very good people that have committed suicide. One didn't do nothing but work in a gas station all his life. Nobody referred to him as a poet, but if you're gonna call people like Robert Frost a poet, then I got to say this gas station boy was a poet, too.

Do you think that publicizing the suicide deaths of famous artists and writers gives the public a distorted understanding of suicide? Do you think that some people commit suicide to emulate a famous person?

SUGGESTED READINGS

American Association of Suicidology. http://www.suicidology.org/index.html

Centers for Disease Control and Prevention. http://www.cdc.gov/ncipc/dvp/suifacts.htm

Durkheim, E. (1951). *Suicide: A study in sociology.* New York: Free Press. (Original work published in 1897)

Kushner, H.I. (1989). *Suicide: A psychocultural exploration.* London: Rutgers University Press.

McIntosh, J.L., Santos, J.F., Hubbard, R.W., & Overholser, J.C. (1994). *Elder suicide: Research, theory and treatment.* Washington, DC: American Psychological Association.

National Institute of Mental Health. http://www.nimh.nih.gov/depression/genpop/su_fact.htm

Shneidman, E.S. (1986). *Definition of suicide.* New York: Wiley.

REFERENCES

Ader, R. (1997). The role of conditioning in pharmacotherapy. In A. Harrington (Ed.), *The placebo effect: An interdisciplinary exploration* (pp. 138–165). Cambridge, MA: Harvard University Press.

Adler, N.E., Boyce, T., Chesney, M., Cohen, S., Folkman, S., Kahn, R.L., & Syme, S.L. (1994). Socioeconomic status and health: The challenge of the gradient. *American Psychologist, 49*(1), 15–24.

Allen-Burge, R., Storandt, M., Kinscerf, D.A., & Rubin, E.H. (1994). Sex differences in the sensitivity of two self-reported depression scales in older depressed inpatients. *Psychology and Aging, 9,* 443–445.

American Psychiatric Association. (1994). *Diagnostic and statistical manual of mental disorders* (4th ed.). Washington, DC: Author.

Appleby, L., Cooper, J., Amos, T., & Faragher, B. (1999). Psychological autopsy study of suicides by people aged under 35. *British Journal of Psychiatry, 175,* 168–174.

Bagby, R.M., Rector, N.A., Bindseil, K., Dickens, S.E., Levitan, R.D., & Kennedy, S.H. (1998). Self-report ratings and informants' ratings of personalities of depressed outpatients. *American Journal of Psychiatry, 155,* 437–438.

Barraclough, B.M. (1971). Suicide in the elderly: Recent developments in psychogeriatrics. *British Journal of Psychiatry, 6*(Suppl.), 87–97.

Barraclough, B.M., Bunch, J., Nelson, B., & Sainsbury, P. (1974). 100 cases of suicide–clinical aspects. *British Journal of Psychiatry, 125,* 355–373.

Bateman, A., & Fonagy, P. (1999). Effectiveness of partial hospitalization in the treatment of borderline personality disorder: A randomized control trial. *American Journal of Psychiatry, 156,* 1563–1569.

Baumeister, R.F. (1990). Suicide as escape from self. *Psychological Review, 97,* 90–113.

Beck, A.T., Steer, R.A., Kovacs, M., & Garrison, B. (1985). Hopelessness and eventual suicide: A 10-year prospective study of patients hospitalized with suicidal ideation. *American Journal of Psychiatry, 142*(5), 559–563.

Bellah, R.N., Madsen, R., Sullivan, W.M., Swidler, A., & Tipton, S.M. (1991). *The good society.* New York: Random House.

Brown, J.H., Henteleff, P., Barakat, S., & Rowe, C.J. (1986). Is it normal for terminally ill patients to desire death? *American Journal of Psychiatry, 143,* 208–211.

Burvill, P.W. (1995). Recent progress in the epidemiology of major depression. *Epidemiologic Reviews, 17,* 21–31.

Callahan, C.M., Nienaber, N.A., Hendrie, H.C., & Tierney, W.M. (1992). Depression of elderly outpatients: Primary care physicians' attitudes and practice patterns. *Journal of General Internal Medicine, 7,* 26–31.

Carney, S.S., Rich, C.L., Burke, P.A., & Fowler, R.C. (1994). Suicide over 60: The San Diego Study. *Journal of the American Geriatrics Society, 42,* 174–180.

Cavanagh, J.T.O., Owens, D.C.G., & Johnstone, E.C. (1999). Suicide and undetermined death in southeast Scotland: A case-control study using the psychological autopsy method. *Psychological Medicine, 29,* 1141–1149.

Centers for Disease Control. (1996). Suicide among older persons—United States, 1980–1992. *Morbidity and Mortality Weekly Report, 45,* 3–6.

Centers for Disease Control and Prevention. (1999, June 30). Deaths: Final data for 1997. *National Vital Statistics Report, 47,* 1–105 [On-line]. Available: http://ww.cdc.gov/nchs/data/nvs47_19.pdf.

Centers for Disease Control and Prevention. (1999, October 5). *U.S. injury mortality statistics: Firearm suicide deaths and rates per 100,000* [On-line]. Available: http://www.cdc.gov/ncipc/osp/usmort.htm

Cheng, A.T.A. (1995). Mental illness and suicide: A case-control study in East Taiwan. *Archives of General Psychiatry, 52,* 594–603.

Chochinov, H.M., Wilson, K.G., Enns, M., Mowchun, N., Lander, S., Levitt, M., & Clinch, J.J. (1995). Desire for death in the terminally ill. *American Journal of Psychiatry, 152,* 1185–1191.

Clark, D.C., & Horton-Deutsch, S. (1992). Assessment in absentia: The value of the psychological autopsy method for studying antecedents of suicide and predicting future suicides. In R.W. Maris, A.L. Berman, J.T. Maltsberger, & R.I. Yufit (Eds.), *Assessment and prediction of suicide* (pp. 144–182). New York: Guilford Press.

Clarke, M., Clarke, S.J., & Jagger, C. (1992). Social intervention and the elderly: A randomized control trial. *American Journal of Epidemiology, 136,* 1517–1523.

Congressional Record. (1997). *Resolution recognizing suicide as a national problem* (CR page S4013, May 6).

Congressional Record. (1998). *Resolution recognizing suicide as a national problem* (CR page H10309, October 9).

Conner, K.R., Duberstein, P.R., Conwell, Y., Herrmann, J.H., Cox, C., Barrington, D.-S., & Caine, E.D. (in press). After the drinking stops: Completed suicide in individuals with remitted alcohol use disorders. *Journal of Psychoactive Drugs.*

Conwell, Y. (1994). Suicide in elderly patients. In L.S. Schneider, C.F. Reynolds, III, B. Lebowitz, & A. Friedhoff (Eds.), *Diagnosis and treatment of depression in late life.* Washington, DC: American Psychiatric Press.

Conwell, Y. (in press). Suicide in later life: A review and recommendations for prevention. In L. Davidson & V. Ross (Eds.), *Suicide prevention now: Linking research to practice.* Atlanta, GA: Center for Disease Control.

Conwell, Y., & Brent, D.A. (1995). Suicide and aging, I: Patterns of psychiatric diagnosis. *International Psychogeriatrics, 7,* 149–164.

Conwell, Y., Caine, E.D., & Olsen, K. (1990). Suicide and cancer in late life. *Hospital and Community Psychiatry, 41,* 1334–1339.

Conwell, Y., Duberstein, P.R., Cox, C., Herrmann, J., Forbes, N.T., & Caine, E.D. (1996). Relationships of age and Axis I diagnoses in victims of completed suicide: A psychological autopsy study. *American Journal of Psychiatry, 153,* 1001–1008.

Conwell, Y., Duberstein, P.R., Cox, C., Herrmann, J., Forbes, N.T., & Caine, E.D. (1998). Age differences in behaviors leading to completed suicide. *American Journal of Geriatric Psychiatry, 6,* 122–126.

Conwell, Y., Lyness, J.M., Duberstein, P.R., Cox, C., Seidlitz, L., DiGiorgio, A., & Caine, E.D. (2000). Suicide among older patients in primary care practices. *Journal of the American Geriatrics Society, 48,* 23–29.

Conwell, Y., Raby, W., & Caine, E.D. (1995). Suicide and aging, II: The psychobiological interface. *International Psychogeriatrics, 7*(2), 165–181.

Costa, P.T., Jr., & McCrae, R.R. (1988). From catalog to classification: Murray's needs and the five-factor model. *Journal of Personality and Social Psychology, 58,* 258–265.

Costa, P.T., Jr., & McCrae, R.R. (1992). *Revised NEO Personality Inventory and NEO Five Factor Inventory: Professional manual.* Odessa, FL: Psychological Assessment Resources.

Coyne, J.C., Schwenk, T.L., & Fechner-Bates, S. (1995). Nondetection of depression by primary care physicians reconsidered. *General Hospital Psychiatry, 17,* 3–12.

Crawford, M.J., Prince, M., Menezes, P., & Mann, A.H. (1998). The recognition and treatment of depression in older people in primary care. *International Journal of Geriatric Psychiatry, 13*(3), 172–176.

De Leo, D., Carollo, G., & Dello Buono, M. (1995). Lower suicide rates associated with a tele-help/tele-check service for the elderly at home. *American Journal of Psychiatry, 152,* 632–634.

Dorpat, T.L., Anderson, W.F., & Ripley, H.S. (1968). The relationship of physical illness to suicide. In H.P.L. Resnik (Ed.), *Suicidal behaviors: Diagnosis and management* (pp. 209–219). Boston: Little, Brown.

Dorpat, T.L., & Ripley, H.S. (1960). A study of suicide in the Seattle area. *Comprehensive Psychiatry, 1,* 349–359.

Drever, F., Whitehead, M., & Roden, M. (1996). Current patterns and trends in male mortality by social class (based on occupation). *Population Trends, 86,* 15–20.

Duberstein, P.R. (1995). Openness to experience and completed suicide across the second half of life. *International Psychogeriatrics, 7,* 183–198.

Duberstein, P.R., & Conwell, Y. (1997). Personality disorders and completed suicide: A methodological and conceptual review. *Clinical Psychology: Science and Practice, 4,* 359–376.

Duberstein, P.R., Conwell, Y., & Caine, E.D. (1994). Age differences in the personality characteristics of suicide completers: Preliminary findings from a psychological autopsy study. *Psychiatry, 57,* 213–224.

Duberstein, P.R., Conwell, Y., & Cox, C. (1998). Suicide in widowed persons: A psychological autopsy comparison of recently and remotely bereaved older subjects. *American Journal of Geriatric Psychiatry, 6,* 328–334.

Duberstein, P.R., Conwell, Y., Seidlitz, L., Denning, D., Cox, C., & Caine, E.D. (2000). Personality traits and suicidal behavior and ideation in depressed inpatients 50 years of age and older. *Journal of Gerontology: Psychological Sciences, 55,* 18–26.

Duberstein, P.R., Conwell, Y., Seidlitz, L., Lyness, J.M., Cox, C., & Caine, E.D. (1999). Age and suicidal ideation in older depressed inpatients. *American Journal of Geriatric Psychiatry, 7,* 289–296.

Duberstein, P.R., Seidlitz, L., & Conwell, Y. (1996). Reconsidering the role of hostility in completed suicide: A lifecourse perspective. In J. Masling & R.F. Bornstein (Eds.), *Psychoanalytic perspectives on developmental psychology* (pp. 257–323). Washington, DC: American Psychological Association.

Durkheim, E. (1951). *Suicide: A study in sociology.* New York: Free Press. (Original work published 1897)

Fawcett, J., Scheftner, W., Fogg, L., Clark, D., Young, M.A., Hedeker, D., & Gibbons, R. (1990). Time-related predictors of suicide in major affective disorder. *American Journal of Psychiatry, 147,* 1189–1194.

Fisher, S., & Greenberg, R.P. (Eds.). (1997). *From placebo to panacea: Putting psychiatric drugs to the test.* New York: Wiley.

Florio, E.R., Jensen, J.E., Hendryx, M.S., Raschko, R., & Mathieson, K. (1998). One year outcomes of older adults referred for aging and mental health services by community gatekeepers. *Journal of Case Management, 7*(2), 1–10.

Florio, E.R., Rockwood, T.H., Hendryx, M.S., Jensen, J.E., Raschko, R., & Dyck, D.G. (1996). A model gatekeeper program to find the at-risk elderly. *Journal of Case Management, 5,* 106–114.

Foster, T., Gillespie, K., & McClelland, R. (1997). Mental disorders and suicide in Northern Ireland. *British Journal of Psychiatry, 170,* 447–452.

Freud, S. (1957). Mourning and melancholia. In J. Strachey, A. Freud, A. Strachey, & A. Tyson (Eds. and Trans.), *The standard edition of the complete psychological works of Sigmund Freud* (Vol. 14, pp. 243–258). London: Hogarth Press. (Original work published 1917)

Gallo, J.J., Anthony, J.C., & Muthen, B. (1994). Age differences in the symptoms of depression: A latent trait analysis. *Journal of Gerontology, 49,* P251–P264.

Gallo, J.J., Rabins, P.V., & Anthony, J.C. (1999). Sadness in older persons: 13-year follow-up of a community sample in Baltimore, Maryland. *Psychological Medicine, 29,* 341–350.

Gallo, J.J., Rabins, P.V., Lyketsos, C., Tien, A.Y., & Anthony, J.C. (1997). Depression without sadness: Functional outcomes of nondysphoric depression in later life. *Journal of the American Geriatrics Society, 45,* 570–578.

Gardner, E.A., Bahn, A.K., & Mack, M. (1964). Suicide and psychiatric care in the aging. *Archives of General Psychiatry, 10,* 547–553.

Goodwin, F.K., & Jamison, K. (1990). *Manic depressive illness.* New York: Oxford University Press.

Gross-Isseroff, R., Biegon, A., Voet, H., & Weizman, A. (1998). The suicide brain: A review of postmortem receptor/transporter binding studies. *Neuroscience & Biobehavioral Reviews, 22*(5), 653–661.

Gunnell, D., & Frankel, S. (1994). Prevention of suicide: Aspirations and evidence. *British Medical Journal, 308,* 1227–1233.

Harper, R.G., Kotik-Harper, D., & Kirby, H. (1990). Psychometric assessment of depression in an elderly general medical population: Over- or underassessment? *Journal of Nervous and Mental Disease, 178,* 113–119.

Harris, E.C., & Barraclough, B.M. (1994). Suicide as an outcome for medical disorder. *Medicine, 73*(6), 281–296.

Harris, E.C., & Barraclough, B.M. (1997). Suicide as an outcome for mental disorders. *British Journal of Psychiatry, 170,* 205–228.

Hawton, K., Appleby, L., Platt, S., Foster, T., Cooper, J., Malmberg, A., & Simkin, S. (1998). The psychological autopsy approach to studying suicide: A review of methodological issues. *Journal of Affective Disorders, 50,* 269–276.

Henriksson, M.M., Marttunen, M.J., Isometsä, E.T., Heikkinen, M.E., Aro, H.M., Kuoppasalmi, K.I., & Lönnqvist, J.K. (1995). Mental disorders in elderly suicide. *International Psychogeriatrics, 7*(2), 275–286.

Henry, B., Moffitt, T.E., Caspi, A., Langley, J., & Silva, P.A. (1994). On the "remembrance of things past": A longitudinal evaluation of the retrospective method. *Psychological Assessment, 6,* 92–101.

Hyman, S., & Arana, G.W. (1989). Suicide and affective disorders. In D. Jacobs & H.N. Brown (Eds.), *Suicide: Understanding and responding* (pp. 171–181). Madison, CT: International Universities Press.

Isometsä, E.T., & Lönnqvist, J.K. (1998). Suicide attempts preceding completed suicide in personality disorders. *British Journal of Psychiatry, 173,* 531–535.

Kagamimori, S., Matsubara, I., Sokejima, S., Sekine, M., Matsukura, T., Nakagawa, H., & Naruse, Y. (1998). The comparative study on occupational mortality, 1980, between Japan and Great Britain. *Industrial Health, 36,* 252–257.

Katon, W., Robinson, P., Von Korff, M., Lin, E., Bush, T., Ludman, E., Simon, G., & Walker, E. (1996). A multifaceted intervention to improve treatment of depression in primary care. *Archives of General Psychiatry, 53,* 924–932.

Keeler, E.M., Solomon, D.H., Beck, J.C., Mendenhal, R.C., & Kane, R.L. (1982). Effect of patient age on duration of medical encounters with physicians. *Medical Care, 20,* 1101–1108.

Kessler, R.C., Borges, G., & Walters, E.E. (1999). Prevalence of and risk factors for lifetime suicide attempts in the National Comorbidity Survey. *Archives of General Psychiatry, 56,* 617–626.

Kraemer, H.C., Kazdin, A.E., Offord, D.R., Kessler, R.C., Jensen, P.S., & Kupfer, D.J. (1997). Coming to terms with the terms of risk. *Archives of General Psychiatry, 54,* 337–343.

Kung, H.-C., Liu, X., & Juon, H.-S. (1998). Risk factors for suicide in Caucasians and in African-Americans: A matched case-control study. *Social Psychiatry, 33,* 155–161.

Kushner, H.I. (1989). *Suicide: A psychocultural exploration.* London: Rutgers University Press.

Kuypers, J.A., & Bengston, V.L. (1973). Social breakdown and competence. *Human Development, 16,* 181–201.

Lewis, G., Hawton, K., & Jones, P. (1997). Strategies for preventing suicide. *British Journal of Psychiatry, 171,* 351–354.

Lin, E.H., Katon, W.J., Simon, G.E., Von Korff, M., Bush, T.M., Rutter, C.M., Saunders, K.W., & Walker, E.A. (1997). Achieving guidelines for the treatment of depression in primary care: Is physician education enough? *Medical Care, 35*(8), 831–842.

Lin, E.H., Katon, W.J., Von Korff, M., Russo, J.E., Simon, G.E., Bush, T.M., Rutter, C.M., Walker, E.A., & Ludman, E.J. (1998). Relapse of depression in primary care: Rate and clinical predictors. *Archives of Family Medicine, 7,* 443–449.

Lin, E.H., Simon, G.E., Katon, W.J., Russo, J.E., Von Korff, M., Bush, T.M., Ludman, E.J., & Walker, E.A. (1999). Can enhanced acute-phase treatment of depression improve long-term outcomes? A report of randomized trials in primary care. *American Journal of Psychiatry, 156*(4), 643–645.

Linehan, M.M. (1993). *Cognitive behavioral treatment of borderline personality disorder.* New York: Guilford Press.

Luborsky, L., Diguer, L., Seligman, D., Rosenthal, R., Krause, E., Johnson, S., Halperin, G., Bishop, M., Berman, J.S., & Schweizer, E. (1999). The researcher's own therapy allegiances: A "wild card" in comparisons of treatment efficacy. *Clinical Psychology—Science & Practice, 6*(1), 95–106.

Lyness, J.M., Cox, C., Curry, J., Conwell, Y., King, D.A., & Caine, E.D. (1995). Older age and the underreporting of depressive symptoms. *Journal of the American Geriatrics Society, 43,* 216–221.

MacMahon, B., & Pugh, T.F. (1965). Suicide in the widowed. *American Journal of Epidemiology, 81,* 23–31.

Mann, J.J., Oquendo, M., Underwood, M.D., & Arango, V. (1999). The neurobiology of suicide risk: A review for the clinician. *Journal of Clinical Psychiatry, 60*(Suppl. 2), 7–11.

Maris, R.W. (1992). The relationship of nonfatal suicide attempts to completed suicide. In R.W. Maris, A.L. Berman, J.T. Maltsberger, & R.I. Yufit (Eds.), *Assessment and prediction of suicide* (pp. 362–380). New York: Guilford Press.

McCleary, R., Chew, K.S., Hellsten, J.J., & Flynn-Bransford, M. (1991). Age- and sex-specific cycles in United States suicides, 1973 to 1985. *American Journal of Public Health, 81,* 494–497.

McCusker, J., Cole, M., Keller, E., Bellavance, F., & Berard, A. (1998). Effectiveness of treatments of depression in older ambulatory patients. *Archives of Internal Medicine, 158,* 705–712.

McDaniel, J.S., Musselman, D.L., Porter, M.R., Reed, D.A., & Nemeroff, C.B. (1995). Depression in patients with cancer: Diagnosis, biology, and treatment. *Archives of General Psychiatry, 52*(2), 89–99.

McIntosh, J.L. (1992). Older adults: The next suicide epidemic? *Suicide and Life-Threatening Behavior, 22,* 322–332.

McIntosh, J.L., Santos, J.F., Hubbard, R.W., & Overholser, J.C. (1994). *Elder suicide: Research, theory, and treatment.* Washington, DC: American Psychological Association.

Musselman, D.L., Evans, D.L., & Nemeroff, C.B. (1998). The relationship of depression to cardiovascular disease: Epidemiology, biology, and treatment. *Archives of General Psychiatry, 55*(7), 580–592.

Niederehe, G., & Schneider, L.S. (1998). Treatments for depression and anxiety in the aged. In P.E. Nathan & J.M. Gorman (Eds.), *A guide to treatments that work* (pp. 270–287). New York: Oxford University Press.

Office of the U.S. Surgeon General. (1999). *The Surgeon General's call to action to prevent suicide* [On-line]. Available: http://www.surgeongeneral.gov/osg/calltoaction/default.htm

Oxman, T.E., Barrett, J.E., Barrett, J., & Gerber, P. (1990). Symptomatology of late-life minor depression among primary care patients. *Psychosomatics, 31,* 174–180.

Pearson, J.L., & Conwell, Y. (1995). Suicide in late life: Challenges and opportunities for research. *International Psychogeriatrics, 7,* 131–136.

Penninx, B.W.J.H., Geerlings, S.W., Deeg, D.J.H., van Eijk, J.T.M., van Tilburg, W., & Beekman, A.T.F. (1999). Minor and major depression and the risk of death in older persons. *Archives of General Psychiatry, 56,* 889–895.

Prigerson, H.G., Frank, E., Kasl, S.V., Reynolds, C.F., III, Anderson, B., Zubenko, G.S., Houck, P.R., George, C.J., & Kupfer, D.J. (1995). Complicated grief and bereavement-related depression as distinct disorders: Preliminary empirical validation in elderly bereaved spouses. *American Journal of Psychiatry, 152,* 22–30.

Reynolds, C.F., III, Frank, E., Perel, J.M., Imber, S.D., Cornes, C., Miller, M.D., Mazumdar, S., Houck, P.R., Dew, M.A., Stack, J.A., Pollock, B.G., & Kupfer, D.J. (1999). Nortriptyline and interpersonal psychotherapy as maintenance therapies for recurrent major depression: A randomized controlled trial in patients older than 59 years. *Journal of the American Medical Association, 281*(1), 39–45.

Rich, C.L., Young, D., & Fowler, R.C. (1986). San Diego Suicide Study I: Young vs. old subjects. *Archives of General Psychiatry, 43,* 577–582.

Robins, E., Murphy, G.E., Wilkinson, R.H., Gassner, S., & Kayes, J. (1959). Some clinical considerations in the prevention of suicide based on a study of 134 successful suicides. *American Journal of Public Health, 49,* 888–889.

Rost, K., Smith, G., Matthews, D., & Guise, B. (1994). The deliberate misdiagnosis of major depression in primary care. *Archives of Family Medicine, 3,* 333–337.

Rutz, W., von Knorring, L., Pihlgren, H., Rihmer, Z., & Walinder, J. (1995). Prevention of male suicides: Lessons from Götland study. *Lancet, 345*(8948), 524.

Rutz, W., von Knorring, L., & Walinder, J. (1992). Long-term effects of an educational program for general practitioners given by the Swedish committee for the prevention and treatment of depression. *Acta Psychiatrica Scandinavica, 85,* 414–418.

Sainsbury, P. (1955). *Suicide in London* (Maudsley Monograph No. 1). London: Chapman and Hall.

Schmutte, P.S., & Ryff, C.D. (1997). Personality and well-being: Reexamining methods and meanings. *Journal of Personality and Social Psychology, 73,* 549–559.

Schulberg, H.C., Block, M.R., Madonia, M.J., Scott, C.P., Rodriguez, E., Imber, S.D., Perel, J., Lave J., Houck, P.R., & Coulehan, J.L. (1996). Treating major depression in primary care practice: Eight month clinical outcomes. *Archives of General Psychiatry, 53,* 913–919.

Schulberg, H.C., Pilkonis, P.A., & Houck, P. (1998). The severity of major depression and choice of treatment in primary care practice. *Journal of Consulting & Clinical Psychology, 66*(6), 932–938.

Shneidman, E.S. (1986). *Definition of suicide.* New York: Wiley.

Simon, G.E., Von Korff, M., & Barlow, W. (1995). Health care costs of primary care patients with recognized depression. *Archives of General Psychiatry, 52,* 850–856.

Tiemens, B.G., Ormel, J., & Simon, G.E. (1996). Occurrence, recognition, and outcome of psychological disorders in primary care. *American Journal of Psychiatry, 153*(5), 636–644.

Valenstein, E.S. (1998). *Blaming the brain: The truth about drugs and mental health.* New York: Free Press.

Von Korff, M., Katon, W., Bush, T., Lin, E.H., Simon, G.E., Saunders, K., Ludman, E., Walker, E., & Unutzer, J. (1998). Treatment costs, cost offset, and cost-effectiveness of collaborative management of depression. *Psychosomatic Medicine, 60,* 143–149.

Waern, M., Beskow, J., Runeson, B., & Skoog, I. (1996). High rate of antidepressant treatment in elderly people who commit suicide. *British Medical Journal, 313*(7065), 1118.

Wallace, J., & Pfohl, B. (1995). Age related differences in the symptomatic expression of major depression. *Journal of Nervous and Mental Disease, 183,* 99–102.

Werth, J.L., Jr. (Ed). (1999). *Contemporary perspectives on rational suicide.* Philadelphia: Brunner/Mazel.

Whitbourne, S.K. (1987). Openness to experience, identity flexibility, and life change in adults. *Journal of Personality and Social Psychology, 50,* 163–168.

Zahner, G.E.P., Hsieh, C.C., & Fleming, J.A. (1995). Introduction to epidemiologic research methods. In M.T. Tsuang, M. Tohen, & G.E.P. Zahner (Eds.), *Textbook in psychiatric epidemiology* (pp. 157–177). New York: Wiley.

CHAPTER 11

Substance Abuse Disorders

EDITH S. LISANSKY-GOMBERG

CASE STUDIES

James, 65, has been admitted to a veterans' facility with a diagnosis of chronic alcoholism and an intense need for detoxification and treatment. This is his twentieth admission and although, as a veteran of World War II, he is eligible, no one—least of all James—is optimistic about his prognosis. He has been drinking heavily for 30+ years, and in this admission, he shows signs of cognitive and liver dysfunction. His family had given him up years ago and has minimal contact with him; his current social group consists of several drinking buddies. James is a compliant patient and within the limits of what medicine and psychiatry offer, he will improve moderately. Inviting him to participate in Alcoholics Anonymous, as was done in the past, may be tried again.

Eleanor is a widow of 72; she keeps reasonably busy by volunteering in a few community organizations. Since her husband died 10 years ago, she has had difficulty sleeping. Her physician, who perceives the sleep difficulties as based on depression and grieving, prescribed antidepressants. Because her insomnia continued, he also prescribed sedatives. She is now a regular user of sedatives and has appeared in the emergency department of the local hospital recently complaining of logginess and fatigue.

Richard, 70, is a "survivor" who has used heroine (injected) for several decades. A middle-level "con man," he has avoided violence and the street drug subculture. A fastidious, well-organized person, he has kept his needles clean, avoided other drugs, and joined a local methadone program, where he socializes. He has arthritis and some pulmonary disorder, based on years of heavy smoking. Although older addicts are good, compliant patients, it is often difficult to find a hospital or nursing home bed when it is needed because health care workers do not like to admit drug-addicted patients.

DIAGNOSIS OF SUBSTANCE ABUSE

s is true of all psychopathologies, substance abuse is not a simple or single phenomenon. It applies to taking a legally banned drug, to side effects of medication, and to toxin exposure; the *Diagnostic and Statistical*

Manual of Mental Disorders (DSM-IV; American Psychiatric Association [APA], 1994) groups substances into 11 classes: alcohol, amphetamines, caffeine, cannabis, cocaine, hallucinogens, inhalants, nicotine, opioids, phencyclidine (PCP), and the group of sedatives, hypnotics, and anxiolytics (p. 175). We discuss here problems related to medications and over-the-counter drugs, nicotine, illegal substances, and alcohol.

The *DSM-IV* divides substance abuse disorders into two major categories. First, *substance dependence* is defined as a combination of cognitive, behavioral, and physiological symptoms "indicating that the individual continues use of the substance despite significant substance-related problems" (APA, p. 176). There are seven criteria for the diagnosis, but three or more must be present in the same year:

1. Tolerance—markedly diminished effects of the substance and/or need for increased amounts.
2. Withdrawal—withdrawal patterns vary for different substances.
3. Substance taken in larger amounts or over a longer time period than intended.
4. Persistent desire or unsuccessful effort to cut down or control substance use.
5. Much time spent on obtaining, using, and recovering from substance.
6. Important social/occupational/recreational activities given up or reduced.
7. Continued use of substance despite substance-related problems, effects, consequences.

These behaviors will occur either with or without physiological dependence.

Second, there is a diagnosis of *substance abuse.* This is manifested by a "maladaptive pattern" of substance use in the face of recurrent and significant consequences. Criteria for this diagnosis are:

1. Failures to fulfill major role obligations at school, work, or home.
2. Continued substance use in situations where it is physically hazardous.
3. Continued substance use related to legal problems.
4. Continued substance use despite persistent/recurrent social or interpersonal problems.

The American Medical Association convened an ad hoc committee on alcoholism among older persons to create guidelines for primary care physicians (AMA, 1995). Barriers to diagnosis and treatment included denial, uncertainty, pessimism, and ageism. Patients may present intoxicated or in withdrawal; they may report physiological or psychological symptoms; they may be worried about their drinking; or they simply come in for a periodic checkup examination. The AMA guidelines suggest taking a medical, drug, and alcohol history, laboratory tests, mental status exam, and a "social inventory." There are many alcohol-related medical consequences: anemia, cardiomyopathy, peripheral neuropathy, alcoholic liver disease or pancreatitis, malignancies of the head and throat, esophagus varices, delirium tremens, and more. It is of some interest that in a follow-up comparison of older treated/rehabilitated heroin addicts and alcoholics (Barr, 1985), mortality rates for alcoholics resulted from disease and violence; for heroin addicts, there were increased mortality rates from violence alone (both groups of patients had persisted in substance abuse after treatment).

DRUGS

A drug is defined as a substance (not food) that may be produced in nature or in a laboratory, which by its chemical nature alters the structure or function of an organism. Drugs may be prescribed, bought in pharmacies over the counter, purchased (as with alcoholic beverages and cigarettes), or bought "on the street." Drugs may be classified in terms of chemical composition, central nervous system action, or social acceptability. The latter classification varies from socially acceptable substances (e.g., caffeine) to Schedule I substances, banned by law. Many drugs, like medications, may be described in terms of *use*. When usage is deviant and/or excessive, we may diagnose drug abuse or dependence.

Pharmacokinetics studies the time course of absorption, tissue distribution, metabolism, and excretion of drugs and their metabolites from the body. There are few age changes in absorption, but there are age changes in distribution and elimination.

Pharmacodynamics is the physiological and psychological response to drugs. Different psychoactive drugs may produce different pharmacodynamic effects among older people; for example, some investigators report that the response to benzodiazepines is enhanced (McCormack & O'Malley, 1986). Adverse drug reactions (ADRs) occur more frequently among older patients, related to multiple drug therapies, drug overdose or misuse, age-related chronic diseases, alcohol intake, and food-drug incompatibilities. Age changes in drug metabolism and elimination are related, and ADRs among older people are not only more frequent but more severe as well. Risk factors for ADRs include being female, living alone, having multiple diseases, multiple drug intake, and poor nutritional status. Although only 3% of people who come to emergency rooms with drug-related episodes are 55 or older, two-thirds of these older people present with "overdose," 10% with "chronic effects," and 6% with "unexpected reaction" (Drug Abuse Warning Network [DAWN], 1996).

EPIDEMIOLOGICAL DATA

MEDICATION

There is a good deal of work by sociologists and anthropologists on group norms about substance use. Ethnicity, religion, nationality and region, tribal affiliation, and community organizations are the group classifications.

Earlier studies reported cultural differences and attitudes toward alcohol of groups such as the Chinese, the Italians, the Jews, and the Irish usually studied in the United States. A favorite subject of study by anthropologists was the American Indian. Although knowledge of ethnicity might have been useful in developing a predictive equation, time has changed the drinking customs and attitudes of many of these groups, possibly because of assimilative processes. It should be noted that study of ethnicity pertains not only to drug use per se but also to marked group differences in educational aspirations, kinship networks, religious participation, group values about sexuality and marriage, and many other elements of socialized behavior.

More recent work has been less ethnographic and more epidemiological. A recent report by the Substance Abuse and Mental Health Services Administration (SAMHSA, 1998) examines substance use in racial/ethnic subgroups within the United States. Overall rate of illicit drug use in the prior year (persons 12 and older) was 11.9% of the total U.S. population. Subgroup rates of illicit drug use included Native Americans (13.1%), Mexican Americans (6.9%), Caucasians (5.3%), other Hispanic Americans (4.9%), and African Americans (4.7%). Regarding smoking, prevalence in the entire United States was estimated at 30.9%; this figure includes everyone 12 and older who smoked within the prior year. Heaviest smoking was reported for Native Americans (52.7%), Puerto Ricans (32.7%), Caucasians (31.5%), and African Americans (29.9%).

Although 13% of the U.S. population is defined as elderly, they account for a third of all prescription drug expenditure. There is increased use of prescription drugs for both chronic and acute illnesses, and the elderly also are more likely to purchase and use over-the-counter (OTC) drugs (Korrapati & Vestal, 1995). The most commonly prescribed drugs are diuretics, cardiovascular drugs, and sedatives-hypnotics; the most commonly purchased OTC drugs include analgesics, vitamins, and laxatives. Types of medications prescribed and purchased OTC is similar in most Western industrialized countries among older people.

The question of psychoactive drugs such as tranquilizers, sedatives, and hypnotics brings up a related question. Not only are such drugs more likely to be prescribed for older persons, but they are also more likely to be prescribed for women.

As noted above, an older person being seen in an emergency room is most likely to present with "misuse of a psychoactive drug" (LaRue, Dessonville, & Jarvik, 1985). Although some treatment facilities report patient intake with drug-associated problems and dependence on psychoactive drugs, this information has not evoked much interest among researchers and gerontologists. Older persons frequently associate their intake of such drugs with problems such as depression and insomnia. However, one study reported that almost half of the older subjects taking such medications respond that they could not perform their daily activities without the medication. The use and misuse of psychoactive substances among older people merits research examination: neuropsychological components, relationship to geriatric medical practice, societal attitudes toward the elderly, and so on.

The use and misuse of psychoactive drugs are also linked with nursing home care; this has come up in several media stories. This stands in contrast to the current wisdom that "successful aging" (Rowe & Kahn, 1998) should involve exercise and activity. It is of course, a small percentage of the elderly who are residents in nursing homes (4%–5%), and the current trend to offer "assisted living" residences to older people will bear watching and study.

Age and gender differences do appear among drug-associated emergency room visits: younger patients are more likely to show up with problems associated with controlled substances (cocaine, heroin, marijuana, etc.) and older patients with problems associated with psychoactive drugs, usually prescribed. As for gender patterns: up to approximately age 65, women are more often prescribed and use more psychoactive drugs than men. But data suggest that older men may be prescribed more antidepressants. This might be related to older males' greater utilization of medical resources than younger men or to loss of power for the aging male (the suicide rate remains stable for aging women but rises for aging men).

One study compared 26 elderly and 33 younger substance abusers: both groups were polydrug users, with alcohol as the most commonly used drug (Solomon & Stark, 1993). Despite the small sample size, some significant differences emerged: the older patients were more likely to have dual diagnoses, to abuse benzodiazepines, and to present with neurological, cognitive, or psychotic symptoms (memory loss, sleep disturbance, disorientation, etc.). The younger subjects were more likely to use "street drugs" (e.g., cocaine) and to have job, housing, and legal problems. Interestingly, the older patients were more likely to be noncompliant with medical care than the younger ones. Although the histories are not given, it is likely that this group of older patients had a longer history of substance abuse than the younger group. Among older substance abusers, a distinction has been made between those with early onset and those with recent/late onset; this will be discussed under the section on alcohol abuse.

The question of compliance is raised frequently in writings about older people in general, primarily in relation to prescribed drugs. Noncompliance includes the following behaviors:

1. Nonuse—not obtaining the drug, perhaps because of inadequate money.
2. Partial use—ceasing before the recommended course is complete, often because of side effects or drug interactions.
3. Incorrect dosage—more/less than prescribed.
4. Improper timing or sequencing of medication.
5. Medication shared with a relative or friend.

Although it has been traditional to attribute noncompliance to cognitive limitation, there are other factors: limited money, denial, issues of autonomy, and the quality of the patient-physician relationship. It is always a good idea to have a patient aware of possible side effects of a given drug and many pharmacies are disseminating the information. Nonetheless, older persons would be wise to ask the prescribing physician about possible side effects.

We have not included epidemiological information about older persons' use of vitamins, herbs, and alternative medicines, largely because the information is limited. Vitamins are among the folk remedies, and most people have clear opinions of the effects of specific foods (e.g., the effects of grits, greens, prunes, chicken soup). Home remedies would make a most interesting research study: Do people use these as a first line of defense, because they have limited funds, as a mechanism of denial, or because of rebellious feelings about the authority of medicine? The phenomenal growth of alternative medicine raises the same questions.

Several relevant classifications have been made of different usages of psychoactive drugs. One classification distinguishes appropriate use, unintentional misuse, and purposeful misuse. Another classification is specifically related to benzodiazepine usage: first, there is *low* or therapeutic dose, as usually prescribed with no withdrawal symptoms when use ceases; second, there is *high* dose therapeutic use, prescribed but usually producing withdrawal symptoms when use ceases; third, there is intake involved in multiple drug use frequently involving alcohol, when the aim is to achieve a "high" or some self-prescribed relief.

Recent reports of OTC sleep aids (Pillitteri, Kozlowski, Person, & Spear, 1994) point to the paucity of studies of OTC drugs or alcohol as sleep aids. Earlier studies (e.g., Balter & Uhlenhuth, 1991) showed the majority of OTC sleep aids to be used by people under the age of 40. Pillitteri et al. state that "elderly individuals tend to use the majority of benzodiazepines" (p. 320). Public health concerns about prescription of benzodiazepines to younger people are apparently based on potential side effects and abuse potential. Nevertheless, very little is known about individual responsiveness and effects of prolonged use of OTC sleep aids. OTC sleep aids might be risky for the elderly because of hepatic and renal insufficiency or because of drug interactions.

NICOTINE

The epidemiology of nicotine use focuses primarily on cigarettes, although some surveys take into account cigars, pipes, chewing tobacco, and other forms. Cigarette consumption rose from the beginning of the 20th century until the 1960s, when the Surgeon General began a campaign for smoking cessation. Although nicotine is, technically, a socially approved drug substance, its status has been changing; from 1974 on, consumption dropped steadily. Smoking is banned in an increasing number of public places, and it could conceivably become a banned substance (Although American experience with prohibiting another socially acceptable substance, alcohol, was not particularly successful). In the 1960s, more than 42% of the adult population were smokers; by 1993, the percentage had dropped to 25% (National Center for Health Statistics, 1996); current increases in adolescents' and young peoples' smoking needs to be monitored.

Men are more likely to smoke than women are, although the gender gap has narrowed. The Public Health Service, tracking the rise in female smoking during and after World War II, has documented the fact that mortality from lung cancer surpassed mortality from breast cancer in 1985. In all countries for which statistics are available, there appear to be more male than female smokers. Among men 65 and older, the percentage of cigarette smokers was 13.5% in 1993; among older women in the United States it was 10.5%. A survey of people 65 and older in Massachusetts showed that those less likely to be smoking currently were respondents living alone or with their children, those who reported their health as poor or fair, and the frail elderly.

The U.S. Center for Disease Control has released data from its 1995 to 1997 Behavioral Risk Factor Surveillance System that confirms a relationship between smoking and toothlessness among persons 65 and older: only 19.9% who never smoked are currently toothless, compared with 41.3% of daily smokers.

BANNED SUBSTANCES

The occasional use of such drugs as marijuana, heroin, and cocaine undoubtedly occurs among older individuals. In a comparison of 169 White and African American older male alcoholics in treatment or clearly diagnosable but not in treatment (Gomberg & Nelson, 1995), respondents were asked about the use of drugs other than alcohol. The African American men ($N = 27$) reported significantly more public drinking and, when queried about other drug use, a significantly higher proportion reported use of drugs other than alcohol and significantly more drug dependence. The White/Black difference might be based on either of two factors: the Black men reported a much earlier age at onset of drug dependence (age 27, compared with White men's report at age 40); and the much greater likelihood that the Black men would be drinking publicly (i.e., on the street). Also, issues of availability and social facilitation may be raised.

That some use of illegal drugs occurs among older people, though considerably less than among younger people, is spelled out in data from Michigan (Michigan Department of Public Health, 1994). When the primary substance of abuse was heroin, treatment admissions were 6% under 60 and 3% older. When the primary substance of abuse was cocaine or crack, treatment admissions showed 18% under the age of 60 and 2% 60 or older.

Although it was believed that opiate addicts did not survive into old age but either died or "matured out," there is apparently a small number who began use of heroin early and survived into old age despite the heroin use. Pascarelli (1985) reported that in 1974, patients 60 and older in the New York City methadone maintenance program constituted .005%; 10 years later, they constituted 2% of patients. These were not recent-onset addicts; they were long-term heroin-dependent people. DesJarlais, Joseph, and Courtwright (1985) studied this group of survivors and reported a number of variables apparently relevant to survival: they avoided violence and were careful about the use of clean needles; they were able to hold some drugs in reserve, used other drugs (e.g., alcohol) moderately, and were generally in reasonable health compared with same aged people in the general population. In fact, Barr (1985), treating aging alcoholics and narcotic drug addicts, comments, "If drug addicts survive the risk of violent death, their medical complication may not be as severe as those of older alcoholics" (p. 195).

ALCOHOL

The most widely available and widely used drug substance is alcohol. Because it is a socially approved substance, a distinction needs to be made between use and misuse, including abuse and dependence. In addition, there are social problems, such as driving while intoxicated, alcohol-related accidents, alcohol-related violence, and alcohol-related university campus problems.

Starting with the question of *use*, usually infrequent or moderate, to what extent are alcoholic beverages used by older people? It has been generally accepted that social drinking declines with age. That may well be true. For one thing, drinking norms change over time; for another, women have greater longevity than men and drink lesser amounts and less often than do men. This question of alcohol usage by older persons is still open. Data from the National Health Interview Survey (NHIS) indicate an increase in alcohol intake among men 65+ and a smaller increase among women in the same age group. However, several regional studies in Boston and in San Francisco do not support the decline in older persons' drinking. Glynn, Bouchard, LoCastro, and Hermos (1984) did not find a decline with a sample of healthy male aging veterans in Boston. Also, Huffine, Folkman, and Lazarus (1989) found that 90% of a sample of healthy retired adults in San Francisco reported having had at least one drink in the prior six months. A recent report about drinking by older persons from the National Health and Nutrition Examination Survey I Epidemiologic Follow-up Study (Moore, Hays, Greendale, Damesyn, & Reuben, 1999) concluded that in their large U.S. probability sample, most older persons who ever drank in their lifetime were currently drinking. They further reported that 16% of the men and 15% of the women who drank were heavy drinkers, placing them at risk of alcohol-related health consequences. Finally, a study of alcohol-related health hospitalizations of elderly people (Adams, Yuan, Barboriak, & Rimm, 1993) found such hospitalizations to be "common with a gender ratio of approximately 3½ males: 1 female" (p. 1223). Interestingly, there was a strong relationship between alcohol-related hospitalizations and per capita consumption of alcohol by state.

In a recent study of a Canadian sample of older adults (Graham & Schmidt, 1999), the amount consumed was related to "poorer psychological well being, especially depression." The role of isolation, loneliness, and depression in older people's drinking (or among younger people, for that matter) is discussed frequently, but there is also evidence of older drinking facilitated by sociability (Alexander & Duff, 1988). It may well be that social drinking by older persons tends to be moderate, whereas those who are isolated and living alone tend to be abstainers or, if they drink, tend to be heavy drinkers. It is a complex issue.

One thing emerges clearly: the linkage between negative affect and alcohol. A recent report (Carpenter & Hasin, 1999) lists reasons for drinking as coping with negative affect, social facilitation, the enhancement of positive affect, perceived social pressure, and celebratory activities. Although all the drinking motives appear to have a positive origin, it is hypothesized that drinking to cope with negative affect places people at more risk for becoming problem drinkers. Using a nonclinical sample of men and women with mean ages in the 30s, the investigators examined three models: risk-factor, generalizing, and epiphenomena. Among alcohol-dependent and no-drinking-problem subjects, comparisons suggested the predictions of a risk-factor model. Although this study did not focus on older subjects, there is no reason to doubt that the findings would apply to them. There is some evidence that negative affect strongly impacts the elderly and that drinking may indeed be a coping mechanism to deal with these negative feelings. In this sense, alcohol may be the self-selected antidepressant of choice.

In general, the impression left after examining the surveys and the reported literature is that, indeed, alcohol abuse and dependency may be more limited in older subsets of the populations than in younger ones. However, the literature also suggests that the numbers may be larger than original estimates, that the number of drinkers and problem drinkers among the elderly is greater than originally estimated, and that the frequency of the problem varies regionally, by gender, and by marital status.

Most of the reports are from hospitals and treatment facilities; it would expedite our understanding of the epidemiology of alcohol-related problems among the elderly if physicians and gerontologists routinely asked in their examinations about clients' use of alcohol. The generation influenced by the Prohibition amendment and the "wet versus dry" controversies has pretty much passed from the scene, and health care workers could ask questions about alcohol consumption as a regular feature of health examinations. There seems to be very modest interest in the behavior of the elderly insofar as alcohol, drugs, and medications go. Most research interest is restricted to adolescent and younger persons.

RELEVANT THEORIES

Most theorizing has focused on the pathological use of alcohol but these theories could be applied to the abuse of and dependence on other drugs. Theories may be divided into developmental, biopsychosocial, genetic, neurophysiological, psychopharmacological, psychological, and classical conditioning/social learning.

DEVELOPMENTAL THEORY

Developmental theory emphasizes the importance of studying earlier behaviors to comprehend later developmental characteristics and stresses the importance of "charting process as well as structure" (Zucker, 1998, p. 5). Recommended is evaluation of "the interplay between contextual and organismic factors, and of timing and sequencing" in creating and maintaining new structures and relinquishing older structures. Developmental analysis requires both specifications of potential maintenance functions of context and intra-individual mechanisms. The interaction of alcohol and aging involves understanding of neurobiological structure as well as contextual factors (i.e., nonspecific causative agents). This viewpoint emphasizes a life span approach.

BIOPSYCHOSOCIAL THEORY

The etiology of alcoholism exists within a longitudinal-developmental framework that includes physiological, behavioral, and sociocultural variables (Zucker & Gomberg, 1986). *Physiological variables* include genetics, and the trend of research evidence shows that a heritable basis for alcoholic etiology does indeed exist. Neurophysiological research seems at the moment more focused on results of excessive alcohol intake rather than etiology, but with the increasing sophistication of brain research, presumably antecedent neurophysiological status before the onset of alcoholic drinking will be explored.

Behavioral/psychological variables review longitudinal etiologic evidence, those reports that study childhood/adolescence through to adult diagnosis of problem drinking. Although most of the subjects in longitudinal studies reviewed are male, recent studies have included females (Gomberg & Schmidt, 1999); a comparison of alcoholic women and a matched control group shows educational achievement to be significantly different, although early family socioeconomic status showed little difference. A review of longitudinal etiologic evidence (Zucker & Gomberg, 1986) indicates:

1. Childhood antisocial behavior appears to be consistently related to later alcoholic outcome.
2. More childhood difficulty in achievement was consistently found in those children who later develop alcohol problems.
3. Several longitudinal studies raise the question of a greater activity level.
4. Males who are prealcoholic appear during childhood and adolescence to be "more loosely tied to others interpersonally" (Zucker & Gomberg, 1986, p. 789).
5. More marital conflict is reported consistently in the homes of prealcoholic children. This is consistent with the report of greater alcoholism in the early family life of problem drinkers.
6. Parenting in the homes of children who will later manifest alcohol-related problems is inadequate, and the parents are more frequently inadequate role models for normalcy.

GENETICS

A recent review of genetics, alcohol, and aging (McClearn, 1998) begins with the simple observation that X or Y "runs in families." This does not separate genetic from environmental influences, but adoption, twins-separated-at-birth, and similar studies indicate that "environmental influences alone cannot account for the observed degree of familiarity of alcoholism" (p. 91). However, genetic effects do not necessarily appear at birth but could have a developmental course (e.g., as in Huntington's disease or alcoholism). Cloninger (1987) has proposed genetic heterogeneity in alcoholism by age of onset. McClearn suggests that twin studies indicate a decline in heritability of alcohol use in older people—an interesting suggestion flowing from the observation that "the genetic contribution to individual differences in the human response to alcohol may be substantially different at different ages" (p. 96). This would account for the recent onset of heavy drinking and alcohol problems among older adults with no previous history of alcohol abuse or dependence.

NEUROPHYSIOLOGICAL THEORY

Neuropathological studies of the relationship between alcohol and aging were reviewed by Harper et al. (1998). They conclude:

1. There is loss of brain tissue with aging and alcoholism.
2. Loss is greater among alcoholics.
3. Loss occurs mainly from the cerebral hemisphere, and mainly white matter.
4. Loss of white matter is greater among alcoholics.
5. A correlation exists between loss of white matter and alcohol intake.
6. A correlation exists between white matter loss and cognitive dysfunction in both aging and alcoholism.

The interaction of aging and alcohol on brain membrane structure and neurotransmitters (Wood, 1998) begins with the observation that aged animals and human beings differ in response to alcohol in vivo when compared with younger subjects. Research in this area is limited, and it is not known whether GABA, NMDA, and dopamine are or are not involved in alcohol sensitivity and tolerance.

Specific neurotransmitters also have a role in the etiology and treatment of addiction (Oslin & Mellow, 1998). Reviewing a variety of systems—dopaminergic, opioid, serotonergic, gluatamatergic, gavaergic system and melatonin, acetylcholine, and norepinephrine—the authors looked at the major neurotransmitter systems involved in addictions and the significance of age-related changes in those systems.

The search for the neurophysiological aspects of aging and alcohol intake/problems has just begun. We may look to the future for further development of the role of etiology in the implications for treatment.

PSYCHOPHARMACOLOGIC THEORY

Kalant's (1998) review of the pharmacological interactions of aging and alcohol raises several questions:

1. Are the elderly more sensitive to alcohol than younger persons?
2. If so, to what extent is that difference due to pharmacokinetics, to pharmacodynamics, or to both?
3. Is the difference based on true increase in sensitivity or on lowered ability to develop tolerance?
4. Does the difference apply to all effects of alcohol, including reinforcing as well as aversive effects?

For both genders in the 60+ age group, the frequency of alcohol-related symptoms is directly proportional to the amount of alcohol consumed. There are differences between older and younger people in blood alcohol concentrations (even when the same amount is consumed). Are there age differences in impairment? To what extent are such age differences due to aging, illness, and/or drug interactions? Pharmacokinetics shows that aging does result in higher blood alcohol levels because of changes in proportion of lean body mass and fat. Rates of absorption and elimination are not apparently affected by age. Pharmacodynamically, the elderly show greater effects at the same blood alcohol concentrations than younger persons do (e.g., in balance and fine motor coordination). There is evidence that age difference in response to different drugs varies; a systematic examination of age-related changes in central nervous system sensitivity to a broad range of depressants is needed. Also to be distinguished are the acute effects of alcohol (i.e., effect on a single drinking situation) and chronic effects of heavy drinking. Among chronic effects, some suggest that alcoholism results in premature brain aging: brain cells are lost in normal aging, but alcoholics lose more brain cells more rapidly. Several studies report greater cell loss in elderly alcoholics than in younger alcoholics, but the weight of evidence does not necessarily support or produce an accelerated rate of loss. There is, however, some support that age diminishes tolerance to alcohol. Whether alcohol results in premature brain aging or change is a result of aging and a result of drinking—independent but additive—is not resolved.

PSYCHOLOGICAL THEORY

One may begin a commentary on psychological theories with a historical approach. Freud himself wrote little about drinking or drug abuse/dependence. He described alcohol as warding off unpleasant feelings; excessive drinking could be explained by an unusual need for a pleasurable effect. Freud therefore anticipated much of the modern view of alcohol and its reinforcements. Later Freudian writers elaborated on the theory, particularly in terms of drinking to relieve distress about homosexual urges or conflicts over dependency, and as a result of self-destructive impulses. In this way, the followers of Freud turned his conception of unusual need for the pleasurable effect of alcohol into alcohol as utilized to deal with negative affect (Barry, 1988).

Although the concept of "the alcoholic personality" is not generally accepted, there has been some evidence of prealcoholic "distinctive personality characteristics" (Cox, 1988). These include impulsivity, independence, social adroitness, and rejection of conventional values; low frustration tolerance and high sensation seeking; and, manifest in treatment, low self-esteem, depression, and anxiety.

CLASSICAL CONDITIONING AND SOCIAL LEARNING THEORIES

Classical conditioning theory is based on Pavlovian principles and deals with acquired preferences/aversions for alcohol-related stimuli, alcohol tolerance, and urge/craving for alcohol (Sherman, Jorenby, & Baker, 1988).

Social learning theory developed from the interest in behavior modification (Wilson, 1988). Learning theory applications to psychopathology and its treatment were narrowly based on animal work, to account for the more complex social behavior of human beings, social learning theory expanded to include symbolic events, vicarious learning, and self-regulatory processes. Inevitably, the theory became more cognitive and became the base of most behavioral therapies.

SUMMARY OF THEORIES

Relevant theories are those that offer some etiological basis for problem drinking. Not only do most theories display modest, if any, interest in the motivations for the use and abuse of alcohol, but most have little to say about the older population. Despite the almost universal interest in alcohol, despite the social problems (e.g., traffic accidents related to alcohol), and despite the frequency with which hospital admissions involve alcohol-related disorders, the theories offer little by way of etiological explanation. Any writing about aging and alcohol misuse have, in the past, cited the stresses of aging (e.g., ill health, depression, social isolation). Yet the surveys and research available to us have indicated that the *stresses* of the aging process *do not act as a major etiological factor*. We must distinguish between early-onset/long-duration alcoholism, and recent-onset/relatively short-duration alcoholism. Whatever has been written about the etiology of alcoholism is relevant to those older people who have a history of early onset. For those who manifest more recent onset, the etiologies are unclear. It is interesting that older female alcoholics are much more likely to be recent, late-onset alcoholics than older men. A recent gender comparison (Gomberg, 1995) shows that women are not only older when first introduced to alcohol but also are significantly older than men when they report their first alcohol problem.

The most sensible theoretical approach to aging and alcohol, it seems to me, is a biopsychosocial approach, which recognizes the complex etiology of alcoholism and encompasses neurophysiology and biochemistry, behavioral and personality variables, and social norms. Experimental studies of the effects of alcohol on cognition and affect are relevant; surely, the effect of alcohol in reducing anxiety, fear, insecurity, and depression is critical.

For the clinician who works with older patients and the researcher who investigates a question of interest about older subjects, awareness of the different theories outlined briefly is a good place to start. Chaudron and Wilkinson's edited work on theories of alcoholism published by the Addiction Research Foundation in Toronto, is another good place to start. Beresford and Gomberg's book on alcohol and aging contains much relevant information on theoretical approaches, and reports about genetics, cognition, epidemiology, medication use, and several biological aspects will be useful to those interested in gerontology and geriatrics. Finally, *Research Monograph 33*, published by the National Institute on Alcohol Abuse and Alcoholism in 1998 and edited by Gomberg, Hegedus, and Zucker covers the most recent contributions to this area. The three recommendations are all listed in Suggested Readings.

TREATMENT

Substance-related disorders, whether at the level of abuse or dependence, involve loss of control, but dependence also involves tolerance and withdrawal. How useful the *DSM-IV* criteria are for older persons or how effective screening tests designed for youthful or middle-aged subjects might be has been questioned. Using a number of measures is good for accurate assessment, for example, collateral information from significant others, blood alcohol or drug toxicology tests, assessment of biochemical markers, review of earlier medical history, and assessment of current medical conditions and psychosocial problems.

A note on comorbidity: Older substance abusers are more likely than younger ones to have medical problems. Age-related illnesses coexisting with substance abuse problems include anemia, arrhythmia, dementia, diabetes, hypertension, incontinence, osteoporosis, liver pathology, and pancreatitis. A demonstration project with medically ill older alcoholics did produce significantly lower age of mortality (Willenbring, Olson, & Bielinski, 1995); however, dual diagnosis involves a psychiatric diagnosis or an organic disorder. It has been reported that more hospitalization and treatment are required and that the relapse rate is higher (Moos, Brennan, & Mertens, 1993).

Regarding withdrawal, it has been reported that older patients take significantly longer to withdraw than younger patients (Brower, Mudd, Blow, Young, & Hill, 1994), in spite of similar duration of drug/alcohol abuse. It is advisable to monitor medically the withdrawal of older patients; they may manifest sleeplessness, cognitive impairment, weakness, and hypertension to a greater extent than younger patients.

Earlier work on elder-specific treatments tended to report negatively; recent work, however, suggests that patients in an elder-specific program are more likely to complete the course of treatment and to be in follow-up (Atkinson, Tolson, & Turner, 1993).

In general, therapists should consider the following factors:

1. Recovery rates, with treatment, tend to be similar for older and younger substance abusers.

2. More patience is required when working with older abusers, related in part to slowed reaction time.
3. Age differential between therapist and patient needs to be discussed.
4. Work with families of older abusers, as with younger abusers, is necessary.
5. Therapists should respect the dignity needs of older persons at all times.

TREATMENT MODALITIES

Chemotherapy

Medications used in general alcoholism treatment (e.g., Antabuse) must be carefully evaluated and are contraindicated for medically ill older alcoholics. Zimberg (1995) has suggested the efficacy of antidepressants with depressed older patients. Naltrexone use with older patients has been reported recently in a study of 44 V.A. Hospital patients (Oslin, Liberto, O'Brien, Krois, & Norbeck, 1997); naltrexone was tolerated well, and "efficacious in preventing relapse in subjects who drank" (p. 324).

Psychosocial Treatment

Although the role of perceived stress is not widely supported as etiology of elderly substance abuse, a recent report (Brennan & Moos, 1995) compared problem drinkers with nonproblem drinkers in an elderly sample drawn from medical facilities. The problem drinkers reported more negative life events, more chronic stress, fewer material resources, and less social support. Where stress exists, it needs to be discussed in a treatment program.

Behavioral Treatment

A day treatment program for late-onset alcoholics in Florida that included a self-management approach, skills acquisition, and reestablishment of social support reported some success (Dupree, Broskowski, & Schonfeld, 1984). Schonfeld and Dupree (1997) make several recommendations with empirical support:

1. Age-specific group treatment with supportive approach; avoiding confrontation.
2. Focus on negative emotional states (e.g., depression, loneliness, overcoming loss).
3. Rebuilding of social networks and social skills.
4. Staff should be experienced/interested in working with the older patient.
5. Linkages with aging services, medical facilities.
6. Pact/content of treatment for the older patient.

Glantz (1995) describes a cognitive therapy approach for older alcoholics, including a thoughtful discussion of establishing goals, problem solving, "homework assignments," and relapse prevention. Graham et al. (1995) describe the Community Older Persons Alcohol program (COPA), an outreach program for older persons with alcohol and/or drug problems. Treatment is divided into three stages: assessment, active treatment, and maintaining follow-up/aftercare. The goals of the program are not merely changing substance-using behavior but improving the person's well-being and maintenance of independence. The approach is nonconfrontational, although the problem areas related to substance abuse need to be identified and addressed. People in treatment need to be aware of their strengths, limited though these may be. Treatment includes direct services to the client (housing, finances, medical/dental needs, nutrition, etc.), direct services to the family, and contact with other agencies. The COPA approach produced "some improvement" for approximately 75% of the clients, improvements that appeared to be stable over time.

Apparently, the programs in this category of behavioral treatment, with their emphasis on the nonconfrontational and the holistic approach, are reasonably effective. Brief intervention (i.e., limited contact with the client) usually uses a behavorial approach; it is currently undergoing wide experimentation, and a few reports suggest that it may work efficaciously.

Group Therapy

Because loss, isolation, and loneliness are frequently part of the clinical picture of elderly substance abusers, group therapy is important. Whether such groups should be age-specific is an unresolved question in need of study. Older patients do well in mixed-age programs, and there are benefits in contacts with younger patients (Atkinson, 1998). On the other hand, Johnson (1989) surveyed recovering older people who expressed preferences for elder-specific groups, large print in written materials, and a slow pace.

Family Therapy

There is not a great deal available on the efficacy of different models of family therapy, nor is there much on family therapy with older clients. One study (Tabisz, Jacyk, Fuchs, & Grymonpre, 1993) raised the question of enabling, particularly among elderly women substance abusers. How the enabling mechanism fits is not clear; many of the older women referred to substance abuse treatment have a history of an alcohol/drug-abusing spouse and a shared usage of substances. When they are widowed, the substance abuse continues, and such women are often diagnosed as using substances in response to loss of a spouse. Much needed, in addition, is study of the rehabilitative role of family therapy with long-term elderly male alcoholics.

Community Outreach

COPA (Graham et al., 1995), a community-based project in Toronto, provided individualized assistance to encourage the maintenance of older people in their homes, improve physical and emotional health, and reduce or eliminate substance dependence. The investigators noted the rather high abuse of prescribed psychoactive drugs. Improvement was measured in 35% to 40% of the participants, and considering the prognosis for the group studied, the results are encouraging.

Self-Help Groups

Membership in Alcoholics Anonymous (AA) among individuals 50 years and older has increased. AA has developed some special groups for the elderly (Zimberg, 1995). As with group therapies in general, the social support aspect and shared histories are very important to the alcohol-dependent. A preference for age peers in one's group has been expressed in the little evidence available.

SUMMARY OF TREATMENT

Recovery rates seem to be as good for older substance abusers as for younger ones. As with all age groups, heterogeneity must be recognized: among older people are the young-old and the old-old (75 years of age is usually the dividing point); the rich, the poor, and the middle class; ethnic and religious subgroups; and the relatively healthy and those with more or less severe health problems. Program planning will vary with the subgroups: the homeless alcoholic, the veterans hospital patient, and the "well-to-do." Treatments will vary from community outreach by the Salvation Army to a residential center in California where movie stars and VIPs go for treatment.

In practice with older substance abusers, the pace must be slower than with younger clients. Patience is needed, and more medical intervention may be necessary. The age differential between patient and therapist needs to be openly discussed because self-disclosure to a much younger therapist may be difficult for an older patient. If possible, families should be brought into the treatment process because the basic social network begins with the family and the patient has usually taxed the anxiety load of family members. At all times, and no matter what the treatment program being followed, the dignity and self-view of the older patient must be prime matters of consideration, as with all patients.

The pros and cons of age-specific treatment of older alcoholics were reviewed by Atkinson (1998). Recommendations include the need for further comparative studies of age-specific community outreach program development and the fact that brief intervention and prevention efforts may also need age-specific considerations to be more effective.

The American Medical Association (AMA, 1995) has published guidelines for primary care physicians on the diagnosis, treatment, and prevention of alcoholism in older persons. After discussing with the client the presenting problems and the procedures of withdrawal, a treatment plan should have a clear goal: harm avoidance versus abstinence (harm avoidance is the goal of therapists who sanction controlled drinking as a goal). The treatment plan may involve referral to an inpatient facility, an outpatient facility, a halfway house, or some other setting, depending on social supports, employment, insurance coverage, and financial resources. Also considered should be health problems, previous history of alcoholism and attempted previous treatments, cognitive status, and "the likelihood of the patient being able to refrain from the use of alcohol and other addicting substances" (p. 14). These guidelines also recommend that AA or a similar support group be utilized. The guidelines note that the prognosis for recovery of elderly alcoholics is good.

CONCLUSION

The major contribution of the study of substance abuse disorders among older people is the understanding that the disorders do not disappear with mature years. Once widely held was the view that heroin addicts "mature out," while there are older addicts, those no longer addicted have probably been exposed to a methadone program or died through violence or illness (e.g., AIDS). There is no particular mystery about older alcoholics. Indeed, the reports suggest that etiology, manifestations, and consequences may vary slightly from the alcoholism of younger patients but not in substantial ways.

In reviewing substance abuse disorders among older people, the substance under study must be specified. Older people probably have more misuse and abuse problems with medication and OTC drugs. On the other hand, street drugs or banned substances and the lifestyle they involve are clearly less frequently an issue for the older groups. Alcohol and tobacco are still used by younger populations. The problem of drug interaction (with medications) must be considered, and the physiological response of the aging organism to various substances needs more exploration. Theories that seek to explain the onset of substance abuse are fundamentally similar for different age groups, although some considerations are relevant to older patients. There is probably more comorbidity, withdrawal is more prolonged and perhaps more difficult, and the fundamental question of elder-specific treatment must be raised: Do these older people do better in age-matched treatment groups? Caution needs to be exercised in chemotherapeutic regimens. The need for rapport and respect and a supportive approach by the therapist is primary; rebuilding social networks and linkages with other services for older people is also primary.

STUDY QUESTIONS

1. In dealing with elderly alcohol/drug abusers, what is the difference between early and later onset?
2. What are the implications of early and later onset for therapy and for prognosis?
3. Using the definitions of the *DSM-IV*, how are substance abuse and substance dependence differentiated?
4. What is pharmacokinetics?
5. What is pharmacodynamics?
6. When older individuals show up in emergency rooms with a drug-related medical emergency, what class of drugs is likely to be involved?
7. What are some of the reasons you believe that use of marijuana, heroin, cocaine, and methamphetamine is more likely among younger than older persons?

8. What is meant when we describe a drug-related behavior as compliant or noncompliant? What are the different ways in which a person can be noncompliant?
9. How do you account for the recent elevation of interest in vitamins and herbal remedies?
10. There are many folk remedies that vary from one subgroup to another. Name a folk remedy you are familiar with and explain its persistence.
11. Both alcoholics and narcotic addicts are more likely than nonaddicted people to die from violence, but medical complications are reported to be more severe among alcoholics. Why?
12. What are the advantages/disadvantages of a biopsychosocial theory of the etiology of drug dependence?
13. Which are the therapy points most supported by behavioral/cognitive therapies?
14. Discuss some of the arguments for/against elder-specific treatments.

SUGGESTED READINGS

American Medical Association. (1995). *Alcoholism in the elderly: Diagnosis, treatment, prevention. Guidelines for primary care physicians.* Department of Geriatric Health: Author.

Beresford, T.P., & Gomberg, E.S.L. (Eds.). (1995). *Alcohol and aging,* New York: Oxford University Press.

Chaudron, C.D., & Wilkinson, D.A. (Eds.). (1988). *Theories on alcoholism.* Toronto, Canada: Addiction Research Foundation.

Gomberg, E.S.L. (1990). Drugs, alcohol and aging. In L.T. Kozlowski, H.M. Annis, H.D. Capella, F.B. Glasser, M.S. Goodstadk, Y. Israel, H. Kalant, E.M. Sellers, & E.R. Vingilis (Eds.), *Research advances in alcohol and drug problems* (pp. 171–213). New York: Plenum Press.

Gomberg, E.S.L. (1995). Older women and alcohol. In M. Galanter (Ed.), *Recent developments in alcoholism* (Vol. 12. pp. 63–79). New York: Plenum Press.

Gomberg, E.S.L., Hegedus, A.M., & Zucker, R.A. (Eds.). (1998). *Alcohol problems and aging.* Research Monograph No. 33, National Institute on Alcohol Abuse and Alcoholism. Washington, DC: U.S. Department of Health and Human Services.

Gottheil, E., Druley, K.A., Skoloda, T.E., & Waxman, H.M. (1985). (Eds.). *The combined problems of alcoholism, drug addiction and aging.* Springfield, IL: Thomas.

Nordhus, I.H., VandenBos, G.R., Berg, S., & Fromholt, P. (1998). (Eds.). *Clinical geropsychology.* Washington, DC: American Psychological Association.

Rowe, J.W., & Kahn, R.L. (1998). *Successful aging.* New York: Pantheon Books.

Zucker, R.A., & Gomberg, E.S.L. (1986). Etiology of alcoholism reconsidered: The case for a biopsychosocial process. *American Psychologist, 41*(7), 783–793.

REFERENCES

Adams, W.L., Yuan, Z., Barboriak, J.J., & Rimm, A.A. (1993). Alcohol-related hospitalization of elderly people. *Journal of the American Medical Association, 270*(10), 1222–1225.

Alexander, F., & Duff, R.W. (1988). Social interactions and alcohol use in retirement communities. *Gerontologist, 28,* 632–636.

American Medical Association. (1995). *Alcoholism in the elderly: Diagnosis, treatment, prevention. Guidelines for primary care physicians.* Chicago: Author.

American Psychiatric Association. (1994). *Diagnostic and statistical manual of mental disorders* (4th ed.). Washington, DC: Author.

Atkinson, R. (1998). Age-specific treatment for older adult alcoholics. In E.S.L. Gomberg, A.M. Hegedus, & R.A. Zucker (Eds.), *Alcohol problems and aging: Research Monograph 33* (pp. 425–438). Washington, DC: National Institute on Alcohol Abuse and Alcoholism.

Atkinson, R.M., Tolson, R.L., & Turner, J.A. (1993). Factors affecting outpatient treatment compliance of older male problem drinkers. *Journal of Studies on Alcohol, 54,* 102–106.

Balter, M.B., & Uhlenhuth, E.H. (1991). The beneficial and adverse effects of hypnotics. *Journal of Clinical Psychiatry, 52,* 16–23.

Barr, H.L. (1985). What happens as the alcoholic and the drug addict get older? In E. Gottehil, K.A. Druley, T.E. Skoloda, & H.M. Waxman (Eds.), *The combined problems of alcoholism, drug addiction and aging* (pp. 193–200). Springfield, IL: Thomas.

Barry, H., III. (1988). Psychoanalytic theory of alcoholism. In C.D. Chaudron & D.A. Wilkinson (Eds.), *Theories on alcoholism* (pp. 103–141). Toronto, Canada: Addiction Research Foundation.

Brennan, P., & Moos, R. (1995). Life context, coping responses, and adaptive outcomes: A stress and coping perspective on late life drinking problems. In T.P. Beresford & E.S.L. Gomberg (Eds.), *Alcohol and aging* (pp. 203–248). New York: Oxford University Press.

Brower, K.J., Mudd, S.A., Blow, F.C., Young, J.P., & Hill, E.M. (1994). Severity and treatment of alcohol withdrawal in the elderly *vs.* younger patients. *Alcoholism: Clinical and Experimental Research, 18,* 196–201.

Carpenter, K.M., & Hasin, D.S. (1999). Drinking to cope with negative affect and *DSM-IV* alcohol use disorders: A test of three alternative explanations. *Journal of Studies on Alcohol, 60*(5), 694–704.

Cloninger, C.R. (1987). Neurogenetic adaptive mechanisms in alcoholism. *Science, 236* 410–416.

Cox, W.M. (1988). Personality theory. In C.D. Chaudron & D.A. Wilkinson (Eds.), *Theories on alcoholism* (pp. 143–172). Toronto, Canada: Addiction Research Foundation.

DAWN (Drug Abuse Warning Network). (1996). *Annual emergency department data 1994* (DHHS Series 1, No. 14-A). Washington, DC: Substance Abuse and Mental Health Services Administration Office of Applied Studies.

DesJarlais, D.C., Joseph, H., & Courtwright, D.F. (1985). Old age and addiction: A study of elderly patients in methadone maintenance treatment. In E. Gottheil, K.A. Grealey, T.E. Skoloda, & H.M. Waxman (Eds.), *The combined problems of alcoholism and aging* (pp. 201–209). Springfield, IL: Thomas.

Dupree, L.W., Broskowski, H., & Schonfeld, L. (1984). The Gerontology Alcohol Project: A behavioral treatment program for elderly alcohol abusers. *Gerontologist, 24,* 510–516.

Glantz, M.C. (1995). Cognitive theory with elderly alcoholics. In T.P. Beresford & E.S.L. Gomberg (Eds.), *Alcohol and aging* (pp. 211–229). New York: Oxford University Press.

Glynn, R.J., Bouchard, G.R., LoCastro, A.S., & Hermos, J.A. (1984). Changes in alcohol consumption behaviors among men in the normative aging study. In G. Maddox,

L.N. Robins, & N. Sosanberg (Eds.), *Nature and extent of alcohol problems among the elderly: Research Monograph 14* (pp. 101–116). Washington, DC: National Institute on Alcohol Abuse and Alcoholism,

Gomberg, E.S.L., & Nelson, N. (1995). Black and White older men: Alcohol use and abuse. In T.P. Beresford & E.S.L. Gomberg (Eds.), *Alcohol and aging* (pp. 307–322). New York: Oxford University Press.

Graham, K., Saunders, S.J., Flower, M.C., Timney, C.B., White-Campbell, M., & Pietropaola, A.Z. (1995). *Addictions Treatment for Older Adults. Evaluation of an innovative client-centered approach.* New York: Haworth Press.

Graham, K., & Schmidt, G. (1999). Alcohol use and psychosocial well-being among older adults. *Journal of Studies on Alcohol, 60*(3), 345–351.

Harper, C., Sheedy, D., Halliday, G., Double, K., Dodd, P., Lewohl, J., & Kril, J. (1998). Neuropathological studies: The relationship between alcohol and aging. In E.S.L. Gomberg, A.M. Hegedus, & R.A. Zucker (Eds.), *Alcohol problems and aging: Research Monograph 33* (pp. 117–134). Washington, DC: National Institute on Alcohol Abuse and Alcoholism.

Huffine, C., Folkman, S., & Lazarus, R.S. (1989). Psychoactive drugs, alcohol, and stress and coping processes in older adults. *American Journal of Drug and Alcohol Abuse, 15,* 101–109.

Johnson, L.K. (1989). How to diagnose and treat chemical dependency in the elderly. *Journal of Gerontological Nursing, 15,* 22–26.

Kalant, H. (1998). Pharmacological interactions of aging and alcohol. In E.S.L. Gomberg, A.M. Hegedus, & R.A. Zucker (Eds.), *Alcohol problems and aging: Research Monograph 33* (pp. 99–116). Washington, DC: National Institute on Alcohol Abuse and Alcoholism.

Korrapati, M.R., & Vestal, R.F. (1995). Alcohol and medications in the elderly: Complex interactions. In T.P. Beresford & E.S.L. Gomberg (Eds.), *Alcohol and aging* (pp. 42–55). New York: Oxford University Press.

LaRue, A., Dessonville, C., & Jarvik, L.F. (1985). Aging and mental disorders. In J.E. Birrin & K.W. Schaie (Eds.), *Handbook of the psychology of aging* (pp. 664–702). New York: Van Nostrand-Reinhold.

McClearn, G.E. (1998). Genetics, aging, and alcohol. In E.S.L. Gomberg, A.M. Hegedus, & R.A. Zucker (Eds.), *Alcohol problems and aging: Research Monograph 33* (pp. 91–98). Washington, DC: National Institute on Alcohol Abuse and Alcoholism.

McCormack, P., & O'Malley, K. (1986). Biological and medical aspects of drug treatment in the elderly. In R.E. Dunkle, G.J. Petot, & A.B. Ford (Eds.), *Food, drugs and aging* (pp. 19–28). New York: Springer.

Michigan Department of Public Health. (1994). *Substance abuse services for older adults* (OA 089/IOM/9–94/NOG). Lansing, MI: Author.

Moore, A.A., Hays, R.D., Greendale, G.A., Damesyn, M., & Reuben, D.B. (1999). Drinking habits among older persons: Findings from the NHANES I Epidemiologic Follow-up Study (1982–1984). *Journal of the American Geriatics Society, 47,* 412–416.

Moos, R.H., Brennan, P.L., & Mertens, J.R. (1993). Patterns of diagnosis and treatment among late middle-aged and older substance abuse patients. *Journal of Studies on Alcohol, 54,* 479–487.

National Center for Health Statistics. (1996). *Health United States 1995* (pp. 173). Hyattsville, MD: Public Health Services.

Oslin, D.W., Liberto, J.G., O'Brien, J.O., Krois, S., & Norbeck, J. (1997). Naltrexone as an adjunctive treatment for older patients with alcohol dependence. *American Journal of Geriatric Psychiatry, 5*(4), 324–332.

Oslin, D.W., & Mellow, A.M. (1998). Neurotransmitter-based therapeutic strategies in late life alcoholism and other addictions. In E.S.L. Gomberg, A.M. Hegedus, & R.A. Zucker (Eds.), *Alcohol problems and aging: Research Monograph 33* (pp. 169–190). Washington, DC: National Institute on Alcohol Abuse and Alcoholism.

Pascarelli, E.F. (1985). The elderly in methadone maintenance. In E. Gottheil, K.A. Druley, T.E. Skoloda, & H.M. Waxman (Eds.), *The combined problems of alcoholism, drug addiction and aging* (pp. 210–214). Springfield, IL: Thomas.

Pillitteri, J.L., Kozlowski, L.T., Person, D.C., & Spear, M.E. (1994). Over-the-counter sleep aids: Widely used but rarely studied. *Journal of Substance Abuse, 6,* 315–324.

Rowe, J.W., & Kahn, R.L. (1998). *Successful aging.* New York: Pantheon Books.

SAMHSA (Substance Abuse Mental Health Services Administration) Office of Applied Studies. (1998, July 6). *Prevalence of substance use among racial and ethnic subgroups in the United States, 1991–1993* [News Release]. Rockville, MD: Author.

Schonfeld, L., & Dupree, L.W. (1997). Treatment alternatives and outcomes for the older alcohol abuser. In A.M. Gurnack (Ed.), *Older adults' misuse of alcohol, medicine, and other drugs* (pp. 112–131). New York: Springer.

Sherman, J.E., Jorenby, D.E., & Baker, T.B. (1988). Classical conditioning with alcohol: Acquired preferences and aversions, tolerance, and urges/craving. In C.S. Chaudron, & D.A. Wilkinson (Eds.), *Theories on alcoholism* (pp. 173–237). Toronto, Canada: Addiction Research Foundation.

Solomon, K., & Srark, S. (1993). Comparison of older and younger alcoholics and prescription drug abusers: History and clinical presentation. *Clinical Gerontologist, 12*(3), 41–56.

Tabisz, E.M., Jacyk, W.R., Fuchs, D., & Grymonpre, R. (1993). Chemical dependency in the elderly: The enabling factors. *Canadian Journal of Aging, 17,* 78–88.

Willenbring, M.L., Olson, D.H., & Bielinski, J. (1995). Integrated outpatient treatment for medically ill alcoholic men: Results from a quasi-experimental study. *Journal of Studies on Alcohol, 56,* 337–343.

Wilson, G.T. (1988). Alcohol use and abuse: A social learning analysis. In C.S. Chaudron, & D.A. Wilkinson (Eds.), *Theories on alcoholism.* (pp. 139–287). Toronto, Canada: Addiction Research Foundation.

Wood, W.G. (1998). Interaction of aging and ethanol on brain membrane structure and neurotransmitters. In E.S.L. Gomberg, A.M. Hegedus, & R.A. Zucker (Eds.), *Alcohol problems and aging: Research Monograph 33* (pp. 135–144). Washington, DC: National Institute on Alcohol Abuse and Alcoholism.

Zimberg, S. (1995). The elderly. In E.M. Washton (Ed.), *Psychotherapy and substance abuse* (pp. 413–427). New York: Guilford Press.

Zucker, R.A. (1998). Developmental aspects of aging, alcohol involvement and their interrelationships. In E.S.L. Gomberg, A.M. Hegedus, & R.A. Zucker (Eds.), *Alcohol problems and aging: Research Monograph 33* (pp. 3–24). Washington, DC: National Institute on Alcohol Abuse and Alcoholism.

Zucker, R.A., & Gomberg, E.S.L. (1986). Etiology of alcoholism reconsidered: The case for a biopsychosocial process. *American Psychologist, 41,*(7), 783–793.

CHAPTER 12

Insomnia in Older Adults

BRANT W. RIEDEL AND KENNETH L. LICHSTEIN

CASE STUDY

Ms. H., a 68-year-old woman who was generally in good health, reported to the sleep clinic with a complaint of insomnia that had persisted for six years. The problem had worsened after her retirement three years previously. As part of a research project conducted during the prior year, Ms. H.'s sleep was assessed via an overnight sleep study (polysomnography), and sleep disorders other than insomnia such as sleep apnea (multiple episodes of breathing cessation during sleep) and periodic limb movements (arm or leg movements that disrupt sleep) were ruled out.

During her initial interview at the sleep clinic, information was gathered regarding her sleep pattern and possible causes of the sleep disturbance. The patient reported obtaining about six hours of sleep per night. Ten years ago, she slept about seven and a half hours per night. For several years, this drop in total sleep time did not bother Ms. H., but recently she was becoming concerned that reduced sleep would have a negative impact on her health. She stated, "When I was younger, my body could probably tolerate six hours of sleep per night, but now I need more rest. I'm worried about my health. I try to eat right, and I'd like to sleep right, too." She was currently averaging about eight hours in bed each night, and she was usually awake for 90 minutes or more during the middle of the night. She experienced mild to moderate chronic lower back pain, which had become more troublesome during the past two years. Her sleep problem started before the back pain, but she did feel that the back pain was adding to her sleep difficulties. She used only one medication regularly, an antihypertensive medication that she began taking one year previously. In general, she reported a reluctance to take medication. She had tried sleep medication for a month, but she discontinued using it because it seemed to lose its effectiveness, and she was worried about becoming dependent on the medication. She only occasionally used an over-the-counter pain medication when her back pain worsened. Questionnaires completed during the interview did not suggest a mood or anxiety disorder. Daytime behaviors that could impact sleep were also explored, and she reported that she did not take naps but did drink about three caffeinated beverages after noon. When asked to think about daytime functioning, her only complaint was that she often felt fatigued.

Global self-reports of functioning may differ from information derived from daily monitoring. Therefore, Ms. H. was asked to complete a sleep diary each morning for two weeks. In the diary, she recorded information about the previous night (time to fall asleep, time in bed, total sleep time, etc.), and she tracked daytime behaviors such as napping, caffeine use, and exercise. In addition to the diaries, she was asked to complete a sleepiness scale and a fatigue scale once during the morning and once during the afternoon each day. After this two-week assessment period, it was apparent that the patient's global self-report and daily self-monitoring were consistent, with one exception. On only one day during the two-week period was there evidence of elevated fatigue, although her global report suggested daytime fatigue was a consistent problem.

The treatment approach chosen consisted of several components. First, the patient would be educated about typical changes in sleep that accompany aging (increased awake time, decreased total sleep time). Also, given her general lack of daytime dysfunction, she would be encouraged to view age-related sleep changes as developmental rather than pathological. Second, she would be encouraged to gradually reduce time in bed over the first few weeks of treatment. This strategy focuses on decreasing unnecessary, frustrating awake time rather than increasing sleep time. Third, she would be trained in a ten-minute passive relaxation procedure that could be used during the day, at bedtime, and also in the middle of the night. The relaxation procedure was introduced to dampen any general arousal that was interfering with sleep and also to reduce her chronic back pain. Fourth, she was asked to abstain from caffeine use after noon.

Ms. H. adhered to most of the treatment recommendations. She eliminated caffeine use during the afternoon, and she enjoyed the relaxation procedure and used it often. She was initially skeptical of the proposal that her reduced sleep time was developmental rather than pathological. She noted that her 65-year-old husband slept about eight hours per night and was rarely awake during the middle of the night. However, after continuing to self-monitor daytime functioning, she began to conclude that she generally functioned well during the day and might require less sleep than her husband. It was recommended that she gradually reduce her time in bed to six and a half hours per night so that time in bed would better match total sleep time. She refused to reduce time in bed to less than seven hours, but she did begin to consistently spend seven hours in bed per night, and she settled on consistent going-to-bed and morning-arising times. She chose to go to bed an hour later than her husband because she would not be able to awaken herself an hour earlier in the morning without also awakening him. She watched taped television shows during the extra hour she was out of bed.

After five weeks of treatment, she was averaging 6 hours and 15 minutes of sleep per night and 40 minutes of awake time during the middle of the night. The time it took her to fall asleep at night had been reduced from 20 minutes to about 5 minutes. It was not clear which strategy or strategies had produced the observed sleep improvement. Ms. H. felt that the relaxation procedure and a more consistent sleep schedule produced most of the improvement. She noted that her sleep had worsened after retirement, when her sleep schedule became less consistent. The patient was contacted one year after treatment, and she reported that her sleep pattern was similar to that observed at posttreatment.

At posttreatment and follow-up, Ms. H. indicated that her satisfaction with her sleep had significantly increased after treatment. Her daytime functioning was also satisfactory. However, she still did not consider herself a "normal" sleeper. She still spent about 40 minutes awake during the middle of the night, and, unlike some of her friends, she had to strictly adhere to a consistent sleep schedule. She noticed that when the regularity of her sleep schedule was disrupted (e.g., on holidays and other special occasions), her sleep became more disturbed. She also continued to be tempted to compare her sleep to that of her husband.

DSM-IV CRITERIA

The *Diagnostic and Statistical Manual of Mental Disorders (DSM-IV)*; American Psychiatric Association [APA], 1994) describes several sleep-related disorders. Insomnia is the most prevalent sleep disorder in older adults, and it is the only sleep disorder for which several psychological treatments have been developed and empirically tested. Treatment approaches for other sleep disorders typically focus on the use of medication, surgery, or medical devices rather than psychological intervention. This chapter focuses on psychological treatment of insomnia, and it includes information on distinguishing insomnia from other sleep disorders.

INSOMNIA

The *DSM-IV* defines four subtypes of insomnia: primary insomnia, insomnia related to another mental disorder, insomnia due to a general medical condition, and substance-induced insomnia. For each of these subtypes, insomnia is defined as difficulty initiating or maintaining sleep or nonrestorative sleep that has persisted for at least one month. The diagnosis of insomnia also requires that the sleep disturbance is not created by another sleep disorder such as narcolepsy or sleep apnea, and there must also be a report of significant distress in social, occupational, or other areas of functioning.

Primary insomnia refers to insomnia that is not produced by another mental disorder, a general medical condition, or the physiological effects of a substance (e.g., alcohol). Primary insomnia may initially be produced by a psychological or medical stressor, but the insomnia persists after the stressor has been removed. For example, upon retirement, an older adult could experience a brief period of depression that precipitates insomnia. After the depression resolves, insomnia could persist because of negative sleep associations and habits formed during the depressive episode (e.g., excessive worry about getting enough sleep, conditioned arousal in response to the bedroom, too much time spent in bed). In other cases, it is difficult to identify any stressor that precipitated primary insomnia.

The remaining types of insomnia are often collectively referred to as "secondary insomnia." If the insomnia appears to be produced and maintained by an Axis I or Axis II diagnosis, it falls under the category insomnia related to another mental disorder. Insomnia due to a general medical condition and substance-induced insomnia refer to sleep disturbance that is precipitated and sustained by a medical disorder or substance. Table 12.1 lists some common causes and examples of secondary insomnia (see Kryger, Roth, & Dement,

Table 12.1 Causes of secondary insomnia.

Medical Disorders
    Cardiovascular disease (e.g., congestive heart failure, hypertension).
    Cerebrovascular disease.
    Chronic pain (e.g., caused by arthritis, cancer, fibromyalgia).
    Endocrine disorders (e.g., hyperthyroidism).
    Gastrointestinal disorders (e.g., peptic ulcer disease).
    Neurological disorders (e.g., Alzheimer's disease, parkinsonism).
    Nocturia.
    Renal disease.
    Respiratory disease (e.g., asthma, COPD).

Psychiatric Disorders
    Adjustment disorders.
    Anxiety disorders (e.g., generalized anxiety disorder, panic disorder).
    Mood disorders (e.g., major depressive disorder).
    Somatoform disorders.

Substances
    Corticosteroids.
    Hypertension medication.
    Opioids.
    Serotonergic agonists and antagonists.
    Stimulants: amphetamines, caffeine, cocaine, nicotine.

1994, for an extensive review). Many medical disorders cause frequent awakenings during the night, and any medical problem causing pain or discomfort can create sleep initiation and/or maintenance difficulties (Aldrich, 1993; Bradley, 1993; Gottlieb, 1990; Moran & Stoudemire, 1992; Wittig, Zorick, Blumer, Heilbronn, & Roth, 1982). Pain may also increase time in bed and daytime napping, thereby fragmenting the circadian sleep/wake cycle (Prinz, Vitiello, Raskind, & Thorpy, 1990).

The incidence of insomnia in anxiety and mood disorders is high; insomnia secondary to psychiatric disorder is the most frequent clinical diagnosis of insomnia patients (Buysse et al., 1994). People with depression typically complain of early morning awakening with an inability to return to sleep (terminal insomnia). Sleep onset and sleep maintenance difficulties are common in anxiety disorders. People with insomnia secondary to an anxiety or mood disorder also complain of daytime tiredness and fatigue (Walsh, Moss, & Sugerman, 1994).

Certain drugs can produce insomnia (Engle-Friedman & Bootzin, 1991; Monane, 1992). Amphetamines, cocaine, caffeine, nicotine, and over-the-counter medications with stimulant properties can disrupt sleep patterns. Alcohol causes lighter sleep and frequent awakenings. Diuretics can cause nocturia, especially when taken near bedtime.

Older adults may be particularly susceptible to secondary insomnia for a number of reasons. Age-related sleep changes predisposing individuals toward lighter sleep may increase the vulnerability to sleep disruption by the influence of illness or drugs (Becker & Jamieson, 1992). Not only are older adults more vulnerable to the effects of illness, but they are also at increased risk for chronic illness. High rates of polypharmacy in older adults also contribute to secondary insomnia. In 1991, 5 of the top 10 drugs prescribed in the elderly had side effects related to insomnia (Becker & Jamieson, 1992). Finally, psychosocial factors in the elderly, such as retirement, bereavement, loneliness, and hospitalization, can increase anxiety, depression, and insomnia.

Insomnia, medical illness, and psychological factors are complexly related. Chronic illnesses create psychological stress that may contribute to secondary insomnia. Pilowsky, Crettenden, and Townley (1985) found chronic pain patients with sleep disruption were more psychologically distressed than pain patients without sleep problems. Behaviors created by the primary disorder (e.g., bedrest, daytime napping) may perpetuate insomnia (Morin, Kowatch, & Wade, 1989). Alternatively, secondary insomnia may negatively impact medical or psychiatric disorders. For example, sleep disruption due to chronic pain may in turn exacerbate perceived pain levels (Wittig et al., 1982). Finally, secondary insomnia may acquire partially independent status and may be sustained by factors unrelated to the primary illness, such as learned behaviors.

The *DSM-IV* insomnia subtypes are based on the perceived cause of the insomnia rather than the pattern of sleep disturbance. However, in clinical practice and research, the following terms are commonly used to further define the type of sleep disturbance being experienced: initial (sleep onset difficulty), maintenance (awakenings during the night), terminal (early morning awakening), and mixed (some combination of the preceding problems) insomnia. The *DSM-IV* does not provide quantitative criteria regarding the severity of sleep disturbance that is required for a diagnosis of insomnia. Common practice in research and clinical settings is to require a sleep-onset latency or middle-of-the-night awake time greater than 30 minutes at least three times per week for a diagnosis of insomnia. These criteria were established in early studies that focused on young and middle-aged adults, and they may be too liberal for an older population that generally experiences greater sleep disruption than do younger adults. Ultimately, insomnia is a diagnosis that is heavily influenced by the subjective sleep perception of the patient. In fact, researchers have sometimes found no significant difference between the sleep of older adults who do and do not complain of insomnia (Fichten et al., 1995; Lichstein & Johnson, 1991).

DIFFERENTIAL DIAGNOSIS OF INSOMNIA AND OTHER SLEEP DISORDERS

For older adults presenting with an insomnia complaint, it is important to rule out obstructive sleep apnea, a sleep disorder that may mimic insomnia but requires a different treatment approach. Obstructive sleep apnea consists of multiple episodes of complete (apnea) or partial (hypopnea) upper airway obstruction during sleep, and it is substantially more prevalent in older adults than in younger populations (Ancoli-Israel et al., 1991b). Although sleep apnea patients and insomnia patients may self-report similar symptoms (e.g., nighttime sleep fragmentation, elevated daytime fatigue), different treatment approaches are indicated for the two disorders. Cognitive-behavioral approaches that improve insomnia would not be expected to reverse upper airway obstruction, and pharmacological agents used to treat insomnia may worsen sleep apnea (Saskin, 1997). Sleep apnea is typically treated through surgery or continuous positive airway pressure (CPAP). The CPAP machine delivers a stream of air into a nasal mask worn during sleep. The positive pressure created by this process acts as a splint that keeps the pharyngeal airway open and thus prevents apneas and hypopneas (see Kryger et al., 1994, and Saskin, 1997, for further information on treatment of sleep apnea).

A definitive diagnosis of OSA requires an overnight sleep study, termed polysomnography (PSG). Standard PSG consists of monitoring EEG (brain activity), EOG (eye movement), and EMG (muscle tension) channels. In addition, respiration, blood oxygenation, and limb movements are assessed. The role of PSG in differential diagnosis of insomnia and OSA is debatable based on current evidence. Some studies suggest that a clinical interview is sufficient for insomnia diagnosis, whereas other investigations indicate that PSG may alter initial clinical impressions. Kales et al. (1982) conducted PSG on 200 consecutive individuals of varied ages referred for insomnia and found no cases of clinically significant apnea. Similarly, Vgontzas, Kales, Bixler, Manfredi, and Vela-Bueno (1995) compared patients presenting with insomnia and noncomplaining sleepers and found that only 2.3% of the insomnia patients and 1.3% of the noncomplaining sleepers had sleep apnea based on PSG. These results suggested that PSG would be unlikely to alter an initial diagnosis of insomnia. A recent review article concludes that PSG should not be used routinely for evaluation of chronic insomnia (Reite, Buysse, Reynolds, & Mendelson, 1995). However, the authors concluded that PSG is more likely to be useful for older adults and should be considered when there are strong clinical indicators of apnea or after a patient has failed to progress in a comprehensive insomnia treatment program.

Other studies have suggested a need for PSG screening, especially for older adults. In a sample of 100 people presenting with insomnia, Edinger et al. (1989) found that apnea and another sleep disorder, periodic limb movements during sleep (PLMS), were more likely to be found by PSG among older individuals (> 40 years). Only one of three apnea cases was suspected by clinical interview, and the interview produced seven false positive diagnoses of apnea. Vgontzas et al. (1995) also found that the rate of apnea in patients presenting with insomnia increased with age.

Particularly high rates of occult (i.e., not detected by self-report) sleep disorders among older adults reporting insomnia have been found among recruited insomnia volunteers. Through PSG screening, Morin, Kowatch, Barry, and Walton (1993) found apnea or periodic limb movements during sleep in 14 (35%) of 40 older adults reporting chronic insomnia. In another sample of 80 older individuals complaining of insomnia, PSG revealed occult apnea in 23 (29%) individuals (Lichstein, Riedel, Lester, & Aguillard, 1999). Males made up 40% of the total sample, but 70% of the apnea cases were male, suggesting that PSG screening is especially important in older males reporting insomnia (Lichstein, Riedel, et al., 1999).

Several studies have attempted to identify clinical predictors of apnea. Increased age, a higher body mass index, male gender, and self- or bed partner report of snoring or breathing difficulty have been identified as significant predictors of apnea in multiple studies (Bliwise et al., 1987; Edinger et al., 1989; Flemons, Remmers, Whitelaw, & Brant, 1993; Hoffstein & Szalai, 1993; Kapuniai, Andrew, Crowell, & Pearce, 1988). Other clinical features that may be associated with apnea include hypertension (Flemons et al., 1993), nocturia (Pressman, Figueroa, Kendrick-Mohamed, Greenspon, & Peterson, 1996), and dry mouth upon awakening (Lichstein, Riedel, et al., 1999). However, with the exception of bed partner observation of apnea, significant clinical predictors have explained only a small proportion of variance in the dependent variable (apnea presence or severity).

There is also a higher prevalence of PLMS in older adults (Ancoli-Israel et al., 1991a). Periodic limb movements during sleep (also called nocturnal myoclonus) involves fragmented sleep produced by repetitive limb movements. Periodic limb movements during sleep is sometimes accompanied by restless legs syndrome, which is characterized by uncomfortable, "crawling" sensations in the legs that interfere with sleep onset. Distinguishing between insomnia and periodic limb movements during sleep may be less crucial than ruling out sleep apnea. The same class of pharmacological agents (benzodiazepines) is often prescribed for periodic limb movements during sleep and insomnia. Also, results from a preliminary study suggested that cognitive-behavioral treatments used for insomnia may also result in subjective sleep improvement for PLMS patients (Edinger et al., 1996).

EPIDEMIOLOGY

Insomnia in older adults is more common and more troublesome than in younger people. Insomnia prevalence in older people exceeds 25% (Bixler, Kales, Soldatos, Kales, & Healey, 1979; Mellinger, Balter, & Uhlenhuth, 1985), and these same surveys found a 30% to 50% higher rate than in younger samples. As with younger adults, among older adults with insomnia, the disorder is more common in women than in men, with a ratio approximating 1.5 to 1. Older adults with insomnia are more likely to have medical illness, physical disability, and elevated anxiety or depression compared to older adults not complaining of insomnia (Bixler et al., 1979; Foley et al., 1995; Mellinger et al., 1985). Older adults with insomnia turn to sleep medication at a disproportionately high rate, risking addiction, polypharmacy interactions, exacerbation of sleep apnea, and multiple other side effects (Mellinger & Balter, 1981; Roth, Zorick, Wittig, & Roehrs, 1982).

Clinical experience indicates that among people with insomnia (PWI), onset insomnia is the modal symptom of middle-aged patients, but maintenance and mixed insomnia are more common among older adults, though there are only modest epidemiological data to document these relationships (Bixler et al., 1979;

Foley et al., 1995). Because the prevalence of medical and psychiatric disorders increases with age, it is not surprising that secondary insomnia is more common than primary insomnia in older adults (Moran, Thompson, & Nies, 1988).

Complaints of insomnia clearly increase with age. Some increase in insomnia complaints could stem from natural age-related changes in sleep pattern and architecture, such as increased awake time and decreased deep sleep (stages 3 and 4). Such changes are not always accompanied by complaints of insomnia or daytime dysfunction, leading some to hypothesize that many sleep changes experienced by older adults represent a normal developmental process rather than pathology.

RELEVANT THEORIES

AROUSAL THEORIES

One hypothesis is that insomnia is produced by excessive physiological arousal. Several studies have documented greater physiological arousal at night in PWI than in people not reporting insomnia (PNI; e.g., Freedman, 1986; Monroe, 1967). Some researchers have proposed that PWI suffer from a 24-hour chronic hyperarousal disorder (Bonnet & Arand, 1997). In support of this hypothesis, Bonnet and Arand (1995) found that PWI had a significantly higher 24-hour metabolic rate than did PNI. These authors propose that chronic hyperarousal could produce the nighttime symptoms of insomnia and daytime symptoms such as fatigue and anxiety. However, several studies have found no evidence of elevated daytime physiological arousal in PWI relative to PNI, including the only study of this sort to focus on older PWI and PNI (Lichstein & Johnson, 1996).

Others have proposed that excessive psychological arousal produces insomnia. Elevated anxiety in PWI relative to PNI is a common finding (e.g., Kales, Caldwell, Soldatos, Bixler, & Kales, 1983; Morin & Gramling, 1989). Also, PWI are more likely to report that excessive cognitive activity rather than somatic arousal is the source of their sleep difficulty (Lichstein & Rosenthal, 1980). Similar to physiological hyperarousal, psychological hyperarousal can also produce the nocturnal symptoms of insomnia and the accompanying daytime dysfunction. In reality, it is difficult to separate physiological arousal from psychological arousal. Anxiety can produce elevated physiological arousal, and chronic physiological arousal can contribute to increased anxiety.

Elevated arousal can emanate from several sources. For example, increased arousal can be produced by an anxiety disorder, a physical disorder such as hyperthyroidism, or a stimulant such as caffeine or nicotine. Bootzin (1972) proposed that elevated arousal in PWI could be a conditioned response to their bedroom or other stimuli associated with attempting to sleep. For example, after a few nights of poor sleep, the bedroom may become associated with being awake and any arousing emotions that accompany sleep difficulty (e.g., frustration, anxiety). Also, the bedroom may become associated with arousal rather than sleep if a person habitually engages in a number of sleep-incompatible activities in the bedroom (e.g., watching television, talking on the phone). Eventually, increased arousal and awake time may become a conditioned response to the bedroom, resulting in chronic insomnia. Bootzin's hypothesis inspired the stimulus control approach to insomnia treatment described below.

Insomnoid Theory

Another possibility is that many insomnia complaints in older adults result from a misperception of sleep needs. An insomnoid state is characterized by a disrupted nighttime sleep pattern but no evidence of significant daytime impairment, suggesting that sleep needs are being met (Lichstein, 1988b). Older adults are at particularly high risk for insomnoid states. Age-correlated deterioration in sleep architecture and pattern creates a normal sleep pattern among older adults that mimics key characteristics of middle-aged insomnia. The typical sleep changes associated with individuals past 60 years of age include an increase in light sleep (sleep stages 1 and 2), a sharp decline in deep sleep (stages 3 and 4, or at least a suppression of its characteristic delta wave), increased sleep fragmentation, and decreased total sleep time (Bliwise, 1993; Miles & Dement, 1980; Morgan, 1987; Williams, Karacan, & Hursch, 1974). As we demonstrated in the case study above, these nocturnal sleep changes are not necessarily accompanied by daytime dysfunction, suggesting the possibility of decreased sleep need in many older adults. Older individuals uninformed as to normal age-related sleep changes and motivated to preserve a middle-aged sleep pattern are destined to extend time in bed in search of elusive sleep. However, increasing time in bed typically increases awake time rather than sleep time, resulting in a fragmented, unsatisfying sleep experience.

The idea that sleep need decreases with age is controversial. Bliwise (1993) carefully reviewed studies providing information on sleep need and aging and found no clear-cut answer to the question of whether sleep need decreases with age. A number of studies suggested reduced sleep need in older adults, but several studies did not. However, clinical experience and studies finding reduced sleep need suggest that there is at least a substantial subset of older adults who experience a decreased sleep need. Education regarding age-related sleep changes and approaches as sleep restriction and sleep compression that reduce time in bed may be especially helpful for these individuals.

TREATMENT

Description of Psychological Treatments

Relaxation
Progressive relaxation is the most widely researched treatment for insomnia (Lichstein & Fischer, 1985); it involves sequentially tensing and relaxing the

body's major muscle groups while concentrating on and contrasting somatic sensations of tension and relaxation. About 16 muscle groups are tensed and released, and significantly less time is spent tensing muscles (about 7 seconds) in comparison to the relaxation phase (45 seconds).

A class of passive relaxation procedures includes progressive relaxation without the tense phase (just passive body focusing), autogenic phrases (focusing on relaxing sensations in the body), and guided imagery (dwelling on peaceful nature scenes). The literature suggests that passive relaxation techniques are more effective for older adults with insomnia than progressive relaxation, possibly because they are less physically demanding and procedurally simpler (for more detailed descriptions of relaxation procedures, see Lichstein, 1988a, 2000).

Stimulus Control

Stimulus control emerged from the belief that some insomnia may be due to the bedroom becoming a poor discriminative stimulus for sleep. The noncomplaining sleeper associates the bedroom with rapid sleep onset, but the bedroom may elicit a wakeful response in PWI. With this philosophy in mind, the following six instructions are given to the patient:

1. Do not use your bed or bedroom for anything but sleep (or sex).
2. Go to bed only when sleepy.
3. If you do not fall asleep within about 15 to 20 minutes, leave the bed and do something in another room. Go back to bed only when you feel sleepy again.
4. If you do not fall asleep quickly on returning to bed, repeat instruction 3 as many times as is necessary. Also, if you do not fall asleep rapidly after an awakening, follow instruction 3 again.
5. Use your alarm to leave bed at the same time every morning.
6. Do not nap.

Within a few weeks, the arousal response to the bedtime environment should be eliminated and replaced with a sleep-compatible response. Stimulus control may be particularly well-suited for older adults with insomnia, as the method has been shown to be effective for maintenance insomnia (Morin & Azrin, 1987, 1988; Turner & Ascher, 1979; further description of the methods of stimulus control is available in Bootzin and Epstein, 2000).

Sleep Restriction and Sleep Compression Therapies

Sleep restriction and sleep compression were developed based on the hypothesis that excessive time in bed perpetuates insomnia. Sleep restriction therapy consists of the following steps (Spielman, Saskin, & Thorpy, 1987):

1. The total subjective sleep time is calculated from two weeks of baseline sleep diaries.
2. The initial time in bed is restricted to this average total sleep time, with a minimum time in bed set at 4.5 hours. Napping is prohibited.

3. Patients choose fixed times to enter and leave bed. A consistent awakening time is emphasized.

4. When mean sleep efficiency (total sleep time / time in bed × 100) over five days is ≥ 90%, a patient's time in bed is increased by 15 minutes. Five days of unaltered sleep schedule always follow a time in bed increase.

5. If sleep efficiency drops below an average of 85% over five days, time in bed is reduced to the mean total sleep time for those five days. No curtailment of total sleep time occurs during the first 10 days of treatment or for 10 days following a sleep schedule change.

6. If mean sleep efficiency falls between 85% and 90% during a five-day period, a patient's sleep schedule remains constant.

Sleep compression differs from sleep restriction in that the former does not immediately reduce time in bed to the baseline total sleep time average. Instead, the patient's time in bed is reduced in stages by delaying the time entering bed and advancing morning arising time. For example, if baseline time in bed exceeds total sleep time by two hours, time in bed will be reduced by one-half hour a week for four weeks.

Most of the clinical trials of sleep restriction and sleep compression have been conducted with older adults with good success. The rationale for their use is consistent with the concept of insomnoid states described above. Like the patient described in the case study above, some individuals will not be willing to strictly adhere to time in bed recommendations. To avoid unnecessary treatment dropouts, clinicals should allow for patient input when designing a sleep schedule. (Further description of the methods of sleep restriction and sleep compression is available in Wohlgemuth and Edinger, 2000.)

Cognitive-Behavior Therapy

CBT encompasses a variety of methods, and the composition of a given CBT regimen will vary across studies. Defined narrowly, CBT refers to methods of cognitive therapy such as rational emotive behavior therapy and Beck's approach to cognitive therapy of depression. In its application to insomnia treatment, CBT is used to alleviate insomnia-causing anxiety that arises from undue worrying and exaggerated fears related to sleep. At other times, the term CBT refers to a broader array of interventions for insomnia that may include cognitive therapy as well as relaxation, sleep education, stimulus control, sleep restriction, and the like. (Further description of the methods of CBT for insomnia is available in Morin, Savard, and Blais, 2000.)

Sleep Education and Sleep Hygiene

The terms sleep education and sleep hygiene are often used interchangeably. When distinctions exist, sleep education refers to didactic presentations about normal sleep patterns. This may have particular salience for older adults reporting insomnia who may misinterpret normal, developmental sleep changes. Sleep hygiene refers to the collection of daytime activities that may impact sleep, such as napping, caffeine consumption, nicotine use, and exercise. It is uncommon to employ sleep education/hygiene as a solitary intervention. More typically, it is administered with a featured intervention to eliminate nuisance factors disrupting sleep. However, as was demonstrated in the case study above, addressing sleep hygiene issues can be an essential component of treatment. (Further description of the methods of sleep hygiene is available in Riedel, 2000.)

PSYCHOLOGICAL TREATMENT OUTCOME

Primary Insomnia

Although the traditional approach to treating insomnia has been pharmacological, effective and safe behavioral and cognitive treatments have emerged over the past three decades. Psychological treatments for insomnia avoid problems common to drug therapies such as tolerance, dependence, and side effects. Since the mid-1980s, attention has shifted toward exploring the effectiveness of these interventions with older adult populations. This focus on treating insomnia in older adults is important for two reasons. First, older adults are more likely than younger adults to experience insomnia, possibly as a result of age-related sleep changes. Second, older adults are particularly susceptible to the detrimental effects of sleep medications (Engle-Friedman & Bootzin, 1991). Metabolic changes as adults age cause increased drug sensitivity. Older adults are also likely to be taking multiple medications, which increases vulnerability to drug interaction effects. The section below on pharmacological treatment explores medication issues in greater detail. Here, we review the effects of psychological treatments on sleep and daytime functioning variables in older adults with primary insomnia.

Early studies using mixed-age samples found that older adults treated with progressive relaxation or passive relaxation (e.g., autogenic training) techniques had less improvement in sleep-onset latency (time to fall asleep) than younger adults (Lick & Heffler, 1977; Nicassio & Bootzin, 1974). Subsequent studies with older adults found progressive relaxation at least moderately effective in decreasing sleep-onset latency, wake time after sleep onset, and number of nightly awakenings (Bliwise, Friedman, Nekich, & Yesavage, 1995; Friedman, Bliwise, Yesavage, & Salom, 1991; Johnson, 1993).

Passive relaxation techniques for geriatric insomnia have been investigated in two published studies. Morin and Azrin (1988) used imagery training to treat sleep maintenance insomnia in eight older adults. After treatment, nighttime awakenings were less frequent and of shorter duration. Additionally, treated participants reduced sleep-onset latency and increased total sleep time, and these sleep gains were maintained at one-year follow-up. Lichstein and Johnson (1993) found passive relaxation reduced number of awakenings and decreased wake time after sleep onset in a sample of older women with insomnia. Overall, it appears that passive forms of relaxation are more effective than progressive relaxation for older adults with insomnia.

Insomnia treatment with stimulus control procedures also has been investigated in older adults. This treatment effectively decreased sleep-onset latency in older adults with sleep-onset insomnia (Puder, Lacks, Bertelson, & Storandt, 1983). Older adults experiencing sleep maintenance insomnia treated with stimulus control or a modified version (countercontrol treatment) experienced increased total sleep time, reduced wake time after sleep onset, and decreased number of awakenings at posttreatment and at one-year follow-up (Davies, Lacks, Storandt, & Bertelson, 1986; Morin & Azrin, 1988).

Sleep restriction also appears to be an effective treatment for older adults with insomnia. Restricting time in bed may be particularly beneficial to older adults because it directly addresses the issue of insomnoid states. Some older adults simply may be staying in bed too long which produces unnecessary awake time.

Ten studies have employed sleep restriction or sleep compression with older adults with insomnia, though five of these comprised package treatments that obscure appraisal of individual treatments (Edinger, Hoelscher, Marsh, Lipper, & Ionescu-Pioggia, 1992; Hoelscher & Edinger, 1988; Morin, Colecchi, Ling, & Sood, 1995; Morin, Colecchi, Stone, Sood, & Brink, 1999; Morin, et al., 1993), and one of these five focused on PWI who were using sleep medication (Morin et al., 1995). Three studies focused nearly exclusively on sleep restriction or sleep compression, and all observed positive treatment effects. Lichstein (1988b) presented a case study of a 59-year-old man who had suffered crippling insomnia most of his life, and Brooks, Friedman, Bliwise, and Yesavage (1993) treated a group of nine older adults with insomnia. Riedel, Lichstein, and Dwyer (1995) conducted a randomized trial comparing sleep education/sleep compression delivered by a self-help video to sleep education/sleep compression provided by a therapist. The video alone improved sleep, but not as much as the video plus therapist intervention. Two studies compared sleep restriction and progressive relaxation. Friedman et al. (1991) found that older adults in both treatment groups experienced reduced sleep-onset latency and wake time after sleep at posttreatment and increased total sleep time at three-month follow-up. Furthermore, the sleep restriction group demonstrated improvements in sleep efficiency not experienced in the progressive relaxation group. The researchers estimate that overall improvement in the sleep restriction group was approximately twice as much as in the progressive relaxation group. Bliwise et al. (1995) also found both sleep restriction and progressive relaxation groups improved sleep-onset latency after treatment. At three-month follow-up, the sleep restriction group demonstrated significant gains in total sleep time compared to the progressive relaxation group. These studies suggest a treatment advantage of sleep restriction over progressive relaxation in older adults.

In an attempt to maximize outcomes, some researchers have tested treatment combinations for older adults with insomnia. In a study combining self-administered relaxation and stimulus control treatments for insomnia, older adults reported improvement in total sleep time but not on sleep-onset latency, number of awakenings, or sleep quality (Alperson & Biglan, 1979). Hoelscher and Edinger (1988) developed a CBT to target sleep maintenance insomnia. This treatment package combines stimulus control, sleep restriction, and sleep education. Two studies investigating this CBT package in small samples of older adults have found it to be effective in reducing wake time after sleep onset, decreasing time spent in bed, and improving sleep efficiency (Edinger et al., 1992; Hoelscher & Edinger, 1988). A similar CBT package provided to older adults with insomnia yielded comparable results (Morin et al., 1993). Engle-Friedman, Bootzin, Hazlewood, and Tsao (1992) compared groups receiving support and sleep hygiene by itself or combined with progressive relaxation or stimulus control against a sleep education control group. All groups, including the control group, reported sleep improvements such as reduced number of awakenings. The stimulus control group reported the shortest sleep latencies and experienced the most treatment gains at the two-year follow-up.

Despite the importance of daytime functioning in insomnia, few outcome studies have included these measures. Thus, results for older adults with primary insomnia should be considered preliminary. In one study, posttreatment questionnaires completed by stimulus control participants suggested improved daytime functioning in some areas (Morin & Azrin, 1988). These findings were corroborated by ratings from significant others. However, measures of depression and anxiety did not change after treatment. Studies of relaxation therapy for late-life insomnia have failed to decrease time spent napping (Lichstein & Johnson, 1993) or improve levels of feeling refreshed on awakening (Johnson, 1993).

Most daytime functioning data for older adults with insomnia have come from studies exploring combination treatments. Preliminary studies of CBT for insomnia suggest an improvement in mood ratings following treatment (Hoelscher & Edinger, 1988; Morin et al., 1993). Cognitive-behavioral studies also reveal trends toward decreased subjective sleepiness levels (Hoelscher & Edinger, 1988) and decreased nap time three months after treatment (Edinger et al., 1992). In the Morin et al. (1993) study, participants in the CBT group and their significant others rated sleep problems as less severe, less noticeable, and less interfering after treatment compared to the control group. These perceptions of improvement remained at thee months. Similarly, in another study, CBT participants reported significantly less daytime functioning interference from sleep problems at posttreatment than a group of placebo participants (Morin et al., 1999).

Similar daytime functioning results were assessed in the Engle-Friedman et al. (1992) study discussed previously. Feeling refreshed on awakening improved for the treatment groups. For all groups, nap time and depression levels decreased. At the end of the study, participants were less concerned about their sleep and felt they had more control over their ability to fall asleep.

In summary, there is a growing literature on the psychological treatment of primary insomnia in older adults. Results so far have been very encouraging, but there are some methodological issues that require attention. One issue is the lack of adequate control groups. Only seven studies included a no-treatment control group (Alperson & Biglan, 1979; Davies et al., 1986; Engle-Friedman et al., 1992; Morin & Azrin, 1988; Morin et al., 1993; Puder et al., 1983; Riedel et al., 1995). Furthermore, only one study focusing on older adults employed a placebo treatment group to investigate the influence of nonspecific treatment effects (Morin et al., 1999).

Most of the studies reviewed above relied on self-report data for screening and classification of participants and therefore, cannot definitively rule out occult sleep apnea and periodic limb movement disorder. Without objective verification of primary insomnia by PSG, the homogeneity of participants cannot be established. Inadequate screening for other sleep disorders may bias outcomes by attenuating treatment effects. Although most of the reviewed studies screened participants for symptoms of other sleep disorders via questionnaire or interview, only three investigations confirmed diagnoses with PSG (Edinger et al., 1992; Morin et al., 1993, 1999).

Subjective measures of sleep were used as dependent variables in all studies. Typically, participants recorded perceptions of their prior night's sleep in a sleep diary kept over a specified time period. Only three studies used PSG to measure objectively treatment outcome. In the Engle-Friedman et al. (1992) study, 55% of participants underwent PSG before and after treatment. PSG did not detect significant changes in sleep and thus did not confirm improvements measured subjectively. Two studies (Morin et al., 1993, 1999) found significant improvements on PSG sleep measures at posttreatment, although the magnitude of improvement was less than that from sleep diaries. These studies suggest that psychological treatments are more effective in altering subjective perceptions of sleep than objective sleep.

SECONDARY INSOMNIA

Treatment for secondary insomnia traditionally has focused on treating the primary disorder. A common assumption is that interventions targeting insomnia will be unsuccessful as long as the primary disorder remains untreated. Although primary and secondary insomnia have been treated differently, the two disorders may share important characteristics. One study compared people with primary and secondary insomnia and found that the two groups did not differ significantly on most self-reported sleep variables (Lichstein & Durrence, 1999). Given the effectiveness of psychological interventions in treating primary insomnia, such interventions may be successful in the treatment of secondary insomnia. Furthermore, treating the complaint of insomnia may facilitate treatment of the primary disorder by alleviating exacerbating factors and symptoms.

Very few studies have addressed the insomnia component associated with primary illnesses. In one case study, relaxation techniques combined with stimulus control procedures improved sleep and reduced tension in a person with severe hemophilia and insomnia (Varni, 1980). Relaxation techniques in cancer patients with insomnia have successfully reduced sleep-onset latency (Cannici, Malcolm, & Peek, 1983; Stam & Bultz, 1986). Morin et al. (1989) treated insomnia secondary to chronic pain with sleep restriction and stimulus control. Patients demonstrated improvements in sleep-onset latency, wake time after sleep onset, and early morning awakenings after treatment and at six-month follow-up. Additionally, these patients reported less depression, anxiety, and fatigue posttreatment.

Two studies of psychological treatment of secondary insomnia have focused on older adults. De Berry (1981–1982) randomly assigned older female widows to a progressive relaxation or control group. Although the participants were selected because they reported stress symptoms such as anxiety and insomnia, they were not clinically diagnosed with an anxiety disorder. Results showed that treated women decreased sleep-onset latency and number of awakenings compared to the control group. The treatment group also reported fewer headaches, less tension, and lower state anxiety after treatment. In a randomized study of older adults with secondary insomnia given a treatment package of passive relaxation, stimulus control, and sleep hygiene, treated participants showed significantly greater improvement on wake time during the night, sleep efficiency percentage, and sleep quality rating than the control group (Lichstein, Wilson, & Johnson, in press). These studies support the idea that sleep complaints and impaired daytime functioning related to secondary insomnia in older adults is amenable to psychological treatment.

PHARMACOLOGICAL TREATMENT

Use of sleep medication, sometimes referred to as hypnotics, is disproportionately high among older adults, and benzodiazepines and zolpidem (a benzodiazepine receptor agonist) are the most frequently employed agents (Walsh & Schweitzer, 1999). Grad (1995) reviewed 10 studies of the efficacy of outpatient benzodiazepine treatment of older adults with insomnia. In general, short-term results were positive, with benzodiazepines decreasing sleep latency by about 30 minutes, increasing total sleep time by about an hour, and reducing number of awakenings. The longest treatment period was four weeks. A more recent study (Morin et al., 1999) compared four treatment conditions: benzodiazepine (temazepam), CBT, benzodiazepine treatment combined with CBT, and placebo. After an eight-week treatment period, participants in all three active treatments reported significantly lower wake time after sleep onset than the placebo group. Although this study conducted a long-term follow-up, the efficacy of long-term benzodiazepine use cannot be determined. Participants were tapered off the benzodiazepine after the treatment period, and only half of the benzodiazepine group and less than half of the combined treatment participants were using sleep medication at one-year follow-up (Morin et al., 1999).

The absence of long-term assessment of benzodiazepine efficacy is problematic because studies with younger adults suggest that tolerance can begin to develop after only a few weeks of continuous use (Gillin & Byerley, 1990; Parrino & Terzano, 1996). Higher dosages encouraged by increasing drug tolerance are associated with a greater frequency of adverse side effects (Gillin & Byerley, 1990), and withdrawal from benzodiazepines may produce rebound (intensification of) insomnia and increased anxiety, particularly with the popular short half-life drugs (Kales, Soldatos, Bixler, & Kales, 1983). Withdrawal effects may encourage chronic use of hypnotics despite their loss of efficacy. Hypnotic-dependent insomnia refers to a state in which a person chronically uses sleep medication and becomes dependent on the medication, but still experiences substantial sleep disruption (American Sleep Disorders Association, 1990).

Other problems are associated with chronic benzodiazepine use. Unsuspected apnea in older adults may be exacerbated by benzodiazepine use. Benzodiazepines may interfere with memory and psychomotor functioning (Roehrs, Merlotti, Zorick, & Roth, 1994). The rate of hospitalization for automobile accident injuries is higher in older adults who use benzodiazepine hypnotics compared to matched nonusers (Neutel, 1995). Sleep medication use increases the risk of polypharmacy effects in older adults already taking multiple medications, and metabolic changes associated with aging slow down elimination of hypnotic agents. Ray, Griffin, and Downey (1989) found that older adults using long half-life benzodiazepines have a significantly higher rate of hip fractures than nonusers. Other researchers observed a higher risk of femur fractures due to falls in older benzodiazepine users, but increased risk was more dependent on a higher dosage rather than a longer half-life (Herings, Stricker, de Boer, Bakker, & Sturmans, 1995). Because of potential problems associated with benzodiazepines, these medications are recommended for treatment of short-term rather than chronic insomnia.

Among the nonbenzodiazepine hypnotic alternatives, zolpidem appears to be the most promising. In contrast to benzodiazepines, zolpidem does not suppress stages 3 and 4 sleep and is not likely to produce rebound insomnia (Parrino & Terzano, 1996). Zolpidem may produce psychomotor and memory deficits comparable to deficits produced by benzodiazepines (Roehrs et al., 1994). Melatonin, a hormone secreted by the pineal gland, has received attention for its hypnotic effects. In a sample of melatonin-deficient older adults with insomnia, Haimov et al. (1995) found that a sustained-release melatonin formula improved sleep efficiency and a fast-release version improved sleep latency during one-week treatment periods. However, the long-term efficacy of zolpidem or melatonin therapy for insomnia has not been established.

SUBSTITUTING PSYCHOLOGICAL TREATMENTS FOR SLEEP MEDICATION

Psychological treatments for nonmedicated PWI produce long-term maintenance of initial treatment gains without the risk of pharmacological side effects (Morin, Culbert, & Schwartz, 1994). Most studies of psychological treatment for chronic insomnia have excluded PWI using hypnotics and thereby ignored the problem of hypnotic-dependent insomnia. A few studies have included hypnotically medicated and nonmedicated PWI without offering a specific, therapist-supervised medication withdrawal program (Lichstein & Johnson, 1993; Morawetz, 1989; Morin & Azrin, 1988; Spielman et al., 1987). In general, medicated PWI experienced modest sleep improvement, whereas nonmedicated PWI showed more substantial treatment progress. Two of these studies concentrated on older adults with insomnia (Lichstein & Johnson, 1993; Morin & Azrin, 1988). Lichstein and Johnson treated hypnotically medicated and hypnotic-free older adults with passive relaxation. Hypnotically medicated participants reduced hypnotic use by 47% from baseline to six-week follow-up. For the hypnotically medicated group, sleep variables at follow-up remained at baseline levels or were slightly improved. The hypnotic-free group showed greater sleep improvement than the hypnotically medicated group at follow-up. Morin and Azrin compared stimulus control with imagery training in a group of hypnotically medicated and nonmedicated older adults with insomnia. Hypnotic use was reduced in both treatment groups at posttreatment, but this reduction was not maintained at follow-up. Regardless of treatment condition, nonmedicated older adults with insomnia exhibited a better treatment response.

Six studies have combined a supervised hypnotic withdrawal program with psychological treatments for insomnia (Espie, Lindsay, & Brooks, 1988; Kirmil-Gray, Eagleston, Thoresen, & Zarcone, 1985; Lichstein, Peterson, et al., 1999; Morin et al., 1995; Morin, Stone, McDonald, & Jones, 1994; Riedel et al., 1998). Reduction of medication use was substantial in each study. In the majority of these studies, a few sleep variables improved significantly, and most sleep variables remained at baseline levels after psychological treatment and medication reduction.

One of these studies focused on older adults (Morin et al., 1995). Morin's study added two methodological improvements over most previous studies of CBT for medicated PWI. PSG was included in addition to sleep diaries, and urine screens were used to verify self-reported medication use. Five chronic users of benzodiazepines as hypnotics received an individualized medication-tapering schedule and CBT that included cognitive therapy, stimulus control, sleep restriction, progressive relaxation, and sleep education. All participants substantially reduced hypnotic consumption. Four individuals were hypnotic-free at posttreatment and three participants were hypnotic-free at three-month follow-up. PSG immediately after medication reduction/treatment indicated moderate sleep deterioration from baseline (e.g., sleep efficiency dropped 6%). By three-month follow-up, sleep efficiency had returned to its baseline level. A weakness of the study was the absence of a control group that received medication withdrawal only. Such a design would allow for distinction of sleep effects due to CBT versus medication withdrawal.

CONCLUSION

Psychological treatment of hypnotic-free older adults with insomnia can be expected to produce substantial subjective sleep improvement. Because of negative side effects and tolerance to therapeutic effects, long-term use of hypnotics for insomnia is not recommended. More research is needed on the psychological treatment of insomnia in older adults who use hypnotics. Psychological treatment of older hypnotic users has resulted in only modest sleep improvement. However, psychological treatments have helped older adults with insomnia reduce sleep medication without long-term sleep deterioration. Another challenge for the future is to continue to develop and evaluate psychological treatments for secondary insomnia in older adults. Although only a few studies have examined psychological treatments for secondary insomnia, preliminary results with this population have been encouraging.

STUDY QUESTIONS

1. Name and describe the four subtypes of insomnia defined by the *DSM-IV*. What characteristics do all of the subtypes share? How are the subtypes different?
2. What symptoms or characteristics would make you suspicious that a patient has sleep apnea rather than insomnia?
3. What are some of the typical changes in sleep that occur as a person moves from being a middle-aged adult to an older adult?
4. Contrast arousal theory with insomnoid theory. What does each theory predict about daytime functioning?
5. How does stimulus control treatment differ from sleep restriction treatment?
6. Describe different relaxation approaches and discuss their effectiveness in treating insomnia in older adults.
7. Name four behaviors that are addressed in sleep hygiene treatment.
8. Name three medical disorders and three substances that may produce secondary insomnia.
9. What are some problems associated with benzodiazepine treatment of insomnia in older adults?
10. Summarize the results of studies that have provided psychological insomnia treatments to older adults using sleep medication.

SUGGESTED READINGS

Bliwise, D.L. (1993). Sleep in normal aging and dementia. *Sleep, 16,* 40–81.

Foley, D.J., Monjan, A.A. Brown, S.L. Simonsick, E.M. Wallace, R.B., & Blazer, D.G. (1995). Sleep complaints among elderly persons: An epidemiologic study of three communities. *Sleep, 18,* 425–432.

Lichstein, K.L., & Morin, C.M. (2000). *Treatment of late-life insomnia.* Thousand Oaks, CA: Sage.

Lichstein, K.L., Riedel, B.W., Lester, K.W., & Aguillard, R.N. (1999). Occult sleep apnea in a recruited sample of older adults with insomnia. *Journal of Consulting and Clinical Psychology, 67,* 405–410.

Morin, C.M. Colecchi, C., Stone, J., Sood, R., & Brink, D. (1999). Behavorial and pharmacological therapies for late-life insomnia: A randomized controlled trial. *Journal of the American Medical Association, 281,* 991–999.

REFERENCES

Aldrich, M.S. (1993). Insomnia in neurological diseases. *Journal of Psychosomatic Research, 37*(Suppl. 1), 3–11.

Alperson, J., & Biglan, A. (1979). Self-administered treatment of sleep onset insomnia and the importance of age. *Behavior Therapy, 10,* 347–356.

American Psychiatric Association. (1994). *Diagnostic and statistical manual of mental disorders* (4th ed.). Washington, DC: Author.

American Sleep Disorders Association. (1990). *The international classification of sleep disorders: Diagnostic and coding manual.* Rochester, MN: Author.

Ancoli-Israel, S., Kripke, D.F., Klauber, M.R., Mason, W.J., Fell, R., & Kaplan, O. (1991a). Periodic limb movements in sleep in community-dwelling elderly. *Sleep, 14,* 496–500.

Ancoli-Israel, S., Kripke, D.F., Klauber, M.R., Mason, W.J., Fell, R., & Kaplan, O. (1991b). Sleep-disordered breathing in community-dwelling elderly. *Sleep, 14,* 486–495.

Becker, P.M., & Jamieson, A.O. (1992). Common sleep disorders in the elderly: Diagnosis and treatment. *Geriatrics, 47,* 41–52.

Bixler, E.O., Kales, A., Soldatos, C.R., Kales, J.D., & Healey, S. (1979). Prevalence of sleep disorders in the Los Angeles metropolitan area. *American Journal of Psychiatry, 136,* 1257–1262.

Bliwise, D.L. (1993). Sleep in normal aging and dementia. *Sleep, 16,* 40–81.

Bliwise, D.L., Feldman, D.E., Bliwise, N.G., Carskadon, M.A., Kraemer, H.C., North, C.S., Petta, D.E., Seidel, W.F., & Dement, W.C. (1987). Risk factors for sleep disordered breathing in heterogeneous geriatric populations. *Journal of the American Geriatric Society, 35,* 132–141.

Bliwise, D.L., Friedman, L., Nekich, J.C., & Yesavage, J.A. (1995). Prediction of outcome in behaviorally based insomnia treatments. *Journal of Behavior Therapy and Experimental Psychiatry, 26,* 17–23.

Bonnet, M.H., & Arand, D.L. (1995). 24-hour metabolic rate in insomniacs and matched normal sleepers. *Sleep, 18,* 581–588.

Bonnet, M.H., & Arand, D.L. (1997). Hyperarousal and insomnia. *Sleep Medicine Reviews, 1,* 97–108.

Bootzin, R.R. (1972). Stimulus control treatment for insomnia. *Proceedings of the American Psychological Association, 7,* 395–396.

Bootzin, R.R., & Epstein, D.R. (2000). Stimulus control. In K.L. Lichstein, & C.M. Morin (Eds.), *Treatment of late-life insomnia.* Thousand Oaks, CA: Sage.

Bradley, T.D. (1993). Sleep disturbances in respiratory and cardiovascular disease. *Journal of Psychosomatic Research, 37*(Suppl. 1), 13–17.

Brooks, J.O., III, Friedman, L., Bliwise, D.L., & Yesavage, J.A. (1993). Use of the wrist actigraph to study insomnia in older adults. *Sleep, 16,* 151–155.

Buysse, D.J., Reynolds, C.F., III, Kupfer, D.J., Thorpy, M.J., Bixler, E., Manfredi, R., Kales, A., Vgontzas, A., Stepanski, E., Roth, T., Hauri, P., & Mesiano, D. (1994). Clinical diagnoses in 216 insomnia patients using the International Classification of Sleep Disorders *(ICSD), DSM-IV* and *ICD-10* categories: A report from the APA/NIMH *DSM-IV* field trial. *Sleep, 17,* 630–637.

Cannici, J., Malcolm, R., & Peek, L.A. (1983). Treatment of insomnia in cancer patients using muscle relaxation training. *Journal of Behavior Therapy and Experimental Psychiatry, 14,* 251–256.

Davies, R., Lacks, P., Storandt, M., & Bertelson, A.D. (1986). Countercontrol treatment of sleep-maintenance insomnia in relation to age. *Psychology and Aging, 3,* 233–238.

De Berry, S. (1981–1982). An evaluation of progressive muscle relaxation on stress related symptoms in a geriatric population. *International Journal of Aging and Human Development, 14,* 255–269.

Edinger, J.D., Fins, A.I., Sullivan, R.J., Marsh, G.R., Dailey, D.S., & Young, M. (1996). Comparison of cognitive-behavioral therapy and clonazepam for treating periodic limb movement disorder. *Sleep, 19,* 442–444.

Edinger, J.D., Hoelscher, T.J., Marsh, G.R., Lipper, S., & Ionescu-Pioggia, M. (1992). A cognitive-behavioral therapy for sleep-maintenance insomnia in older adults. *Psychology and Aging, 7,* 282–289.

Edinger, J.D., Hoelscher, T.J., Webb, M.D., Marsh, G.R., Radtke, R.A., & Erwin, C.W. (1989). Polysomnographic assessment of DIMS: Empirical evaluation of its diagnostic value. *Sleep, 12,* 315–322.

Engle-Friedman, M., & Bootzin, R.R. (1991). Insomnia as a problem for the elderly. In P.A. Wisocki (Ed.), *Handbook of clinical behavior therapy with the elderly client* (pp. 273–298). New York: Plenum Press.

Engle-Friedman, M., Bootzin, R.R., Hazlewood, L., & Tsao, C. (1992). An evaluation of behavioral treatments for insomnia in the older adult. *Journal of Clinical Psychology, 48,* 77–90.

Espie, C.A., Lindsay, W.R., & Brooks, D.N. (1988). Substituting behavioural treatment for drugs in the treatment of insomnia: An exploratory study. *Journal of Behavior Therapy and Experimental Psychiatry, 19,* 51–56.

Fichten, C.S., Creti, L., Amsel, R., Brender, W., Weinstein, N., & Libman, E. (1995). Poor sleepers who do not complain of insomnia: Myths and realities about psychological and lifestyle characteristics of older good and poor sleepers. *Journal of Behavioral Medicine, 18,* 189–223.

Flemons, W.W., Remmers, J.E., Whitelaw, W.A., & Brant, R. (1993). The clinical prediction of sleep apnea. *Sleep, 16*(Suppl. 8), 10.

Foley, D.J., Monjan, A.A., Brown, S.L., Simonsick, E.M., Wallace, R.B., & Blazer, D.G. (1995). Sleep complaints among elderly persons: An epidemiologic study of three communities. *Sleep, 18,* 425–432.

Freedman, R.R. (1986). EEG power spectra in sleep onset insomnia. *Electroencephalography and Clinical Neurophysiology, 63,* 408–413.

Friedman, L., Bliwise, D.L., Yesavage, J.A., & Salom, S.R. (1991). A preliminary study comparing sleep restriction and relaxation treatments for insomnia in older adults. *Journal of Gerontology: Psychological Sciences, 46,* P1–P8.

Gillin, J.C., & Byerley, W.F. (1990). The diagnosis and management of insomnia. *New England Journal of Medicine, 322,* 239–248.

Gottlieb, G.L. (1990). Sleep disorders and their management: Special considerations in the elderly. *American Journal of Medicine, 88*(Suppl. 3A), S29–S33.

Grad, R.M. (1995). Benzodiazepines for insomnia in community-dwelling elderly: A review of benefit and risk. *Journal of Family Practice, 41,* 473–481.

Haimov, I., Lavie, P., Laudon, M., Herer, P., Vigder, C., & Zisapel, N. (1995). Melatonin replacement therapy of elderly insomniacs. *Sleep, 18,* 598–603.

Herings, R.M.C., Stricker, B.H.C., de Boer, A., Bakker, A., & Sturmans, F. (1995). Benzodiazepines and the risk of falling leading to femur fractures. *Archives of Internal Medicine, 155,* 1801–1807.

Hoelscher, T.J., & Edinger, J.D. (1988). Treatment of sleep-maintenance insomnia in older adults: Sleep period reduction, sleep education, and modified stimulus control. *Psychology and Aging, 3,* 258–263.

Hoffstein, V., & Szalai, J.P. (1993). Predictive value of clinical features in diagnosing obstructive sleep apnea. *Sleep, 16,* 118–122.

Johnson, J. (1993). Progressive relaxation and the sleep of older men and women. *Journal of Community Health Nursing, 10,* 31–38.

Kales, A., Bixler, E.O., Soldatos, C.R., Vela-Bueno, A., Caldwell, A.B., & Cadieux, R.J. (1982). Biopsychobehavioral correlates of insomnia, part 1: Role of sleep apnea and nocturnal myoclonus. *Psychosomatics, 23,* 589–600.

Kales, A., Caldwell, A.B., Soldatos, C.R., Bixler, E.O., & Kales, J.D. (1983). Biopsychobehavioral correlates of insomnia II: Pattern specificity and consistency with the Minnesota Multiphasic Personality Inventory. *Psychosomatic Medicine, 45,* 341–355.

Kales, A., Soldatos, C.R., Bixler, E.O., & Kales, J.D. (1983). Rebound insomnia and rebound anxiety: A review. *Pharmacology, 26,* 121–137.

Kapuniai, L.E., Andrew, D.J., Crowell, D.H., & Pearce, J.W. (1988). Identifying sleep apnea from self-reports. *Sleep, 11,* 430–436.

Kirmil-Gray, K., Eagleston, J.R., Thoresen, C.E., & Zarcone, V.P. (1985). Brief consultation and stress management treatments for drug-dependent insomnia: Effects on sleep quality, self-efficacy, and daytime stress. *Journal of Behavioral Medicine, 8,* 79–99.

Kryger, M.H., Roth, T., & Dement, W.C. (Eds.). (1994). *Principles and practice of sleep medicine* (2nd ed.). Philadelphia: Saunders.

Lichstein, K.L. (1988a). *Clinical relaxation strategies.* New York: Wiley.

Lichstein, K.L. (1988b). Sleep compression treatment of an insomnoid. *Behavior Therapy, 19,* 625–632.

Lichstein, K.L. (2000). Relaxation. In K.L. Lichstein & C.M. Morin (Eds.), *Treatment of late-life insomnia.* Thousand Oaks, CA: Sage.

Lichstein, K.L., & Durrence, H.H. (1999). An analysis of the differences between primary insomnia and secondary insomnia on sleep and daytime functioning variables [Abstract]. *Sleep, 22*(Suppl. 1), S-207.

Lichstein, K.L., & Fischer, S.M. (1985). Insomnia. In M. Hersen & A.S. Bellack (Eds.), *Handbook of clinical behavior therapy with adults* (pp. 319–352). New York: Plenum Press.

Lichstein, K.L., & Johnson, R.S. (1991). Older adults' objective self-recording of sleep in the home. *Behavior Therapy, 22,* 531–548.

Lichstein, K.L., & Johnson, R.S. (1993). Relaxation for insomnia and hypnotic medication use in older women. *Psychology and Aging, 8,* 103–111.

Lichstein, K.L., & Johnson, R.S. (1996). The utility of pupillometric assessment in older adults with insomnia. *Journal of Clinical Geropsychology, 2,* 337–352.

Lichstein, K.L., Peterson, B.A., Riedel, B.W., Means, M.K., Epperson, M.T., & Aguillard, R.N. (1999). Relaxation therapy to assist sleep medication withdrawal. *Behavior Modification, 23,* 379–402.

Lichstein, K.L., Riedel, B.W., Lester, K.W., & Aguillard, R.N. (1999). Occult sleep apnea in a recruited sample of older adults with insomnia. *Journal of Consulting and Clinical Psychology, 67,* 405–410.

Lichstein, K.L., & Rosenthal, T.L. (1980). Insomniacs' perceptions of cognitive versus somatic determinants of sleep disturbance. *Journal of Abnormal Psychology, 89,* 105–107.

Lichstein, K.L., Wilson, N.M., & Johnson, C.T. (in press). Psychological treatment of secondary insomnia. *Psychology and Aging.*

Lick, J.R., & Heffler, D. (1977). Relaxation training and attention placebo in the treatment of severe insomnia. *Journal of Consulting and Clinical Psychology, 45,* 153–161.

Mellinger, G.D., & Balter, M.B. (1981). Prevalence and patterns of use of psychotherapeutic drugs: Results from a 1979 national survey of American adults. In G. Tognoni, C. Bellantuono, & M. Lader (Eds.), *Epidemiological impact of psychotropic drugs* (pp. 117–135). Amsterdam, The Netherlands: Elsevier.

Mellinger, G.D., Balter, M.B., & Uhlenhuth, E.H. (1985). Insomnia and its treatment. *Archives of General Psychiatry, 42,* 225–232.

Miles, L.E., & Dement, W.C. (1980). Sleep and aging. *Sleep, 3,* 119–220.

Monane, M. (1992). Insomnia in the elderly. *Journal of Clinical Psychiatry, 53*(Suppl.), 23–28.

Monroe, L.J. (1967). Psychological and physiological differences between good and poor sleepers. *Journal of Abnormal Psychology, 72,* 255–264.

Moran, M.G., & Stoudemire, A. (1992). Sleep disorders in the medically ill patient. *Journal of Clinical Psychiatry, 53*(Suppl.), 29–36.

Moran, M.G., Thompson, T.L., & Nies, A.S. (1988). Sleep disorders in the elderly. *American Journal of Psychiatry, 145,* 1369–1378.

Morawetz, D. (1989). Behavioral self-help treatment for insomnia: A controlled evaluation. *Behavior Therapy, 20,* 365–379.

Morgan, K. (1987). *Sleep and aging: A research-based guide to sleep in later life.* Baltimore: Johns Hopkins University Press.

Morin, C.M., & Azrin, N.H. (1987). Stimulus control and imagery training in treating sleep-maintenance insomnia. *Journal of Consulting and Clinical Psychology, 55,* 260–262.

Morin, C.M., & Azrin, N.H. (1988). Behavioral and cognitive treatments of geriatric insomnia. *Journal of Consulting and Clinical Psychology, 56,* 748–753.

Morin, C.M., Colecchi, C.A., Ling, W.D., & Sood, R.K. (1995). Cognitive behavior therapy to facilitate benzodiazepine discontinuation among hypnotic-dependent patients with insomnia. *Behavior Therapy, 26,* 733–745.

Morin, C.M., Colecchi, C.A., Stone, J., Sood, R., & Brink, D. (1999). Behavioral and pharmacological therapies for late-life insomnia. *Journal of the American Medical Association, 281,* 991–999.

Morin, C.M., Culbert, J.P., & Schwartz, S.M. (1994). Nonpharmacological interventions for insomnia: A meta-analysis of treatment efficacy. *American Journal of Psychiatry, 151,* 1172–1180.

Morin, C.M., & Gramling, S.E. (1989). Sleep patterns and aging: Comparison of older adults with and without insomnia complaints. *Psychology and Aging, 4,* 290–294.

Morin, C.M., Kowatch, R.A., Barry, T., & Walton, E. (1993). Cognitive-behavior therapy for late-life insomnia. *Journal of Consulting and Clinical Psychology, 61,* 137–146.

Morin, C.M., Kowatch, R.A., & Wade, J.B. (1989). Behavioral management of sleep disturbances secondary to chronic pain. *Journal of Behavior Therapy and Experimental Psychiatry, 20,* 295–302.

Morin, C.M., Savard, J., & Blais, F. (2000). Cognitive therapy. In K.L. Lichstein & C.M. Morin (Eds.), *Treatment of late-life insomnia.* Thousand Oaks, CA: Sage.

Morin, C.M., Stone, J., McDonald, K., & Jones, S. (1994). Psychological management of insomnia: A clinical replication series with 100 patients. *Behavior Therapy, 25,* 291–309.

Neutel, C.I. (1995). Risk of traffic accident injury after a prescription for a benzodiazepine. *Annals of Epidemiology, 5,* 239–244.

Nicassio, P., & Bootzin, R. (1974). A comparison of progressive relaxation and autogenic training as treatments for insomnia. *Journal of Abnormal Psychology, 83,* 253–260.

Parrino, L., & Terzano, M.G. (1996). Polysomnographic effects of hypnotic drugs. *Psychopharmacology, 126,* 1–16.

Pilowsky, I., Crettenden, I., & Townley, M. (1985). Sleep disturbance in pain clinic patients. *Pain, 23,* 27–33.

Pressman, M.R., Figueroa, W.G., Kendrick-Mohamed, J., Greenspon, L.W., & Peterson, D.D. (1996). Nocturia: A rarely recognized symptom of sleep apnea and other occult sleep disorders. *Archives of Internal Medicine, 156,* 545–550.

Prinz, P.N., Vitiello, M.V., Raskind, M.A., & Thorpy, M.J. (1990). Geriatrics: Sleep disorders and aging. *New England Journal of Medicine, 323,* 520–526.

Puder, R., Lacks, P., Bertelson, A., & Storandt, M. (1983). Short-term stimulus control treatment of insomnia in older adults. *Behavior Therapy, 14,* 424–429.

Ray, W.A., Griffin, M.R., & Downey, W. (1989). Benzodiazepines of long and short elimination half-life and the risk of hip fracture. *Journal of the American Medical Association, 262,* 3303–3307.

Reite, M., Buysse, D., Reynolds, C., & Mendelson, W. (1995). The use of polysomnography in the evaluation of insomnia. *Sleep, 18,* 58–70.

Riedel, B.W. (2000). Sleep hygiene. In K.L. Lichstein & C.M. Morin (Eds.), *Treatment of late-life insomnia.* Thousand Oaks, CA: Sage.

Riedel, B.W., Lichstein, K.L., & Dwyer, W.O. (1995). Sleep compression and sleep education for older insomniacs: Self-help *vs.* therapist guidance. *Psychology and Aging, 10,* 54–63.

Riedel, B.W., Lichstein, K.L., Peterson, B.A., Epperson, M.T., Means, M.K., & Aguillard, R.N. (1998). A comparison of the efficacy of stimulus control for medicated and nonmedicated insomniacs. *Behavior Modification, 22,* 3–28.

Roehrs, T., Merlotti, L., Zorick, F., & Roth, T. (1994). Sedative, memory, and performance effects of hypnotics. *Psychopharmacology, 116,* 130–134.

Roth, T., Zorick, F., Wittig, R., & Roehrs, T. (1982). Pharmacological and medical considerations in hypnotic use. *Sleep, 5*(Suppl. 1), 46–52.

Saskin, P. (1997). Obstructive sleep apnea: Treatment options, efficacy, and effects. In M.R. Pressman & W.C. Orr (Eds.), *Understanding sleep: The evaluation and treatment of sleep disorders* (pp. 283–297). Washington, DC: American Psychological Association.

Spielman, A.J., Saskin, P., & Thorpy, M.J. (1987). Treatment of chronic insomnia by restriction of time in bed. *Sleep, 10,* 45–56.

Stam, H.J., & Bultz, B.D. (1986). The treatment of severe insomnia in a cancer patient. *Journal of Behavior Therapy and Experimental Psychiatry, 17,* 33–37.

Turner, R.M., & Ascher, L.M. (1979). Controlled comparison of progressive relaxation, stimulus control, and paradoxical intention therapies for insomnia. *Journal of Consulting and Clinical Psychology, 47,* 500–508.

Varni, J.W. (1980). Behavioral treatment of disease-related chronic insomnia in a hemophiliac. *Journal of Behavior Therapy and Experimental Psychiatry, 11,* 143–145.

Vgontzas, A.N., Kales, A., Bixler, E.O., Manfredi, R.L., & Vela-Bueno, A. (1995). Usefulness of polysomnographic studies in the differential diagnosis of insomnia. *International Journal of Neuroscience, 82,* 47–60.

Walsh, J.K., Moss, K.L., & Sugerman, J. (1994). Insomnia in adult psychiatric disorders. In M.H. Kryger, T. Roth, & W.C. Dement (Eds.), *Principles and practice of sleep medicine* (2nd ed., pp. 500–508). Philadelphia: Saunders.

Walsh, J.K., & Schweitzer, P.K. (1999). Ten-year trends in the pharmacological treatment of insomnia. *Sleep, 22,* 371–375.

Williams, R.L., Karacan, I., & Hursch, C.J. (1974). *Electroencephalography (EEG) of human sleep: Clinical applications.* New York: Wiley.

Wittig, R.M., Zorick, F.J., Blumer, D., Heilbronn, M., & Roth, T. (1982). Disturbed sleep in patients complaining of chronic pain. *Journal of Nervous and Mental Disease, 170,* 429–431.

Wohlgemuth, W.K., & Edinger, J.D. (2000). Sleep restriction therapy. In K.L. Lichstein & C.M. Morin (Eds.), *Treatment of late-life insomnia.* Thousand Oaks, CA: Sage.

CHAPTER 13

General Principles of Therapy

Gregory A. Hinrichsen and Leah P. Dick-Siskin

CASE STUDY

Betty is a 68-year-old married woman who lives with her husband and 37-year-old son, who has multiple sclerosis. Betty has been caring for her son, Paul, for two years since his physical condition worsened and he could no longer live independently. Betty's 69-year-old husband, Jerry, continues to work as an accountant. Betty recently saw her primary care physician complaining of extreme fatigue, irritability, and sad mood. The doctor suggested that Betty see a psychologist for psychotherapy because he felt she was "stressed" by caring for her son.

Betty left the doctor's office feeling insulted that her doctor said she had a "psychological problem." She stuffed the psychologist's name and number in the back of her kitchen junk drawer. A few weeks later, as she seemed to get more depressed, her husband urged her to see the psychologist. Reluctantly, Betty agreed.

During the first session with the psychologist, Betty was anxious and distracted. The psychologist inquired about this, and Betty explained that she was uncomfortable being an hour away from her son because he needed constant care and there was no one else to help him. In fact, Betty said she only left her son for short periods of time to go to the grocery store or to the pharmacy. Betty explained that over the past two to three months, she had grown increasingly sad, irritable, and tired, slept poorly, and had little appetite. She tearfully told the psychologist she felt worthless and that she was doing a bad job as a caregiver for her son. She had isolated herself from her friends and no longer pursued her favorite hobbies of painting and gardening. Her relationship with Jerry was strained: "He doesn't understand me anymore."

The psychologist asked Betty to tell him a bit about her life. She explained that she was the oldest of three sisters. When she was growing up, her father was a gentle, generous, and loving man. Her mother was "always sickly" and was intermittently ill and in bed for most of Betty's childhood. By the time Betty was 16, her mother was quite sick and needed constant attention. As the oldest child, Betty became the person with primary responsibility for the care of the house, her sisters, and her mother. Betty arranged for a cousin and neighbors to look in on her mother during the day, and, after finishing her high school classes, she returned home to care for her mother in the late afternoon and evening.

Her relationship with her sisters was close in their early years, but as her mother's health deteriorated, she became more like a parent than a sibling. Recently, Betty's middle sister had died of cancer. Her youngest sister lived in Florida with her husband. She and her youngest sister have become closer since their sister's death, and they speak frequently by phone.

Following graduation from high school, Betty took a part-time job as a receptionist, where she met her future husband, whom she married a few years later. Although her mother's health condition was stable in those years, her mother continued to need help from Betty. After Betty's father's death, she and Jerry moved to their first house and Betty's mother moved with them. Betty continued to care for her mother until she died.

Betty explained to the psychologist that she had three grown children: a daughter and two sons. Her daughter lived nearby with her family, and her youngest son lived out of state. Betty's middle child, Paul was diagnosed with multiple sclerosis about 10 years previously. His physical condition was fairly stable until a serious decline two years earlier. In addition to physical deterioration, Paul also experienced a loss of mental abilities that is often associated with multiple sclerosis. Paul moved into his parents' home six months ago. As her caregiving duties increased, Betty began to slowly withdraw from her friends and other social activities. She now cares for Paul 24 hours a day, taking him to medical appointments and physical therapy and on short outings.

PROBLEMS THAT BRING OLDER PEOPLE TO PSYCHOTHERAPY

It is important to note at the outset that most older people do not need mental health services. Despite the many challenges of later life, older people cope quite well with the problems that may arise in later late. Further, only a minority of older people actually have diagnosable psychiatric disorders. Rates of most psychiatric disorders are actually lower in persons 65 years and older when compared with younger people (Weissman, Bruce, Leaf, Florio, & Holzer, 1991). Also, in large surveys of the emotional well-being of the elderly, most older people indicate that they are reasonably happy and have satisfying relationships with their families and friends.

As our case illustrates, however, some older people face difficult and complex life problems and seek the services of a mental health care professional. As with younger adults, many older people in need of mental health care do not receive it. Some studies indicate that only a small proportion of those who could benefit from care actually obtain it (Estes, 1995). Psychiatric disorders often accompany these problems. Psychiatric disorders are characterized in the *Diagnostic and Statistical Manual of Psychiatric Disorders* (DSM-IV; American Psychiatric Association [APA], 1994). Disorders that are the most frequent focus of mental health care in older adults include depressive disorders, anxiety disorders, loss of mental abilities as seen in dementia, and adjustment disorder. Many older people with psychiatric disorders benefit from treatment with psychotherapy, psychiatric medications, or both. Although the primary focus of this chapter is on psychotherapy and older adults, we review basic issues in the psychopharmaco-logical treatment of late-life psychiatric disorders.

Although the problems that older people confront are as varied and complex as older people themselves, there are several issues that are most commonly the focus of psychotherapy with this age group. These problems usually reflect difficulties that appear with increasing frequency as people age. They include physical health problems, coming to terms with the death of persons who are important, relationship issues, and the stresses of caring for an infirm relative. Also seen in psychotherapy are older people who have had mental disorders throughout their lives. In addressing these problems, psychotherapy can play an important role in improving older clients' emotional well-being and ability to function day-to-day.

PHYSICAL HEALTH PROBLEMS

A central reality of aging is that physical health problems increase in frequency as people age. This is especially true for people 75 years of age and older. The probability of having one or more chronic health problems increases with age, for example, arthritis, high blood pressure, heart problems, diabetes, and osteoporosis. Most older people successfully contend with these problems and go about daily life with few restrictions on activities. For others, health problems impose formidable practical and emotional burdens for which psychotherapeutic assistance is needed.

For some individuals, the onset of a health problem is a shock. Most younger people take for granted that their bodies will function efficiently and without discomfort. Although most older people well understand that health problems come with later life, some may hope that they will be the exception. When health problems do arise, they can threaten one's view of self and expectations about life. Health problems force people to come to terms with the reality that their physical selves have changed. Some people resist these changes and may experience complex feelings of anger, grief, and depression. Some persons may deny health problems and then fail to seek adequate medical care or follow prescribed medical regimens. For example, one older woman was sent by her medical doctor for psychotherapy after a recent diagnosis of kidney problems that required hemodialysis. In hemodialysis, she was to receive twice-weekly treatments in which she was tethered to a machine that cleansed toxins from her system. She appeared irregularly for these treatments, which resulted in several hospitalizations. At the onset of psychotherapy, she claimed that "the doctors got it all wrong," and she expressed anger at medical staff who treated her. She was also depressed and anxious. The focus in psychotherapy was on helping her to come to emotional terms with her medical condition.

Some medical conditions prevent people from doing things they previously had done. Physical restrictions, reduced energy, or the need for ongoing medical appointments mean that daily life must be restructured. Some may be uncertain how to make these changes, become depressed, and fail to take advantage of many opportunities to live a full, albeit different, life. One very independent older client was diagnosed with a seizure disorder in late life. Because of this, the law prohibited her from driving a car unless she was free of seizures for one year. This created considerable inconvenience for her, as she was a very active person and now had to rely on her husband and friends to drive her. Almost a year passed during which she had no seizures and she eagerly anticipated reclaiming her driving license. Much to her disappointment, she had another seizure, and she grew depressed. In therapy, the focus was on reckoning with this disappointment and creatively reviewing her options so that she could be as socially active as possible even if she could not drive.

Some older persons resent their dependence on others or find that others are weary of their dependence. Illness may require a restructuring of some parts of a relationship with a significant other. A wife who had previously been the major force in running the household and organizing social relationships for herself and her husband must now rely on him to do these things. He may resent these new responsibilities or she may be annoyed that he does not do them in the same way she had done them. This may lead to conflict between them at a time when she may especially need his love and support. Friends may not be as interested in socializing with the woman because her disability means additional effort on their part or it makes them uncomfortable. This may result in feelings of disappointment, abandonment, or anger.

For others, health problems result in physical discomfort or pain. Pain is often tied to depressive symptoms that add to a person's feelings of discouragement and hopelessness. Depression can make pain worse. There are several techniques by which pain can be made more tolerable and that can be learned in psychotherapy.

DEATH OF FRIENDS AND FAMILY

Advancing age is associated with increased health problems not only for oneself but also for one's contemporaries. Because life expectancy is greater for women than men, and because this generation of older women tended to marry men older than themselves, most older women will become widowed. Widowhood is one of life's most stressful events (Zisook, Shuchter, Sledge, Paulus, & Judd, 1994). Marriages or life partnerships of 50 years or more sometimes end abruptly, sometimes after a considerable period of illness. Widowhood requires reckoning with the loss and change in some or many aspects of one's daily routines. Widowers may find that they now are responsible for cooking and cleaning, whereas previously their wives did these tasks. Widows, particularly of this generation of older people, may have relied on their husbands to care for finances, the house, and the car and now must deal with these tasks themselves. Many widowed people report changes in some aspects of their social relationships with others. They may have socialized previously with couples but now find they or others are uncomfortable socializing as a single person.

As with most late-life problems, the majority of older people successfully maneuver the tasks of widowhood. For some, things are more difficult, and they may benefit from psychotherapy. One older woman seen in psychotherapy had severe problems with depression a year and a half after the death of her husband. She said she could not accept her husband's death, kept her husband's room just as it was at the time of his death, and made daily trips to the cemetery, where she stood by his grave and wept. When the first winter came after his death, she became panicked when snow covered her husband's gravesite because she could not "see" where he was buried. The goal of the psychotherapy was to help her come to terms emotionally with her husband's death and to then reestablish a new daily life for herself.

Relationship Issues

Research has demonstrated that, compared with younger couples, older couples appear to develop more successful ways to deal with differences and conflict in their relationships (Carstensen, Gottman, & Levenson, 1995). Further, most gerontological studies have found that, on the whole, older people have satisfying relationships with their adult children (Shanas, 1979). Some older people, however, come to psychotherapy because of difficulties with family members and sometimes with friends. For this generation of older adults, in which the husband typically worked and the wife was the homemaker, his retirement from paid employment can be stressful for both. Some wives report that after their husband's retirement, they resent his presence in the household throughout the day. Husbands are dismayed that "their" home is really *her* domain. Older couples may find that longstanding issues that were kept at bay because they spent only a few hours each day in face-to-face contact reemerge after the man's retirement. One older man sought psychotherapy because during a verbal dispute with his wife, he threw her to the floor and began to choke her. He was horrified by his own behavior. He felt that, in retrospect, he and his wife of 50 years probably should not have married in the first place, but he wanted to engage in marital therapy so that they could "live in peace."

Another common relationship issue seen in psychotherapy is problems between the older adult and an adult child. Sometimes, longstanding disputes between older parents and adult children come to the fore or new problems arise. Some problems include differences over financial issues or frequency of visits by the adult child or grandchildren, or when the older person or adult child has psychiatric problems. Some older people are deeply distressed over a poor relationship with a daughter or son-in-law or are disappointed that some of their children do not get along well with each other. One older couple sought psychotherapy because they were deeply distressed that their adult daughter visited and telephoned much less often than she had previously.

They could not understand her behavior and scolded her, which only made the daughter angry. The daughter agreed to attend family meetings, during which she disclosed that she was recovering from an episode of major depression. The focus in therapy was on educating the older parents about major depression and helping them to establishing a schedule of visiting that was agreeable to all parties.

CAREGIVING ISSUES

As noted earlier, health problems increase in later life, and many older adults, especially older women, provide care to an infirm relative, most commonly a spouse. In addition to physical health problems, older people are at increased risk for dementia, a global and usually progressive loss of mental abilities, the most common form of which is Alzheimer's disease. In contrast to the stereotype that older people are abandoned by their families, the vast majority of family members provide care to infirm older relatives (Cantor, 1994). Providing care to an older relative, especially one with chronic illness, can be quite stressful, and some studies have found high rates of psychiatric symptoms and an elevated risk for psychiatric disorders (depressive, anxiety, and adjustment disorders) in dementia caregivers (Schultz & Williamson, 1990). Issues that are common in psychotherapy with caregivers include coming to terms emotionally with the reality of what has happened; managing practical matters, including the need to provide hands-on care; negotiating with formal care providers; handling the financial pressures that often accompany illness; and dealing with changed behavior in the ill family member, including depression, anxiety, and disruptive behavior. Problems may also arise in relationships with other family members over differing expectations about the amount and kind of help they will provide. Those who provide care for long periods may stop working and cease activities or relationships that previously had given them pleasure.

ADAPTATION TO CHRONIC MENTAL ILLNESS

Some older people have struggled with mental illness throughout most of their lives (Light & Lebowitz, 1991). Recurrent episodes of depression, bipolar disorder, and schizophrenia are the most common problems seen. Other older people suffer from personality disorders in which they evidence maladaptive patterns of relating to other people and to themselves.

It is well established that psychiatric illness damages family and other interpersonal relationships (Coryell et al., 1993). Therefore, some older adults with chronic mental illness do not have close family ties or have troubled relationships. This is particularly unfortunate because research has found that family relationships are important in the sustained recovery from psychiatric illness of younger and older adults (Hinrichsen & Hernandez, 1993).

In psychotherapy, several issues relating to chronic mental illness share a common focus, including educating and reeducating about psychiatric illness, managing psychiatric symptoms, following medication regimens, structuring daily life, and better handling of interpersonal relationships. It is important to note that for some older persons with chronic mental illness, late life may bring a lessening of symptoms. Those who were unable to work in younger years may now find greater ease in affiliating with their age peers, many of whom are retired. They may also feel less stigmatized by their conditions as it becomes increasingly normative for older adults to contend with one or more illnesses.

GENERAL PRINCIPLES IN DOING PSYCHOTHERAPY WITH OLDER ADULTS

In psychotherapy, there are many similarities between younger and older people. It appears that with some adaptation, most of the major psychotherapies that have been used with younger people can be successfully conducted with older people. Gerontologists have found, however, that social and historical experiences influence each age cohort's values and views of self and world. The current generation of older adults grew up in the economic depression of the 1930s and entered adulthood when the world went to war. The now middle-aged "baby boom" generation was raised during a time of more economic affluence, and most were young adults during an era of dramatic social change, including dissent over the Vietnam War. When baby boomers are old, they will be different in some noticeable ways from the current generation of older adults. Like the current generation of older people, however, old baby boomers will face common issues that are part and parcel of late life, notably increasing health problems. Knowledge about old age and specific information about cohort characteristics of a particular generation of older people are important to optimize communication between therapist and client. Surveys demonstrate that the public accepts misinformation about what life is like for most older people (usually viewing it as grimmer than it really is). Even mental health professionals may be ignorant of basic facts on the emotional and social well-being of older adults. Geropsychologist Bob Knight has called a gerontologically informed and sensitive approach to doing psychotherapy with older people the contextual, cohort-based, maturity/specific challenge model (Knight, 1996).

SOCIALIZATION TO PSYCHOTHERAPY

This generation of older people's understanding of mental illness was conditioned by the way mentally ill people were treated in an earlier era. In the past, there were few effective treatments for serious mental disorders. Extended confinement to state psychiatric institutions was common for people with schizophrenia, bipolar disorder, and severe depressive disorders. Making contact with the psychiatric establishment might mean losing one's freedom. Mental disorders were often equated with personal or moral failings and stigmatized both patient and family. For an independent generation that weathered the Great

Depression and fought World War II at home and abroad, seeking mental health assistance can be seen as a failure. Older people are more likely to understand behavior as a reflection of character, values, and morality, whereas younger generations are more prone to understand behavior in more neutral psychological language that has entered the culture through the media. When they were young, today's generation of older adults had no Dr. Laura, Oprah, or Joyce Brothers. Because of this, there are often generational differences in the vocabulary for describing internal states such as depression and anxiety.

Many older people come for mental health care at the behest of a family member or another health care provider. Engagement of older clients is the first task and includes understanding why they have come to see a therapist in the first place. "I came to see you for my daughter" is a comment we sometimes hear. Without some basic motivation on the older client's part, it is unlikely that engagement in psychotherapy will take place. Motivation can be built by the therapist by establishing himself or herself as professionally sensitive and knowledgeable about older adults, educating the older person about the problem he or she is experiencing (e.g., "You have what is called a major depressive disorder, which is a severe form of depression"), explaining the treatment that is proposed, and establishing goals and a plan for treatment.

For example, many older people find it patronizing to be referred to by their first names. At a first meeting, one older woman made it clear that when her daughter was invited in at the end of the session, the therapist must make eye contact with her and not just with her daughter. She explained, "When I see my medical doctor and my daughter is present, he talks to her and not me. Who is the patient here, anyway?" Some therapists inexperienced with older adults forget that some older people may not have a clue as to what psychotherapy is. Some older people are puzzled by why psychotherapeutic meetings are weekly: "But I only see my doctor four times a year!" They may question why talking about a problem can be helpful. They may believe that what they tell the therapist will be shared with their children. Of course, permission must be granted by the older person to share information with other family members. Even older people who have received or are currently receiving mental health services may not understand why. A woman on antidepressant medication for many years remarked to one of the authors, "I always wondered why I had to take those pills."

ACCOMMODATING TO SENSORY OR OTHER IMPAIRMENTS

Most older people have varying degrees of difficulty with seeing or hearing. These may or may not be remediated with glasses or hearing aides. Some older people may be reluctant to tell the therapist of their impairment. One woman who was seen by one of the authors for several months in psychotherapy asked one day if he would close the shades on the window. It turned out that for all those months, she could barely see the therapist because of glare from the window behind him. Out of embarrassment, some older people will try to disguise hearing loss and answer questions as if they had been heard. Not uncommonly, people who would benefit from a hearing aide actually have one but do not use it. Some persons with orthopedic or arthritic problems cannot sit comfortably in the type of chair available in the office. Some older people cannot ambulate well and may need a first-floor office in close proximity to the building's entrance. Others with incontinence problems may need bathroom breaks during the session. The bottom line is that the therapist needs to have a conversation with the older client about these issues so that an optimal environment is created for psychotherapy.

Some older adults may present with mild cognitive impairments that may or may not be immediately apparent to the therapist. Notebooks used to record important information, frequent summaries during the session, and even audiotapes of sessions (for the patient to review in between sessions) can be useful strategies to reinforce what is learned in psychotherapy. Evidence of cognitive impairment may be poor recall of material discussed in previous sessions, incomplete psychotherapy "homework," or confusion over appointment times. Therapists should be very cautious of overinterpreting these as reluctance to engage in treatment. Inability to accurately understand and remember rather than lack of motivation to participate in therapy may be the cause of the difficulties.

INTERPERSONAL PROCESSES IN PSYCHOTHERAPY

In the language of psychodynamic psychotherapy, transference and countertransferential phenomena may enter psychotherapy. Transference may reflect older clients' propensity to view the therapist in ways that reflect experiences with other persons in their lives. Younger therapists may been seen as a "good child" whom the older person wishes were his or her own. Some older adults may view the therapist as having qualities of a spouse at an earlier stage of life. Erotic transferences occur. An older woman seen in psychotherapy learned from another staff member that her therapist was unmarried. She confessed her love for the therapist and suggested that they might marry. She had even consulted her minister about the difference in her age and that of the therapist. The minister, apparently unaware that the object of her affections was her therapist, was quoted as saying, "Age is no bar when there is love between two people."

In countertransference, therapists may similarly project issues onto the older client. Some therapists may find it gratifying to take on the role of the "good child," which can cloud understanding of the often complex issues that exist between dissatisfied older clients and their "ungrateful" children. Some therapists with little experience in working with older adults may grow uncomfortable about aging-related issues raised by older clients and avoid the discussion of them in psychotherapy. Because all of us will grow old, health and related late-life problems may resonate personally for the therapist. Some therapists have or have had complicated relationships with their older parents, elements of which can be projected onto the client. One of our psychology trainees conveyed her dislike for a frail older client who reminded her of "my mother's endless complaining at the end of her life." Some therapists may see older adults as "cute" or "feisty" and treat them in caricatured ways. The plight of the older adult may cloud a therapist's judgment about appropriate professional boundaries. One therapist inexperienced with older people saw a widowed woman in her 80s who had no children. The older woman felt overwhelmed by unpaid bills and other financial issues. The therapist volunteered to go to her home to help her with her finances, and soon the relationship developed into what was described as a "friendship." The therapist felt that she was doing the older person a good deed but seemed unaware of the poor boundaries that were set. When asked about this, the therapist said, "Oh, but I told her that if she wanted my undivided attention, then she would have to pay me for an hour of therapy."

TREATMENT PLAN AND GOALS

As with clients of any age, treatment goals need to be delineated and a plan for achieving them developed. We find that many older people are comforted by knowing that there is a plan of action that will guide weekly meetings. Many older people are pragmatic about what they want from therapy: "I want to feel better"; "I want my daughter and I to get along better"; "I just want to get back to my old self." Congruence of individual and therapeutic goals enhances motivation for treatment. Typical goals include a reduction in psychiatric symptoms (e.g., depression, anxiety) and improvement in the life problem that brought the older person for psychotherapy. Client goals may be quite circumscribed or more ambitious. We believe that it is important to review intermittently treatment goals with the older client. Standardized symptom rating scales can be helpful in concretely marking progress in symptom reduction.

It is often useful to have a time frame for the length of treatment. For example, client and therapist may agree to meet for eight sessions, at the end of which progress will be reviewed. At that point, a joint decision will be made about continued therapy.

TREATMENT SETTINGS

As discussed earlier, older adults may have problems that involve their physical, psychological, and social well-being (Zeiss & Steffen, 1996). An exacerbation in one of these problems areas creates difficulties in other areas. For example, the pain of arthritis may make it more difficult for someone to care for herself and socialize with friends. These difficulties my lead to depression, which makes it even more difficult to cope with arthritis pain, socialize, and function as a homemaker. Zeiss and Steffen propose that the best way to deliver services to older patients with complex problems is the simultaneous management of all problems in what they call the interdisciplinary team model. The interdisciplinary team consists of members from different disciplines who collaborate to evaluate, plan, and treat the patient. In our example, this patient would likely receive psychotropic medication from a psychiatrist, psychotherapy from a psychologist, consultation from a medical internist to help her manage arthritis, an evaluation from a physical therapist to identify devices to enhance her independence, and linkage to transportation services from a social worker.

The fact is that most older adults receive mental health services from the family doctor in the form of psychiatric medication. There is a concern, however, that family doctors often fail to diagnose psychiatric disorders or fail to refer older patients to psychologists or psychiatrists when needed. Below is a brief outline of some of the most common settings in which older people receive mental health services.

COMMUNITY MENTAL HEALTH CENTER

Community mental health centers are outpatient settings that generally serve all age groups. Staff often include doctoral psychologists, social workers, and psychiatrists. Typically, patients receive once-weekly individual or group psychotherapy and/or once-monthly medication management. It is rare that community mental health centers have staff formally trained to provide services to older adults.

GEROPSYCHIATRY CLINIC

A geropsychiatry clinic is an outpatient service with multidisciplinary staff specifically trained to deal with the complex problems of late life. Like community mental health centers, these clinics provide psychiatric, psychological, and social work services. These clinics are often associated with medical schools and frequently provide opportunities for training of students.

INPATIENT SERVICE

An inpatient setting provides services to more acutely mentally ill older adults than are seen in an outpatient setting. There is intensive treatment with psychiatric medication management, group therapy, family therapy, and linkages to social services following discharge.

GERIATRIC PARTIAL HOSPITAL

A partial hospital is a daily outpatient treatment program that provides intensive, structured multidisciplinary services to older adults who have been recently discharged from a psychiatric inpatient setting, or as an alternative to hospitalization. Treatment focuses on medication management and compliance, social functioning, discharge planning, and relapse prevention.

Geriatric Continuing Day Treatment

Continuing day treatment is a less intense program than that offered by a geriatric partial hospital program. Older patients generally attend a day treatment program three days each week, with an emphasis on their independent functioning on nonprogram days.

Nursing Home

There is a high prevalence of psychiatric disorders and psychiatric symptoms in nursing homes. Increasingly, psychologists are providing individual and group psychotherapies to nursing home residents, often in conjunction with psychiatric medications prescribed by psychiatrists.

THE THEORY AND PRACTICE OF COGNITIVE-BEHAVIORAL THERAPY WITH OLDER ADULTS

Cognitive-behavioral therapy (CBT) views psychiatric disorders as the result of cognitive and behavioral disturbances and their interaction with emotional and physical factors (Beck, Rush, Shaw, & Emery, 1979; Lewinsohn, Hoberman, Teri, & Hautzinger, 1985; Lewinsohn, Munoz, Youngren, & Zeiss, 1978). For example, an older depressed man with a flare-up of arthritis (physical) may choose not to attend his social club (behavior), and while at home, think (cognition), "I'll never make new friends. No one will ever want to get close to someone who is handicapped like me." Consequently, these catastrophic thoughts result in negative emotions such as depression or anxiety, which further exacerbate physical symptoms (pain, tension) and negative behaviors (social isolation). Ways to intervene in this downward spiral include *cognitive strategies* to identify, challenge, and restructure negative thought patterns and *behavioral techniques* to both introduce new activities and to manage the physical symptoms associated with negative emotions.

Key elements of CBT include: (1) a good collaborative relationship between the patient and the therapist; (2) a short-term treatment that focuses on well-defined, measurable goals; (3) the use of inductive reasoning to identify themes and patterns of cognitions and behaviors; and (4) the use of regular homework assignments. CBT is divided into early, middle, and late stages of therapy. The tasks and goals at each of these stages are individualized for the patient (Beck et al., 1979; Dick, Gallagher-Thompson, & Thompson, 1996;

Thompson, Gallagher-Thompson, & Dick, 1997). CBT works well with older adults and requires few adaptations from the way it was developed for younger adults (Dick et al., 1996; Thompson, Davies, Gallagher, & Krantz, 1986; Thompson et al., 1991; Zeiss & Lewinsohn, 1986).

EARLY PHASE (SESSIONS 1–3)

The development of a collaborative relationship between the therapist and the patient is critical at the outset of CBT. A collaborative relationship rests on an accurate understanding of what psychotherapy is and the likelihood of success. A collaborative relationship also develops through a discussion of what each party can expect from treatment and how CBT differs from other psychotherapies (Dick et al., 1996; Dick et al., 1997; Thompson et al., 1997; Zeiss & Lewinsohn, 1986). From the beginning, the therapist teaches the patient the CBT model, discusses the role of homework, and contracts for length of treatment.

Specific, measurable goals are identified in the initial phase of treatment. For example, a depressed widow may state that she wishes to manage anxiety better, increase social activities, and decrease the tendency to "jump to conclusions" about situations involving her family. Patients are introduced to basic cognitive techniques including the Dysfunctional Thought Record (DTR), which patients use to monitor cognitive perceptions and emotional consequences of stressful situations (Beck et al., 1979). The patient's current frequency of pleasant events and magnitude of pleasure derived from each event are assessed. Often, older adults who have lost pleasure in activities may find it difficult to generate spontaneously a list of pleasant events. The Older Person's Pleasant Events Scale (OP-PES; Teri & Lewinsohn, 1982) can be very helpful to generate an accurate profile of these events.

MIDDLE PHASES (SESSIONS 4–16)

The focus of the middle phase of treatment is to work toward goals established in the first phase by teaching the patient the cognitive and behavioral skills needed to achieve the goals. Cognitive skills include identifying unhelpful thought patterns (using the DTR), challenging these patterns, and developing more adaptive ways to perceive and to respond to stressful situations. Behavioral skills are implemented to develop new pleasant activities or reintroduce activities that have been abandoned. Patients learn the direct relationship between the frequency and the pleasure of activities.

Patients are also taught to recognize the interaction between cognitive and behavioral domains; hesitation to engage in new activities may be based on cognitions. Consider the earlier example. The older gentleman may not attend his social club unless there is substantial change in his beliefs about himself and his disability. As the middle phase of treatment progresses, patients become more independent in generating hypotheses about thought patterns and begin to develop exercises to challenge the validity of assumptions. In this phase, patients are taught additional skills such as assertiveness, relaxation, and anger management. In CBT, large-print handouts, notebooks, and frequent summaries of material are often used to enhance learning and are especially useful for older adults with sensory impairments (Dick et al., 1996; Thompson et al., 1986, 1991).

END PHASE (SESSIONS 17–20)

In the end phase, patient and therapist discuss thoughts and feelings about termination and, as part of the collaborative spirit of CBT, discuss what each party has learned from the other. In this phase of treatment, progress is reviewed and strategies to manage independently manage future stressful situations are identified. Dick and colleagues recommend the use of a written "maintenance guide" that outlines what was accomplished in CBT as well as the steps to prevent relapse (Dick et al., 1996; Dick et al., 1997; Thompson et al., 1997).

TREATMENT OF CASE EXAMPLE: CBT

Early Phase
During the initial session of CBT, Betty said she had little interest in psychotherapy. Betty's beliefs about psychotherapy were immediately explored. She believed that the need for psychotherapy meant she was a failure as a mother and a caregiver. She was anxious about attending weekly sessions, as they would take too much time away from her son. She reluctantly agreed to return the next week.

At the next meeting, Betty arrived in tears, explaining that she recently found herself yelling, almost "uncontrollably," at her son. She explained that this behavior frightened her, and she reconsidered her need for help. Betty was aware that she needed help but felt hopeless about change in her stressful problems. The therapist said that it was important that he and Betty work together to identify treatment goals and the means to achieve them. The therapist explained, "I have been specially trained to assist older people with their unique problems. In our treatment, I will be on time for sessions, come with a clear memory of what we previously discussed, and offer creative ideas to help you manage stress. Your role in this work is to discuss your experiences, actively work with me in sessions to develop new skills, and then practice these new skills in between sessions." The therapist went on to explain the CBT model.

Following this discussion, Betty identified three goals: (1) reduce the frustration and guilt she felt toward her son; (2) stop "blowing small details out of proportion"; and (3) restart some of her old hobbies and interests. Although these goals were set, Betty expressed skepticism about achieving them.

The therapist noted that Betty presented with an episode of major depression. He discussed with Betty the importance of monitoring her depressed mood on a weekly basis to track improvement. The therapist gave Betty the brief version of the Beck Depression Inventory (BDI), and she scored 27 (out of a possible 39) indicating a moderate-to-severe level of depression. Betty was asked to complete this measure before every session.

Middle Phase

Behavioral Interventions. Betty was first taught a brief relaxation exercise to manage her physical experience of tension and frustration and was encouraged to use an audio recording of the exercise at home. However, at first, Betty did not practice the exercise because she could not find the time to do it. In discussion with the therapist, Betty revealed that she did not believe that she was entitled to a few moments to herself—an issue that was addressed later in therapy. She said that her only time alone was running errands. Therefore, it was suggested that she do the relaxation exercise in her car on the way to and from errands. Betty tried this for one week and was pleased with the results.

Betty could not remember things she had enjoyed previously in her spare time other than a life-long interest in painting. With the aid of the OP-PES (Teri & Lewinsohn, 1982), Betty identified enjoyable activities from several areas about which the OP-PES inquires, including nature, social, recognition from others, and leisure activity (see Figure 13.1). From her OP-PES profile, Betty and

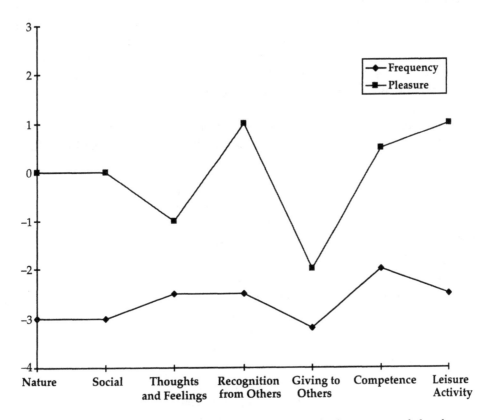

Figure 13.1 Betty's OP-PES: The relationship between the frequency and the pleasure of pleasant events.

the therapist generated a daily activity plan designed to increase Betty's pleasant events. Betty was taught to record the relationship between the daily frequency of her pleasant events and a self-rating of her daily mood (on a scale of 1–10: 1 = very depressed, 10 = not at all depressed). Initially, Betty had difficulty engaging in pleasant events every day. As a result, Betty learned that when she engaged in few events (0–2), her mood was quite low (2–3). Because Betty's participation in this behavioral plan was inconsistent, therapy shifted to cognitive interventions to address Betty's beliefs that prevented her from finding time for herself and reorganizing her caregiving duties.

Cognitive Interventions.   Betty's DTR revealed perfectionistic and inflexible thinking, particularly in terms of caregiving. For example, she believed that as a mother, she should be her son's only caregiver. To take time for herself would mean neglecting her son's needs, which meant she was a bad caregiver and a bad mother. Betty also believed that no one could care for her son the way she did, and she often criticized the help she received from either her husband or her daughter: "They just do not do things correctly. It's not worth fixing their mistakes." This belief led to conflict with her husband and daughter, and, not surprisingly, offers of help from them grew less frequent, leaving Betty to believe "I am all alone."

While Betty evidenced inflexible thinking about how to care for her son, she was also overwhelmed by the amount of responsibility she had. In discussion with the therapist, she realized how angry she was at Paul for needing care, especially after sacrificing so much of her life to care for her mother. However, this realization generated tremendous guilt for Betty. Betty's painful experience of guilt motivated her to examine carefully and challenge her beliefs about caregiving.

In the language of CBT, she evidenced patterns of *all-or-nothing thinking, catastrophizing, emotional reasoning,* and *jumping to conclusions* (see Table 13.1). Using

Table 13.1   Betty's DTR documenting her beliefs about caregiving.

Describe the event that led to your unpleasant emotions.	What are your negative thoughts? Identify your unhelpful thought patterns.	What are you feeling? (sad, angry, anxious, etc.)?
Jerry calls to say he will be late, which delays my food shopping. He suggests that I leave Paul for 1 hour. I yell at him, "You don't know what you are talking about!"	He never helps me. He doesn't care about how much I do for Paul.	Anger
	If I leave Paul alone and he needs something, he may hurt himself.	Resentment
	Dysfunctional thought patterns: Jumping to conclusions, mind-reading, and catastrophizing.	Depression

another CBT technique, Betty examined the costs (disadvantages) and benefits (advantages) of her beliefs. She identified a benefit of being the sole caregiver: it gave her an opportunity to be close to her son. She also identified many costs to believing she must be the sole caregiver. She had set up a "no-win" situation: if she needed help from others, it meant that she failed as a caregiver, yet when she did not receive offers of help, she felt alone, overwhelmed, irritable, and depressed. She realized that by her behavior, she had inadvertently encouraged her husband and daughter not to help in the care of her son.

Betty's anger toward Paul was another cost she experienced by being the sole caregiver. Betty eventually understood that although she wanted to be close to him, her caregiving burden did not provide "quality time." Betty also began to understand that being a "good" mother required more than performing care tasks. She also realized that if she began to alleviate her responsibilities and have some time for herself, her energy and mood would increase so that she could be with Paul in a more enjoyable way.

Betty agreed to conduct a small experiment designed to help practice asking her husband for help as well as to restart a pleasant activity that she had abandoned. She scheduled lunch with a friend over the weekend while Jerry and Paul were home together. She utilized relaxation techniques to manage the anxiety of leaving Paul alone and a DTR to monitor critical thoughts about how Jerry cared for Paul. Although initially anxious during lunch, when she returned home, Paul and Jerry were watching a baseball game and Jerry was helping Paul eat ice cream. They invited her to join them: "It was the first relaxing moment in a long time." Following this, Betty briefly struggled with beliefs that she was "no longer needed," but she carefully weighed the benefit of the outing with her friend and the enjoyable time shared by her husband and son against the costs of believing that she "must do it all."

Prior to the ending phase, the therapist suggested that Jerry come to the next session. Jerry conveyed his concern about how overwhelmed Betty had been. He suggested that Paul could provide more self-care than he had, which might enhance both his physical and emotional independence. Betty feared her son would hurt himself or would be disappointed if he failed at trying new tasks. At the therapist's suggestion, Betty arranged for an evaluation of Paul's functioning by an occupational therapist. Paul was responsive to this recommendation.

End Phase

At termination, Betty's BDI score was 0, indicating that she was symptom-free. She was taking regular outings away from the house and had enrolled in a community center art class. She was more accepting of the help she received from her husband and daughter. Jerry offered to hire a part-time home health care aide, to which Betty agreed for at least a trial period. Betty's energy increased concurrent with the improvement in her relationship with Paul. They now spent more time in shared pleasant activities than struggling over his care needs. Similarly, Betty and Jerry argued less and enjoyed each shared social activity more.

The therapist and Betty constructed a maintenance guide summarizing Betty's gains in treatment. This document highlighted (1) change in Betty's perception of the problems that brought her to treatment, (2) development of new skills to manage stress, and (3) danger signals that would indicate that she might be experiencing a relapse of her depression. At the final session, Betty conveyed her pleasant surprise at the effectiveness of psychotherapy and the pleasure she reclaimed from her family life.

INTERPERSONAL PSYCHOTHERAPY WITH OLDER ADULTS

Interpersonal psychotherapy (IPT) is a time-limited, manualized psychotherapy originally developed for the treatment of major depressive disorder (MDD). IPT is based on theory and research that indicate that interpersonally relevant events often influence the development and course of depression. IPT has been found effective in the treatment of MDD in several acute and longer-term studies of depression in younger individuals (Frank & Spanier, 1995) and in recent years has been studied in older adults (see section on "Do Older Adults Respond to Psychotherapy?" for a brief review of research). It appears that IPT requires little or no adaptation when conducted with depressed elderly, and clinical reports indicate that it has been successfully used with elderly persons with a variety of depressive disorders (Hinrichsen, 1997).

IPT is manualized; that is, the rationale, focus, goals, and structure of therapeutic sessions are outlined (Klerman, Weissman, Rounsaville, & Chevron, 1984). IPT is typically conducted in 16 sessions in three phases of treatment.

INITIAL PHASE (SESSIONS 1–3)

In this phase, several issues are reviewed. First, patient symptoms are assessed using the *DSM-IV* (APA, 1994) system to diagnose the psychiatric condition. The patient is told the name of the condition and is educated about MDD and its treatment. MDD is characterized as a medical illness, and it is emphasized that MDD impairs an individual's ability to function. By viewing MDD as an illness, temporary reduction in daily obligations is sanctioned until the patient is feeling better. An evaluation is made to determine if the patient should be referred for antidepressant medication. Although in research studies, IPT alone has been found to be effective in the treatment of MDD, in clinical practice, both psychotherapy and antidepressant medication are often combined.

Next, current and past interpersonal relationships are reviewed because they may be associated with onset of the depressive episode or its continuation. A review of relationships includes an examination of differences in expectations within relationships, satisfying and unsatisfying aspects, and changes that the patient would like to make in the relationships.

An interpersonal problem area is then identified from one or two of the four problem areas that are a focus of IPT: grief, interpersonal dispute, role transition, and interpersonal deficits. Finally, the therapist recaps his or her understanding of the problem. Treatment goals are established in conjunction with the patient. Finally, the specifics of IPT are explained to the patient (e.g., the focus of IPT on the here-and-now, the need for the patient to discuss important issues of concern, the duration of treatment sessions, and the 16-week length of the treatment).

SECOND PHASE (SESSIONS 4–13)

The majority of treatment sessions are in Phase 2. Therapeutic strategies are implemented in one or two of IPT's four interpersonal problem areas.

Role Transition
Role transition is a major life change. Goals of treatment include helping patients to mourn and accept the loss associated with the change and to see their new role or roles as more positive by restoring patient self-esteem and developing a more solid sense of mastery of the new role. IPT outlines specific strategies that the therapist uses to achieve goals in this and the other three possible treatment foci.

Grief
Grief reflects problems in adjustment to the death of an important person or persons. Treatment goals include facilitating the mourning process and then helping the patient to reestablish relationships with others.

Interpersonal Dispute
Interpersonal dispute is conflict with a significant other, often with a spouse, but it may also involve a friend, coworker, employer, or adult child.

Social Skills Deficits
Social skills deficits are evident in people who lack the requisite skills to establish satisfying relationships with others or, if established, are unable to sustain those relationships. Goals of treatment are to reduce the patient's social isolation and encourage the development of new relationships.

THIRD PHASE (SESSIONS 14–16)

In the third and final phase of treatment, termination issues are discussed. There is discussion about the end of treatment, an acknowledgment that ending therapy can be difficult for some, and encouragement of the patient's independent functioning once the therapy has ended.

PSYCHODYNAMIC PSYCHOTHERAPY WITH OLDER ADULTS

Psychodynamic theory postulates that behavior is shaped by unconscious forces that evolve throughout an individual's early development, coping strategies used to manage stress, and current interpersonal difficulties (Strupp & Binder, 1984; Weiner, 1975). A central concept in psychodynamic psychotherapy is *defenses*. Defenses are unconscious processes that people use to shield them from anxiety. Yet, defenses often result in further emotional distress because they distort or block important information that is needed to deal with life problems. One goal of psychotherapy is the reduction of emotional distress by uncovering the underlying forces driving the individual's problematic behavior and experiences. Hence, psychotherapy makes the unconscious conscious.

Traditional psychodynamic psychotherapy does not limit the number of sessions. The process of therapy varies greatly among patients, but there are roughly three stages of therapy: early, middle, and late (Weiner, 1975).

EARLY PHASE

The initial phase of treatment begins with an evaluation of the patient's presenting problems as well as an assessment of the patient's insight into problems and potential for psychotherapy. The therapist must explore the background of the presenting complaints together with gaining an understanding of the patient as a person. This information assists the therapist to develop a *working formulation* of the patient's situation. The working formulation consists of the diagnostic impression as well as the *dynamic* impression. The dynamic impression summarizes the nature of the patient's internal conflicts, defensive strategies, coping styles, social relationships, and influences from early life experiences (Weiner, 1975; Zweig & Hinrichsen, 1996). The final step of this phase is for the therapist and patient to agree to proceed with treatment.

MIDDLE PHASE

The goal of the middle phase of treatment is to enhance the patient's psychological understanding of the therapist's formulation. The therapist's understanding is communicated through the use of *interpretation*. Interpretive comments are designed to expand the patient's conscious awareness of the unconscious factors that influence his or her behavior. Learning rarely occurs after one interpretation and multiple interpretations are offered on the same theme.

The processes of resistance, transference, and countertransference impede the uncovering of these unconscious forces. *Resistance* is the patient's temporary reluctance to engage in the treatment process, while overtly stating that he or she wants continued help. Patient resistance can be evident in silence, in "chatting" about trivial matters, and/or in frequent negation of the therapist's statements.

For treatment to proceed, the therapist must explore the patient's resistant conduct. In psychodynamic therapy, *transference* is the displacement of feelings and attitudes experienced toward the therapist that have no basis in reality. Transference has been traditionally viewed as a crucial source of information about the patient's interpersonal relationships, but it can also interfere with therapy. Transference is fostered by the nonreciprocal nature of the therapeutic relationship and the therapist's ambiguous, neutral presence. In essence, the therapist becomes a blank screen onto which the patient projects these feelings and attitudes. A patient's transference reaction is often interpreted as a reenactment of interpersonal conflicts that must be resolved in therapy (Levenson, 1995; Strupp & Binder, 1984). In contrast, *countertransference* involves feelings and thoughts of the therapist toward the patient, which may interfere with the therapist's objectivity. Therapists are often advised to resolve countertransferential issues either in their own therapy or during case consultations (Levenson, 1995).

END PHASE

Unlike structured psychotherapies, termination occurs when the therapist recognizes that the patient has achieved an adequate level of self-observation or self-awareness to continue independent goal attainment, usually concurrent with reduction in psychiatric symptoms. Once termination begins, the process includes reviewing the work that has been accomplished and preparing the patient to independently manage future stressful situations.

FAMILY THERAPY

Many of the changes associated with the aging process affect not only the individual, but also family members. An older adult who loses a spouse often has children who have lost a parent. An older adult's depression and isolation may be exacerbated by the perception that family members do not attend to emotional needs. Adaptation to chronic illness frequently affects a family's social functioning as well and may change family roles. An overburdened caregiver who feels guilty about asking the children for help may make them feel excluded from his or her life. Adult children who might have viewed a parent as "invincible" may become deeply distressed watching him or her become disabled by chronic illness, and also face the reality that they are "parenting a parent." Treatment of the whole family can elucidate these issues and help each member to better cope with these changes.

Adaptation to aging can be enhanced by family therapy. As adult children raise their own families, expectations regarding frequency of contact can cause conflict between the generations. Whereas in the past, it was common for an older adult's extended family to live in the same locale, families are now geographically more distant. Geographical distance between family members can elicit fear about who can be called on when help is needed. The necessity to adapt to these changes may challenge older adults' core beliefs about what they can expect from their children.

In family therapy, therapists are encouraged to consider whether the identified patient is the older adult or the entire family (Qualls, 1988). If the consequences of the older adult's decline in functioning are exacerbated by the family's ineffective problem solving, it may be more useful to work with the entire family rather than the patient alone. The process of family therapy with older adults can proceed as with younger families, but the issues usually differ from those that are the focus of therapy in younger families.

One issue that can arise in late-life family therapy is that some older people assume that the younger therapist has a natural alliance with children who may be the same age as the therapist (Qualls, 1988). Adult children may similarly assume that the therapist will side with them because of age similarity. This issue can be addressed by the therapist in a way that builds trust in both the older person and the adult children.

GROUP THERAPY

Group therapy informed by cognitive-behavioral, interpersonal, or psychodynamic perspectives can be very useful for older adults. Many older people with psychiatric problems are socially isolated, which can exacerbate psychiatric symptoms and further erode relationships with family and friends. Although the primary goal of group psychotherapy is to improve psychiatric symptoms and problem solving, it nonetheless offers the opportunity to increase contacts with people and thus enhance social confidence. We have found that as depressed older adults in group therapy begin to improve, they also evidence greater interest in others, which is generally recognized and reinforced by their group peers.

Group psychotherapy also provides older members with an opportunity to offer support and help to others, which runs counter to the common perception among depressed older adults that they have little to offer to anyone. This serves, then, to enhance their sense of social worth. Another therapeutic effect of group psychotherapy for older people is to reduce the sense of being alone in their own distress. It is often observed that when a depressed group member discloses specific difficulties to which friends or family have responded with dismay or irritation, other group members empathically disclose that they too have suffered from the same difficulties.

Several issues must be taken into account when conducting group therapy. Careful attention must be paid to balancing participation among all members. As in group therapies with all age groups, a group member often emerges who tends to monopolize the group. Therapists must address this problem early and consistently or else other members of the group may lose confidence in the therapist.

Older adults often approach group therapy with beliefs and behaviors that can reduce their participation. Some older people believe that one should not disclose painful personal issues to persons other than family (Yost, Beutler, Corbishley, & Allender, 1986). Others avoid open expressions of emotion that can also hamper the process of therapy. A well-defined sense of social etiquette may inhibit some elderly from offering frank feedback to a group peer or disagreeing with the therapist. Explicit attention to these issues must be addressed by the therapist early in treatment.

Young and middle-aged therapists working with older adults may also have to contend with issues tied to generational differences between themselves and older group members. Older people may view the therapist as in the "prime of life," with little personal understanding of the reality of challenges of older adulthood, and as a result raise questions about the therapist's potential to be empathic. One strategy is for younger therapists to acknowledge their lack of personal experience with late-life problems in a way that invites group members to share their lives. This strategy may engender the belief in older people that sharing perspectives on late-life problems helps not only group members but also enhances the therapist's knowledge and understanding of older adults.

DO OLDER ADULTS RESPOND TO PSYCHOTHERAPY?

Nearly two decades of research has demonstrated that depressed older adults respond quite well to both individual and group psychotherapy (Futterman, Thompson, Gallagher-Thompson, & Ferris, 1995; Gatz et al., 1998; Scogin & McElreath, 1994; Teri, Curtis, Gallagher-Thompson, & Thompson, 1994). For the most part, older adults respond well to psychosocial treatments regardless of the therapeutic orientation of the intervention (Futterman et al., 1995; Gatz et al., 1998; Scogin & McElreath, 1994; Thompson, Gallagher, & Breckenridge, 1987). This was first illustrated in a study comparing cognitive therapy (CT), behavior therapy (BT), and a form of psychodynamic psychotherapy called brief relational therapy (BRT), in which all three therapies showed comparable and significant improvement in depressive symptoms for older adults (Gallagher & Thompson, 1982). Six-month follow-up assessments of these participants demonstrated that older patients treated with BT and CT remained symptom-free, and those in the BRT modality evidenced a small increase in symptoms.

In a group of older adults with MDD, Thompson et al. (1987) compared the efficacy of 20 sessions of individual CT, BT, or psychodynamic therapy (PT) with a wait-list control group and found similar results. That is, older adults significantly improved with treatment compared to a wait-list control, with no significant differences among the three modalities. Further, two-year posttreatment results were equivalent across the therapeutic modalities (Gallagher-Thompson, Hanley-Peterson, & Thompson, 1990).

The impact of different modalities did differ, however, in a study by Gallagher-Thompson and Steffen (1994). They compared 66 depressed caregivers who received either individual CBT or brief psychodynamic therapy (BPT). They found that although both groups improved at study end, caregivers who had been in this role for greater than four months showed greater improvement with CBT and caregivers in this role for a shorter time showed more improvement with BPT.

Although less well studied than CBT, IPT appears useful in the treatment of depression in older adults. An initial study found that IPT was as effective as the antidepressant nortriptyline in the treatment of acute depression (Schneider, Sloane, Staples, & Bender, 1986). In another investigation, interpersonal counseling, which is a brief form of IPT, was associated with a reduction of depressive symptoms in older adults who were hospitalized with medical problems and who evidenced clinically significant depressive symptoms (Mossey, Knott, Higgins, & Talerico, 1996). In the most recent investigation of IPT, Reynolds and colleagues (Reynolds et al., 1999) examined whether nortriptyline, IPT, or the combination was effective in preventing the recurrence of MDD in older adults. After initial treatment with IPT and nortriptyline, older patients were randomized to several treatments or treatment combinations. After randomization, IPT patients received monthly IPT. The study found that, over a three-year study period, both nortriptyline and IPT reduced the recurrence rates of MDD and that the combination of IPT and nortriptyline appeared optimal in reducing recurrence. The researchers felt it was notable that, after initial treatment, even monthly IPT significantly reduced recurrence of MDD.

There are limitations to these studies. Most treatment outcome studies of older adults included community-dwelling volunteers who were physically healthy, well-educated, and cognitively intact. These participants may not be representative of most clinical populations. Few studies have examined the efficacy of psychotherapy with chronically ill elderly (Godbole & Verinis, 1974; Lovett & Gallagher, 1988; Steuer et al., 1984) or older adults with a dementing illness (Teri, 1994). Also, disorders other than major depression are largely underrepresented in the literature.

PSYCHOPHARMACOLOGICAL TREATMENT OF LATE-LIFE PSYCHIATRIC DISORDERS

It is common that older adults with serious psychiatric disorders—depression, bipolar illness, anxiety disorders, and psychotic disorders—are treated with psychiatric medications. A wide range of medications have been shown in clinical trials to significantly reduce symptoms of these disorders. Often, they are prescribed without psychotherapy, a practice frequently criticized by psychologists and other mental health care providers. This is because the psychosocial stress that prompted the onset of these disorders or that result from them are psychosocial stresses that can benefit from psychotherapy. Of equal concern is that most older adults are prescribed psychiatric medications from nonpsychiatric physicians who may not have the requisite expertise to diagnose or adequately treat psychiatric problems. Others have argued, however, that only a fraction of older adults with psychiatric problems get treatment and that many are deprived of the potential benefit of pharmacological treatment. On the whole, psychiatric medications often play a critical role in the treatment of serious late-life mental health problems.

A first step before prescribing psychiatric medications is a thorough diagnostic assessment of the presenting problem. As noted earlier, psychiatric problems are diagnosed within the *DSM-IV* psychiatric nosology. Older adults may present particularly difficult diagnostic challenges. Many older adults have one or more medical problems, some of which may be the cause of psychiatric symptoms. Further, many older adults take one of more prescribed medications that may also precipitate psychiatric symptoms. In prescribing psychiatric medications, physicians must also take into account the fact that older adults metabolize medications differently than younger adults, which often means prescribing psychiatric medications in lower doses than for younger persons. Older adults with dementia, most commonly Alzheimer's disease and vascular dementia, may not be able to adequately describe psychiatric symptoms and may be more sensitive to side effects of psychiatric medications than those without cognitive loss.

DEPRESSIVE DISORDERS

Until recently, the most widely prescribed medications for depressive disorders were tricyclic antidepressants (TCAs). Although the efficacy of these medications was clearly demonstrated in research studies (Gerson, Plotkin, & Jarvik, 1988), they were known to be associated with a variety of side effects, including cardiac and blood pressure changes, sedation, and anticholinergic effects such as dry mouth, blurry vision, constipation, and falling. If taken in overdose, TCAs can result in death. Another class of antidepressant medications is monoamine oxidase inhibitors (MAOIs). MAOIs have also been found effective in the treatment of late-life depression, but a major drawback to their use is that they require a restricted diet because of the possibility of a hypertensive crisis. MAOIs interact with certain foods and can cause a high elevation of blood pressure, which can result in stroke. Because of this, careful monitoring of the individual's diet is imperative. Recently, selective serotonin reuptake inhibitors (SSRIs) have been developed that differ in chemical structure from TCAs and MAOIs. Although these medications have side effects, the most common of which are nausea and sexual dysfunction, they are fewer in number than that of TCAs. As a result, SSRIs are generally safer and easier to prescribe than TCAs. They are increasingly the treatment of choice for depression in younger and older individuals.

Electroconvulsive therapy (ECT) may be given to individuals with serious depression. ECT induces a brain seizure and is often repeated two to three times a week for a total of four to eight treatments. Although the notion of electrical current passing through the brain is unsettling to some, ECT has been found to be safe and effective in the treatment of serious depression in older adults (Sackheim, 1994). After an ECT treatment, individuals are often confused and disoriented. During treatment, and for a few weeks afterward, they may experience some memory problems. For the vast majority, memory function returns to normal. The reason ECT improves depressive symptoms is not well understood, but it is thought to favorably change the balance of neuro-transmitters involved in the regulation of mood. ECT is usually provided to individuals who are not responding to standard antidepressant medication therapy, have psychotic symptoms associated with depression, or whose depressive symptoms are so severe that they are life-threatening and require immediate treatment.

BIPOLAR DISORDER

Some individuals who experience episodes of depression may later have episodes of mania in which they may feel especially cheerful or "high," or sometimes, irritable—a condition called bipolar disorder. They may also evidence psychotic symptoms such as hearing or believing things that do not exist. In the 1950s, it was found that the drug lithium significantly reduced symptoms of bipolar disorder. Lithium remains the mainstay of the treatment of bipolar disorder (Young, 1998). Because an adequate concentration of lithium in the blood is tied to its therapeutic efficacy, individuals taking lithium must have regular blood tests. Blood monitoring is also important because too much lithium in the blood, called lithium toxicity, may be life-threatening. Not uncommonly, there are side effects from lithium that may include kidney problems, thyroid difficulties, gastrointestinal symptoms, and skin disruptions.

Older persons with bipolar disorder are often treated with neuroleptics or more recently developed antipsychotic medications, called novel or atypical antipsychotics, during the acute phase of the illness. Another medication that may be used to treat bipolar disorder is the drug carbamazepine. ECT may also be used during acute episodes of illness.

ANXIETY DISORDERS

Like younger individuals, older persons may also experience anxiety disorders, including panic disorder, phobias, obsessive-compulsive disorder, and generalized anxiety disorder. Benzodiazepines are often used to treat generalized anxiety disorder, panic disorder, and phobias. Benzodiazepines are part of a group of medications called sedatives, hypnotics, and anxiolytics. As noted, older people metabolize medications differently than younger persons, and as a result, they eliminate benzodiazepines more slowly from the body and are more vulnerable to possible side effects from them. Common side effects include sedation, fatigue, and drowsiness (Lader & Ancill, 1998). When benzodiazepines are taken for extended periods of time, individuals may become tolerant of them and need higher doses to achieve the same effect, thus increasing the risk of dependence. Other medications used in the treatment of generalized anxiety disorder include beta-adrenergic blocking agents, buspirone, and some antidepressants. Obsessive-compulsive disorder is often treated with SSRIs.

PSYCHOTIC DISORDERS

Psychosis is a state in which the individual may see, hear, or believe things that are not true, evidence impaired thinking processes, or display aggressive or disorganized behavior. Common examples of psychotic disorders include schizophrenia and delusional disorder. Psychotic symptoms may also accompany other disorders, including MDD and bipolar disorder. Older adults with dementia often evidence psychotic symptoms at one time or another during the course of this condition. The pharmacologic mainstay in the treatment of psychotic disorders and symptoms has been neuroleptics (Jeste, Lacro, Gilbert, Kline, & Kline, 1993). There are a number of possible side effects from neuroleptics, including orthostatic hypertension (drop in blood pressure), sedation, anticholinergic and extrapyramidal effects (e.g., muscle spasms), restlessness, reduced motivation, and Parkinson-like symptoms (drooling, shuffling walk). Tardive dyskinesia (TD) is a common side effect of neuroleptics that may be irreversible. TD is characterized by a range of involuntary muscle movements. Older adults are especially prone to the development of TD. When neuroleptics are prescribed to older people, they must be carefully monitored because of the high risk of TD and altered metabolism associated with aging.

In recent years, novel or atypical antipsychotics are often used to treat psychotic symptoms. Novel antipsychotics have fewer side effects than neuroleptics and, most notably, appear to be much less likely to induce TD. Because of these advantages, atypical antipsychotics are now common treatment for psychotic disorders.

CONCLUSION

As this chapter has illustrated, older adults experience a wide range of health, caregiving, and relationship issues that, for some, can result in psychiatric disorder or psychiatric symptoms. Research evidence indicates that psychotherapy can be quite helpful for many problems that older adults bring to psychotherapy and that pharmacotherapy is also effective. When doing psychotherapy with older adults, the psychologist needs to take into account a number of issues, including cohort or generational differences between psychologist and older client, sensory and other impairments often evident in older people, and the need to develop a treatment plan and goals. When prescribing psychiatric medication, physicians must ascertain whether medical illness or medications are the cause of the psychiatric symptoms and take into account the altered metabolism of older adults.

Psychotherapeutic services are delivered in a wide range of settings, including inpatient services, outpatient clinics, continuing day treatment, partial hospitals, and nursing homes. A slowly growing number of specialized settings for older adults have developed, as well as settings that employ mental health care practitioners with training in geriatrics and geropsychology. The most well-established psychotherapies for the treatment of both younger and older adults include cognitive-behavioral therapy, interpersonal psychotherapy for depression, and psychodynamic psychotherapy. The theoretical underpinnings and treatment techniques differ among these therapies, but there are also many common elements. A wide range of effective and less side-effect-inducing psychiatric medications is available. Research suggests that, on the whole, psychotherapy and pharmacotherapy demonstrate usefulness for younger and older adults.

STUDY QUESTIONS

1. Using the case example, if Betty hadn't improved from psychotherapy, what other treatment options might be considered?
2. In what ways are cognitive-behavioral therapy, interpersonal psychotherapy, and psychodynamic therapy alike and different in the treatment of depression?
3. What are some reasons an older adult with a psychiatric disorder would not use mental health services?
4. If Betty also had severe arthritis, how might her psychotherapy be different?
5. What factors should a therapist consider in beginning treatment with an older adult with no history of psychotherapy?

SUGGESTED READINGS

Duffy, M. (Ed.). (1999). *Handbook of counseling and psychotherapy with older adults.* New York: Wiley.

Frazer, D.W., & Jongsma, A.E. (1999). *The older adult psychotherapy treatment planner.* New York: Wiley.

Knight, B.G. (1996). *Psychotherapy with older adults* (2nd ed.). Thousand Oaks, CA: Sage.

Molinari, V. (Ed.). (2000). *Professional psychology in long term care: A comprehensive guide.* New York: Hatherleigh Press.

Rosowky, E., Abrams, R.C., & Zweig, R.Z. (Eds.). (1999). *Personality disorders in older adults: Emerging issues in diagnosis and treatment.* Mahwah, NJ: Erlbaum.

Scogin, F., & Prohaska, M. (1993). *Aiding older adults with memory complaints.* Sarasota, FL: Professional Resources Press.

Zarit, S.H., & Knight, B.G. (1996). *A guide to psychotherapy and aging.* Washington, DC: American Psychological Association.

Zarit, S.H., & Zarit, J.M. (1998). *Mental disorders in older adults: Fundamentals of assessment and treatment.* New York: Guilford Press.

REFERENCES

American Psychiatric Association. (1994). *Diagnostic and statistical manual of mental disorders* (4th ed.). Washington, DC: Author.

American Psychological Association's Working Group on the Older Adult. (1998). What practitioners should know about working with older adults. *Professional Psychology: Research and Practice, 29*, 413–427.

Beck, A.T., Rush, J., Shaw, B., & Emery, G. (1979). *Cognitive therapy of depression*. New York: Guilford Press.

Cantor, M. (Ed.). (1994). *Family caregiving: Agenda for the future*. San Francisco: American Society on Aging.

Carstensen, L.L., Gottman, J.M., & Levenson, R.W. (1995). Emotional behavior in long-term marriage. *Psychology and Aging, 10*, 140–149.

Coryell, W., Scheftner, W., Keller, M., Endicott, J., Maser, J., & Klerman, G. (1993). The enduring psychosocial consequences of mania and depression. *American Journal of Psychiatry, 150*, 720–727.

Dick, L.P., Gallagher-Thompson, D., Powers, D.V., Coon, D., & Thompson, L.W. (1997). *Cognitive-behavioral therapy for late life depression: A client manual*. Unpublished manuscript, Palo Alto VA Health Care System and Stanford University Medical Center at Palo Alto, CA.

Dick, L.P., Gallagher-Thompson, D., & Thompson, L.W. (1996). Cognitive-behavioral therapy. In R.T. Woods (Ed.), *Handbook of the clinical psychology of ageing* (pp. 509–544). Chichester, England: Wiley.

Estes, C.L. (1995). Mental health services for the elderly: Key policy elements. In M. Gate (Ed.), *Emerging issues in mental health and aging* (pp. 303–327). Washington, DC: American Psychological Association.

Frank, E., & Spanier, C. (1995). Interpersonal psychotherapy for depression: Overview, clinical efficacy, and future directions. *Clinical Psychology: Science and Practice, 2*, 349–369.

Futterman, A., Thompson, L.W., Gallagher-Thompson, D., & Ferris, R. (1995). Depression in later life: Epidemiology, assessment, etiology and treatment. In E. Beckham & R. Leber (Eds.), *Handbook of depression* (2nd ed.). New York: Guilford Press.

Gallagher, D., & Thompson, L.W. (1982). Treatment of major depressive disorders in older outpatients with brief psychotherapies. *Psychotherapy: Research and Practice, 19*, 482–490.

Gallagher-Thompson, D., Hanley-Peterson, P., & Thompson, L.W. (1990). Maintenance of gains versus relapse following brief psychotherapy for depression. *Journal of Counseling and Clinical Psychology, 58*, 371–374.

Gallagher-Thompson, D., & Steffen, A. (1994). Comparative effects of cognitive/behavioral and brief psychodynamic psychotherapies for depressed family caregivers. *Journal of Counseling and Clinical Psychology, 62*, 543–549.

Gatz, M., Fiske, A., Fox, L.S., Kaskie, B., Kasl-Godley, J.E., McCallum, T.J., & Wetherell, J.L. (1998). Empirically-validated psychological treatments for older adults. *Journal of Mental Health and Aging, 4*, 9–46.

Gerson, S.C., Plotkin, D.A., & Jarvik, L.F. (1988). Antidepressant drug studies, 1964 to 1986: Empirical evidence for aging patients. *Journal of Clinical Psychopharmacology, 8*, 311–322.

Godbole, A., & Verinis, J.S. (1974). Brief psychotherapy in the treatment of emotional disorders in physically ill geriatric patients. *Gerontologist, 14*, 143–148.

Hinrichsen, G.A. (1997). Interpersonal psychotherapy for depressed older adults. *Journal of Geriatric Psychiatry, 30*, 239–257.

Hinrichsen, G.A., & Hernandez, N.A. (1993). Factors associated with recovery from and relapse into a major depressive disorder in the elderly. *American Journal of Psychiatry, 150*, 1820–1825.

Jeste, D.V., Lacro, J.P., Gilbert, P.L., Kline, J., & Kline, N. (1993). Treatment of late-life schizophrenia with neuroleptics. *Schizophrenia Bulletin, 19*, 817–830.

Klerman, G.L., & Weissman, M.M. (1993). *New applications of interpersonal psychotherapy.* Washington, DC: American Psychiatric Press.

Klerman, G.L., Weissman, M.M., Rounsaville, B.J., & Chevron, E.S. (1984). *Interpersonal psychotherapy of depression.* New York: Basic Books.

Knight, B.G. (1996). *Psychotherapy with older adults* (2nd ed.). Thousand Oaks, CA: Sage.

Lader, M., & Ancill, R. (1998). The treatment of generalized anxiety disorder, panic disorder, and obsessive-compulsive disorder in the elderly. In J.C. Nelson (Ed.), *Geriatric psychopharmacology* (pp. 259–272). New York: Marcel Dekker.

Levenson, H. (1995). *Time-limited dynamic psychotherapy.* New York: Basic Books.

Lewinsohn, P.M., Hoberman, H., Teri, L., & Hautzinger, M. (1985). An integrative theory of depression. In S. Reiss & R.R. Bootzin (Eds.), *Theoretical issues in behavior therapy* (pp. 331–359). New York: Academic Press.

Lewinsohn, P.M., Munoz, R.F., Youngren, M.A., & Zeiss, A.M. (1978). *Control your depression.* Englewood Cliffs, NJ: Prentice Hall.

Light, E., & Lebowitz, B.D. (Eds.). (1991). *The elderly with chronic mental illness.* New York: Springer.

Lovett, S., & Gallagher, D. (1988). Psychoeducational interventions for family caregivers: Preliminary efficacy data. *Behavior Therapy, 19*, 321–330.

Mossey, J.M., Knott, K.A., Higgins, M., & Talerico, K. (1996). Effectiveness of a psychological intervention, interpersonal counseling, for subdysthymic depression in medically ill elderly. *Journal of Gerontology: Medical Sciences, 51A*, M172–M178.

Qualls, S.H. (1988). Problems in families of older adults. In N. Epstein, S.E. Schlesinger, & W. Dryden (Eds.), *Cognitive-behavioral therapy with families* (pp. 215–253). New York: Brunner/Mazel.

Reynolds, C.F., Frank, E., Perel, J.M., Imber, S.D., Cornes, C., Miller, M.D., Mazumdar, S., Houck, P.R., Dew, M.A., Stack, J.A., Pollock, B.G., & Kupfer, D.J. (1999). Nortriptyline and interpersonal psychotherapy as maintenance therapies for recurrent major depression: A randomized controlled trial in patients older than 59 years. *Journal of the American Medical Association, 281*, 39–45.

Sackheim, H.A. (1994). Use of electroconvulsive therapy in late-life depression. In L.S. Schneider, C.F. Reynolds, B.D. Lebowitz, & A.J. Friedhoff (Eds.), *Diagnosis and treatment of depression in late life: Results of the NIH consensus development conference* (pp. 259–278). Washington, DC: American Psychiatric Press.

Schneider, L.S., Sloane, R.B., Staples, F.R., & Bender, M. (1986). Pretreatment orthostatic hypotension as a predictor of response to nortriptyline in geriatric depression. *Journal of Clinical Psychopharmacology, 6*, 172–176.

Schultz, R., & Williamson, G.M. (1990). Psychiatric and physical morbidity effects of caregiving. *Journals of Gerontology: Psychological Sciences, 45*, 181–191.

Scogin, F., & McElreath, L. (1994). Efficacy of psychosocial treatments for geriatric depression: A quantitative review. *Journal of Counseling and Clinical Psychology, 62*, 69–74.

Shanas, E. (1979). Social myth as hypothesis: The case of the family relations of old people. *Gerontologist, 19*, 3–9.

Steuer, J.L., Mintz, J., Hammen, C.L., Hill, M.A., Jarvik, L.F., McCarley, T., Motoike, P., & Rosen, R. (1984). Cognitive-behavioral and psychodynamic group psychotherapy in treatment of geriatric depression. *Journal of Consulting and Clinical Psychology, 52,* 180–189.

Strupp, H.H., & Binder, J.L. (1984). *Psychotherapy in a new key.* New York: Basic Books.

Teri, L. (1994). Behavioral treatment of depression in patients with dementia. *Alzheimer's Disease and Related Disorders, 8,* 66–74.

Teri, L., Curtis, J., Gallagher-Thompson, D., & Thompson, L. (1994). Cognitive-behavioral therapy with depressed older adults. In L.S. Schneider, C.F. Reynolds, B.D. Lebowitz, & A.J. Friedhoff (Eds.), *Diagnosis and treatment of depression in late life: Results of the NIH consensus development conference* (pp. 279–291). Washington, DC: American Psychiatric Press.

Teri, L., & Lewinsohn, P. (1982). Modification of the pleasant and unpleasant events schedules for use with the elderly. *Journal of Consulting and Clinical Psychology, 50*(3), 444–445.

Thompson, L.W., Davies, R., Gallagher, D., & Krantz, S.E. (1986). Cognitive therapy with older adults. *Clinical Gerontologist, 5*(3/4), 245–279.

Thompson, L.W., Gallagher, D., & Breckenridge, J. (1987). Comparative effectiveness of psychotherapies for depressed elders. *Journal of Consulting and Clinical Psychology, 55,* 385–390.

Thompson, L.W., Gallagher-Thompson, D., & Dick, L.P. (1997). *Cognitive-behavioral therapy for late life depression: A therapist's manual.* Unpublished manuscript, Palo Alto VA Health Care System and Stanford University Medical Center at Palo Alto, CA.

Thompson, L.W., Gantz, F., Florsheim, M., DelMaestro, A., Rodman, J., Gallagher-Thompson, D., & Bryan, H. (1991). Cognitive/behavioral therapy for affective disorders in the elderly. In W. Myers (Ed.), *New techniques in the psychotherapy of older patients* (pp. 3–19). Washington, DC: American Psychiatric Association Press.

Weiner, I.B. (1975). *Principles of psychotherapy.* New York: Wiley.

Weissman, M.M., Bruce, M.L., Leaf, P.J., Florio, L.P., & Holzer, C. (1991). Affective disorders. In L.N. Robins & D.A. Regier (Eds.), *Psychiatric disorders in America: The epidemiologic catchment area study.* New York: Free Press.

Yost, E.B., Beutler, L.E., Corbishley, M.A., & Allender, J.R. (1986). *Group cognitive therapy: A treatment approach for depressed older adults.* New York: Pergamon Press.

Young, R.C. (1998). Use of lithium in bipolar disorder. In J.C. Nelson (Ed.), *Geriatric psychopharmacology* (pp. 259–272). New York: Marcel Dekker.

Zeiss, A.M., & Lewinsohn, P.M. (1986). Adapting behavioral treatment for depression to meet the needs of the elderly. *Clinical Psychologist, 39,* 98–100.

Zeiss, A.M., & Steffen, A.M. (1996). Interdisciplinary health care teams: The basic unit of geriatric care. In L.L. Carstensen, B.A. Edelstein, & L. Dornbrand (Eds.), *The practical handbook of clinical gerontology* (pp. 423–450). Thousand Oaks, CA: Sage.

Zisook, S., Shuchter, S.R., Sledge, P.A., Paulus, M., & Judd, L.L. (1994). The spectrum of depressive phenomena after spousal bereavement. *Journal of Clinical Psychiatry, 55*(Suppl. 4), 29–36.

Zweig, R.A., & Hinrichsen, G.A. (1996). Insight-oriented and supportive psychotherapy. In W.E. Reichman & P.R. Katz (Eds.), *Psychiatric care in the nursing home* (pp. 188–208). New York: Oxford University Press.

Author Index

Subject Index